Metaboost Diet

Supercharging Your Health and Transforming Your Body

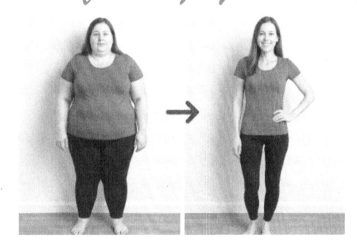

Meredith Shirk

No book can replace the diagnostic expertise and medical advice of a trusted physician. Please be certain to consult with your doctor before making any decisions that affect your health, particularly if you suffer from any medical conditions or have any symptoms that may require treatment.

Published in the United States by Meridian Publishing, an imprint of Lumino House, a division of Crestline Books LLC, New York.
Crestline Books.com
Lumino House.com
Meridian Publishing is a registered trademark, and the Circle colophon is a trademark of Crestline Books LLC.
Library of Congress Cataloging-in-Publication Data has been applied for.
ISBN 1-86197-876-9
Ebook ISBN 0-306-40615-2
Print book design by Cal Morgan
Cover design by Henry Ellison
Cover photograph by Cassie Hartwell /Getty Images

Table Of Content

Vegetables 253

Foreword

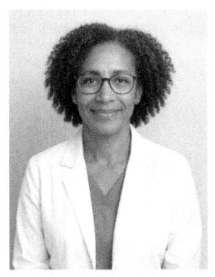

DR. EVELYN CARTER, MD, IFMCP
Integrative Medicine Physician &
Functional Health Educator

By Dr. Evelyn Carter, MD, IFMCP
Integrative Medicine Physician & Functional Health Educator

In my two decades as a physician specializing in integrative medicine and metabolic health, I've seen countless women enter my office carrying the same frustration: "I'm doing everything right, but my body just won't cooperate anymore." For women over 40—navigating hormonal changes, metabolic slowdown, and emotional exhaustion—traditional approaches often fall short.

That's why Meredith Shirk's work is not only revolutionary—it's essential.

Meredith is the founder and CEO of **Svelte Training**, a wellness company that has helped over one million women around the world transform their bodies and reclaim their energy. With a background in biology and behavioral coaching, and certifications as a NASM-Certified Personal Trainer (CPT), Fitness Nutrition Specialist (FNS), and Weight Loss Specialist (WLS), Meredith brings both science and soul to the table. But beyond her credentials, what sets her apart is her **uncanny ability to simplify complex health concepts into powerful, practical strategies**—and her sincere empathy for women who feel forgotten by mainstream fitness.

In *The Metaboost Connection*, Meredith delivers a complete, easy-to-follow blueprint tailored for women in midlife and beyond. Her program is rooted in **targeted nutrition**—including specific "MetaInfluencer" superfoods like flaxseed, avocado, ginger, lentils, and cinnamon—and **short, low-impact workouts** designed to activate lean muscle and ignite metabolism. But what really stands out is her focus on **hormonal balance, anti-inflammatory healing**, and **mind-body alignment**. She understands that weight loss isn't just about calories—it's about restoring harmony within the body's systems.

Meredith's program empowers women to reconnect with their bodies—not through punishment or restriction, but through nourishment, movement, and mindfulness. Her signature Metaboost method is backed by real science, real results, and real stories from thousands of women who have experienced dramatic shifts in their energy, weight, confidence, and vitality.

What I admire most about Meredith is that she doesn't just preach healthy living—she lives it. Her personal journey through injury, stress, and burnout led her to create a method that works *with* your body, not against it. And her relentless commitment to her community—through coaching, content, and compassion—is a testament to the authenticity behind the brand.

To the woman reading this who feels stuck, tired, or invisible—this book is your roadmap back to yourself. Trust the process. Trust your body. And trust that Meredith, through her words and wisdom, will walk alongside you every step of the way.

With respect and gratitude,
Dr. Evelyn Carter, MD, IFMCP
Functional Medicine Practitioner
Women's Health Advocate
Founder, Resilience Wellness Center

Introduction

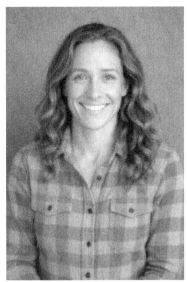

By Meredith Shirk, CPT, FNS, WLS
Founder of Svelte Training & Creator of The Metaboost Connection

If you're holding this book, I want you to know something right away: **this is not just another diet book.** This is a transformation guide. A proven system built on science, simplicity, and self-belief. And most importantly—it's created *for you*.

For over a decade, I've worked with thousands of women around the world—from busy moms to burned-out professionals to women over 40 who thought their metabolism had given up for good. I've seen firsthand what doesn't work: cookie-cutter plans, 1,200-calorie starvation diets, hours of cardio, and toxic weight-loss pressure that leads nowhere. That's not health. That's punishment.

I created the **Metaboost Diet** to change that.

This book is built around a simple truth: **your body is capable of incredible change at any age**—when you feed it the right nutrients, move with intention, and reset your internal systems. The Metaboost Method is not about restriction—it's about **replenishment, rebalancing,** and **reigniting your metabolism from the inside out.**

Inside these pages, you'll find:

☑ A full **120-day roadmap** to reset your body

☑ Over **1,000 clean, delicious recipes** that support hormone health, gut healing, and fat loss

☑ My signature **Metaboost "Superfood" system**, focused on targeted ingredients like flaxseed, cinnamon, lentils, ginger, and avocado

☑ Weekly meal plans, shopping lists, and prep strategies designed to fit real life

☑ Supportive tools to boost your mindset, manage stress, and stay consistent

What makes the Metaboost Diet different is that it's **designed for women's real lives.** It works *with* your body—especially during stages like perimenopause, menopause, or post-menopause when your needs shift. This isn't about achieving some Instagram fantasy—it's about **feeling strong, energized, and empowered in your own skin.**

As someone who's experienced injury, stress, hormonal imbalance, and burnout myself—I get it. That's why everything in this book is here to make your journey doable, motivating, and lasting. Whether you're just starting out or ready to take your wellness to the next level, this is your invitation to commit—not to a diet, but to yourself.

Let this book be your blueprint. Let every recipe be a step toward your strength. And let every day in the next 120 be a powerful reminder: **you are never too old, too tired, or too far gone to start fresh**.

Let's unlock your best, healthiest, most confident self—together.

With strength and gratitude,

Meredith Shirk

Certified Personal Trainer, Fitness Nutrition Specialist, and Founder of Svelte Training

CHAPTER 1

Your Changing Body, Your Changing Needs

Describing my journey from perimenopause to menopause as difficult doesn't quite capture it—it was downright miserable. Hot flashes, night sweats, thinning hair, dry skin, and unexpected weight gain made it a tough time. I couldn't wait for it to be over.

Now that I reflect on that period, I recognize a lot I didn't understand back then. For instance, I wish I had known that symptoms can begin as early as your thirties, and that starting hormone replacement therapy sooner might have significantly eased my experience. Also, feeling moody, anxious, or depressed doesn't mean you're losing your mind—it's just part of the process.

Yes, your body is changing, but it's a natural phase every woman goes through due to hormonal shifts. This transitional time includes three phases: perimenopause, menopause, and postmenopause, and each woman experiences them differently. Let's explore what each stage entails.

Perimenopause

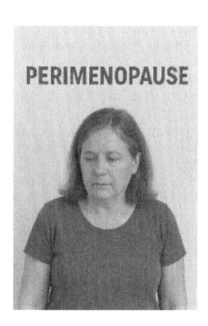

In your late thirties to early forties, you may notice subtle changes that are hard to ignore. Clothes may fit differently, even if the scale hasn't changed. Your skin gets drier, wrinkles start to appear, and fatigue becomes more noticeable. You might feel like a stranger when you look in the mirror.

These changes usually indicate the start of perimenopause—the initial phase of hormonal shifts that happens several years before menopause. This stage can last from just a few months to up to a decade, as your body gradually produces less estrogen. As your estrogen levels fall, your menstrual cycle becomes irregular. Eventually, after going a full year without a period, you've officially entered menopause.

Common Symptoms During Perimenopause

Every woman's experience is different. Some breeze through with minimal symptoms, while others face intense challenges. Many symptoms that begin in perimenopause can persist into menopause, though they often ease by postmenopause. Here's a closer look at the most common ones:

Weight gain.

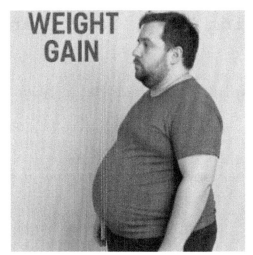

This might be the symptom that led you to this book! Foods you once devoured with no consequence now seem to add pounds overnight. You may find yourself shopping for stretchy waistbands instead of skinny jeans.

This weight gain usually stems from hormonal changes affecting your appetite, metabolism, and fat storage. Extra pounds can worsen other symptoms, like night sweats, joint discomfort, and bladder issues.

Hot flashes, in particular, have been linked to the "thermoregulatory theory," which suggests that higher body fat makes it harder for your body to release heat, leading to more frequent and intense hot flashes.

Studies support this. A 2017 study found that women who are overweight or obese typically face more severe menopause symptoms, including worse night sweats, joint pain, and vaginal dryness.

Another issue is the build-up of visceral fat around your internal organs—what I call the "menopause middle." This is linked to increased androgen (testosterone) activity and is reflected in a higher waist-to-hip ratio (WHR), a marker for fat distribution.

Besides affecting your appearance, this fat is tied to serious health risks, including heart disease, diabetes, certain cancers, and sleep apnea.

Managing your weight can help reduce these symptoms and lower your risk for these conditions. Midlife weight gain isn't just about appearance—it's a significant health concern.

Hot flashes.

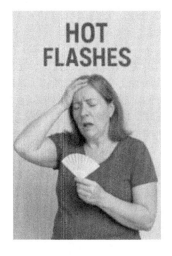

You could be all dressed up, makeup done, and suddenly—bam—an intense wave of heat surges through your body. These episodes might last seconds or minutes, and they often feel overwhelming. Some women experience them occasionally, others every day. Night sweats, their nighttime counterpart, can disrupt sleep and leave you exhausted.

Hair changes.

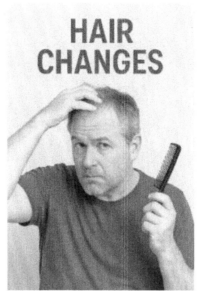

Hair tends to thin out at the crown during midlife, and you might notice more shedding during brushing or showering. These changes are linked to dropping estrogen levels and increased testosterone activity.

You may also spot new facial hair—thanks again to heightened testosterone.

Sleep issues.

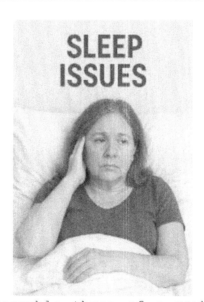

Your nights may begin to resemble those of a newborn—waking every couple of hours, hungry, needing to use the bathroom. You may struggle to fall asleep or wake too early. Hormonal fluctuations, particularly in estrogen and progesterone, are often to blame.

Brain fog and memory lapses.

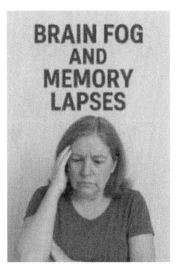

Can't recall a word that's right on the tip of your tongue? Find yourself forgetting why you walked into a room? Repeating stories to family members? Welcome to brain fog—a common result of reduced estrogen levels that affect memory and focus.

Vaginal and bladder changes.

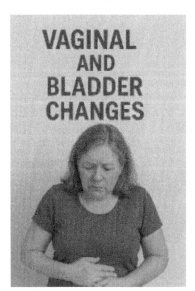

Lower estrogen causes the vaginal walls to become thinner, drier, and less flexible. One woman even described the sensation as having "cobwebs" down there. These changes can make sex uncomfortable and increase the risk of infections.

The bladder, being close to the vagina, is also affected. Thinning tissues can lead to urinary incontinence and frequent infection

Sexual changes.

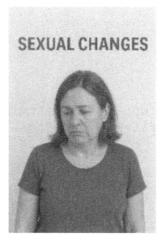

Hormonal dips in midlife can decrease sexual desire and arousal. However, if you were sexually active before, chances are your sex drive will continue. And yes, sex after 50 or 60 is very much possible—if that's what you want.

Mood swings.

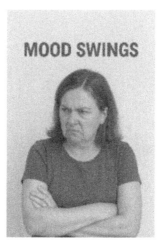

"Irritable" doesn't even come close. Your emotions may feel wildly unpredictable, and small annoyances can set off major reactions. Combined with sleep disruption, this can be particularly tough.

Estrogen plays a big role here too—it influences serotonin production, a key chemical in mood regulation. As estrogen decreases, so does serotonin, often leading to mood instability.

It's important to remind yourself that these emotional changes are biological—not your fault. Explaining this to your partner can help them understand and offer more support when you're feeling overwhelmed.

Other Symptoms

Perimenopause can bring a variety of symptoms—many of which women aren't often warned about. These can include:

- Breast tenderness
- Itchy or dry skin
- Heart palpitations

- Panic attacks
- Constipation
- Dizziness
- Dry mouth
- Urinary leakage
- Intense anger
- Elevated blood pressure
- Increased cholesterol
- Dry eyes
- Feeling light-headed
- Headaches or migraines

The Metaboost Diet's focus on food and lifestyle choices can help you manage not only weight gain but many of these symptoms as well.

Menopause

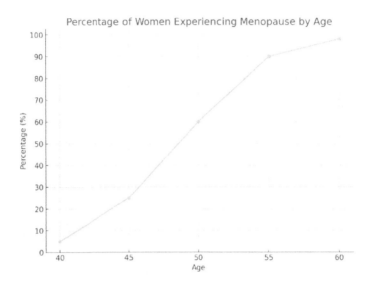

Following perimenopause is menopause, the stage when your ovaries stop producing reproductive hormones and you no longer menstruate for a full 12 months. While the average onset age is 51, some women may enter menopause as early as 45 or as late as 55.

During this time, weight gain often becomes more noticeable and harder to lose. Most women gain between 12 to 15 pounds between the ages of 45 and 55. Hunger may also increase due to shifting hormones, which can make it more difficult to resist overeating.

Additionally, this phase may bring metabolic challenges such as insulin resistance and disruptions in the way your body processes glucose and fats. Your risk for chronic conditions like type 2 diabetes, heart disease, cancer, and osteoporosis also rises.

A significant study tracking 35,000 women over four years found that those consuming diets high in refined carbohydrates—like white rice, chips, pasta, and pretzels—entered menopause roughly 1.5 years earlier than those who primarily ate fish and nutrient-rich foods like fruits, vegetables, and eggs.

Researchers suspect that high-carb diets elevate insulin levels, which may lead to insulin resistance and disrupt hormonal function.

This research sends a clear message: adopting healthy eating habits early can significantly impact your menopause experience and long-term health. The Metaboost Diet is designed to help you do just that.

Moreover, menopause increases vulnerability to other health risks. Before menopause, estrogen provides some protection against heart attacks and strokes. But as estrogen production declines, so does that protection. Midlife often comes with added heart disease risk factors—like high blood pressure, increased cholesterol, and reduced physical activity.

The Metaboost Diet can help you manage or reduce these symptoms and risks.

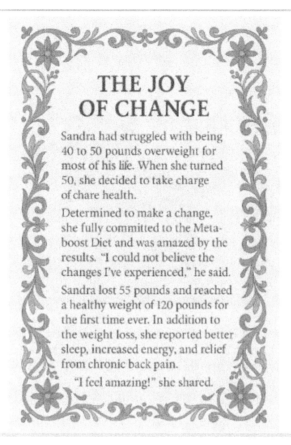

THE JOY OF CHANGE

Sandra had struggled with being 40 to 50 pounds overweight for most of his life. When she turned 50, she decided to take charge of chare health.

Determined to make a change, she fully committed to the Metaboost Diet and was amazed by the results. "I could not believe the changes I've experienced," he said.

Sandra lost 55 pounds and reached a healthy weight of 120 pounds for the first time ever. In addition to the weight loss, she reported better sleep, increased energy, and relief from chronic back pain.

"I feel amazing!" she shared.

Postmenopause

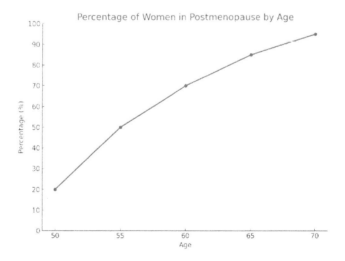

Percentage of Women in Postmenopause by Age

Postmenopause begins after you've gone 12 consecutive months without a period. During this stage, fat tends to accumulate more easily and is harder to lose. Women in postmenopause are almost five times more likely to store visceral fat compared to those who are premenopausal.

Additionally, muscle mass tends to decrease, slowing your metabolism and reducing your body's calorie-burning efficiency. Hormone levels stabilize at a consistently low level in this phase.

This stage brings several potential health concerns, so it's important to understand these risks and take steps—like following proper nutrition—to protect your health.

Osteoporosis

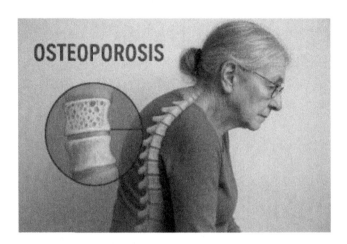

  This condition causes bones to become weak and brittle, increasing the risk of fractures—especially in the hips, spine, and wrists. Bone loss accelerates after menopause due to declining estrogen levels, and you could lose up to 25% of your bone density by age 60.

One in three postmenopausal women will develop osteoporosis, and the lifetime risk of a serious fracture is even higher than the risk of breast cancer.

The good news: you're not helpless. Treatments exist, and one of the most effective is engaging in weight-bearing activities, such as resistance training. Weight training strengthens both muscles and bones by challenging them against gravity.

Nutrition is also vital, and the Metaboost Diet supports bone health through targeted dietary strategies.

Cardiovascular Disease

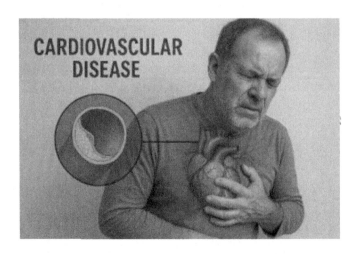

  Contrary to popular belief, heart disease isn't just a men's issue—it's the leading health threat for American women, especially during and after menopause.

While menopause itself doesn't directly cause heart disease, the drop in hormones contributes to risk factors like high blood pressure, elevated LDL (bad) cholesterol, and increased triglycerides. According to the American Heart Association, one in three women will develop cardiovascular disease during menopause.

Ten years after menopause, the likelihood of experiencing a heart attack rises sharply.

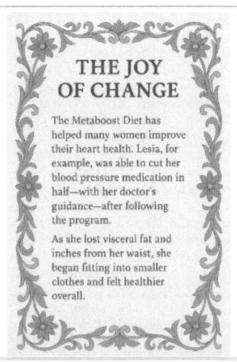

THE JOY OF CHANGE

The Metaboost Diet has helped many women improve their heart health. Lesia, for example, was able to cut her blood pressure medication in half—with her doctor's guidance—after following the program.

As she lost visceral fat and inches from her waist, she began fitting into smaller clothes and felt healthier overall.

Depression and Mental Health

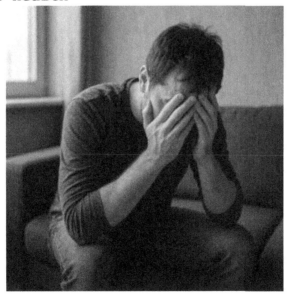

Depression is more common in postmenopause than earlier in life, likely due to both hormonal changes and life transitions, such as children moving out, relationship losses, retirement stress, and age-related health challenges.

A 2019 study examining 371 women not using hormone therapy found that only 21% of premenopausal women experienced mild depression, while nearly 60% of postmenopausal women suffered from major depression, which can be serious and requires medical attention.

Symptoms of depression include sadness, irritability, lack of motivation, and a diminished sense of joy in daily activities. If you're experiencing these feelings, speak to a healthcare provider. Depression is treatable—and you don't have to suffer in silence.

Increased Vaginal Dryness

Vaginal dryness often begins in perimenopause, continues through menopause, and may become more severe after. With lower estrogen levels, the vaginal walls thin and shrink, reducing natural moisture. This can cause discomfort during sex, more frequent UTIs, and greater urinary incontinence.

There's no reason to let these symptoms ruin your sex life. Regular use of vaginal lubricants—especially those free of scents and dyes—can reduce dryness and discomfort. Uberlube and KY Silk-E are recommended options.

Begin using lubricants proactively to maintain vaginal health and enhance intimacy. Additionally, you might want to ask your doctor about estrogen-based treatments like creams or vaginal rings that help restore moisture directly to the affected tissues.

The nutritional and lifestyle tools in the Metaboost Diet can support a smoother, healthier, and more vibrant postmenopausal experience.

Where Are You on Your Hormonal Journey?

If you're unsure where you fall in the hormonal transition—whether it's perimenopause, menopause, postmenopause, or somewhere in between—the short quiz below can help. It evaluates the severity of common symptoms and offers insights into which phase you may be in. You can share your results with your healthcare provider and use them as a reference as you follow the Metaboost Diet.

Instructions: For each symptom, rate how intensely you experience it by circling one of the options: *None, Mild, Moderate,* or *Severe.*

1. Hot flashes
2. Feeling light-headed
3. Headaches
4. Irritability
5. Feelings of depression
6. Feeling unloved or disconnected
7. Anxiety or emotional shifts
8. Trouble sleeping
9. Persistent fatigue
10. Back pain
11. Joint discomfort
12. Muscle aches
13. New or increased facial hair
14. Dry skin
15. Sensations like crawling under the skin
16. Low sex drive
17. Discomfort during sex
18. Vaginal dryness
19. Frequent urination
20. Forgetfulness or mental fog

Scoring:
- *None* = 0

- *Mild* = 1

- *Moderate* = 2

- *Severe* = 3

Total your points:
- **0-20:** Your symptoms may not be clearly related to perimenopause or menopause, but you could be in the early stages.
- **21-40:** There's a good chance your symptoms are linked to perimenopause or menopause.
- **41 or higher:** It's highly likely your symptoms are associated with perimenopause or menopause.

Three Steps to Take Back Control — The Metaboost Diet

After personally navigating perimenopause and menopause, and guiding nearly 100,000 women through the Metaboost Diet online program, I've identified key strategies to overcome weight gain—especially stubborn belly fat—and manage midlife health challenges.

Here's a sumMeredithof the three foundational elements of the Metaboost Diet you'll be adopting:

1. Intermittent Fasting

As discussed in the introduction, intermittent fasting plays a vital role in this plan, especially during menopause. While it might sound daunting at first, it's surprisingly easy to adopt and sustain!

So, what is intermittent fasting? It involves fasting for roughly 16 hours a day (most of which happens while you sleep) and eating all your meals within an 8-hour window. This technique offers numerous benefits for women in midlife, and we'll dive deeper into this in Chapter 4.

2. Anti-Inflammatory Eating

Inflammation is often a defense mechanism that helps our bodies fight illness—but when it lingers too long, it can cause health issues. Chronic inflammation is linked to weight gain and can make losing weight much harder.

The Metaboost Diet helps by cutting out foods that increase inflammation and encouraging foods that reduce it. Sugars—especially added or refined—and processed carbohydrates are major inflammation triggers. If possible, cut them out completely. Doing so can reduce the intensity and frequency of menopausal symptoms. That's a big win for your health and well-being. Learn more about this in Chapter 5.

3. Fuel Refocus

When you eat a diet heavy in carbs, your body burns those for energy and stores the excess as fat. To reverse that process and encourage fat burning, you need to limit carbs.

The Fuel Refocus phase of the Metaboost Diet shifts your macronutrient intake to:

- **70% healthy fats**

- **20% lean proteins**

- **10% complex carbs**

This approach is *not* a keto diet. In fact, many traditional keto plans increase inflammation, which is why the Metaboost Diet intentionally avoids that. Instead, we focus on eating nutrient-rich, anti-inflammatory carbs like quinoa, sweet potatoes, oats, blueberries, and apples. More guidance is provided in Chapter 7.

When you move into the **Metaboost Diet for Life**—the maintenance phase—your macro balance shifts again to a sustainable long-term ratio:

- **40% healthy fats**

- **20% protein**

- **40% carbohydrates**

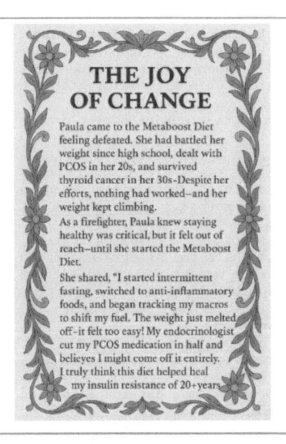

THE JOY OF CHANGE

Paula came to the Metaboost Diet feeling defeated. She had battled her weight since high school, dealt with PCOS in her 20s, and survived thyroid cancer in her 30s–Despite her efforts, nothing had worked–and her weight kept climbing.

As a firefighter, Paula knew staying healthy was critical, but it felt out of reach–until she started the Metaboost Diet.

She shared, "I started intermittent fasting, switched to anti-inflammatory foods, and began tracking my macros to shift my fuel. The weight just melted off–it felt too easy! My endocrinologist cut my PCOS medication in half and believes I might come off it entirely. I truly think this diet helped heal my insulin resistance of 20+years

HOT FLASH TIP: DON'T SKIP EXERCISE

Regular physical activity is a core part of the Metaboost Diet lifestyle. A mix of cardio (brisk walking, jogging, machines—whatever you like) and strength training is ideal.

Don't shy away from lifting weights—even light ones help. As we age, we naturally lose muscle mass through a process called sarcopenia. Without strength training, this muscle loss can slow your metabolism, making weight gain more likely.

Incorporating both cardio and strength workouts also increases post-exercise calorie burn—another great reason to move your body consistently!

Approach This Phase with the Right Mindset

Throughout our lives, we as women pass through meaningful milestones. Getting our first period marks the beginning of womanhood; for many, pregnancy and raising children represent the transition into motherhood. These events are often celebrated as incredible achievements. In contrast, menopause is too often seen as a loss—a loss of fertility, attractiveness, sexuality, and even personal value.

But I believe menopause is actually a gateway to a new and fulfilling chapter. Consider this: around 40% of a woman's life is spent in postmenopause. Let that really sink in.

Think of the possibilities that come with all that time! Often, menopause aligns with a stage in life when your children—if you have them—are becoming independent or have already left home. This shift gives you more time to focus on yourself and explore what brings you joy. Whether it's launching a business, volunteering, writing, creating art, reconnecting with loved ones, spending time outdoors, or even running for office—the options are endless.

In this light, menopause becomes something to appreciate. It means you've lived a long life—something not everyone gets the chance to do. Personally, I make a point to celebrate my birthday every year as a reminder to be thankful for my life, even if it comes with a few more wrinkles, gray hairs, or achy joints.

This phase can be a time for self-discovery. Instead of being discouraged by the changes, use this time to be mindful in your decisions. Learn how your body responds to different foods, movement, and even relationships. Then, put your energy into what uplifts you. When you shift your mindset around menopause—and live by the core ideas in the Metaboost Diet—you may find that this chapter is one of the most rewarding yet.

CHAPTER 2

Understanding and Managing Your Hormones

For too long, women have been misled to believe that losing weight and maintaining it is all about willpower—just push through, resist temptation, and the pounds will drop. But when a diet "fails," the blame often lands unfairly on the person.

Here's the reality: **you are not the problem.** If you've struggled with diets, it's not a reflection of your strength or self-discipline. Those diets failed *you*. And the root of the problem? It's not about willpower—it's about hormones. Hormonal imbalances and related metabolic issues are key drivers of midlife weight gain.

When you can't lose weight despite your best efforts, it's easy to feel defeated or to criticize yourself. This emotional cycle of weight loss and regain only adds more stress. But gaining weight has nothing to do with who you are—it's **hormonal**, plain and simple.

Rethinking the Science Behind Weight Gain

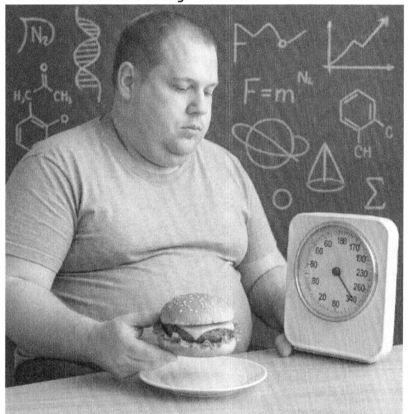

For decades, the standard explanation for weight gain has been based on a simple formula: calories in vs. calories out. According to the World Health Organization, obesity is caused by an imbalance in energy intake and energy expenditure. That's the model I was taught in medical school—and believed. But modern research has shifted this narrative. A pivotal 2020 study published in the *American Journal of Clinical Nutrition*, led by top obesity scientists, revealed that **obesity isn't primarily about calorie balance—it's a hormonal condition.** Hormones govern how fat is stored and how energy is used, regardless of how many calories you consume.

In simpler terms, your weight is influenced more by **hormones**—and especially by the **type and quality** of carbohydrates you eat—than by how much you eat. Carbs, particularly processed or refined ones, can create a hormonal environment that encourages fat gain.

Add to this the natural drop in estrogen that comes with age, and you'll often see new fat accumulation—particularly around the midsection—despite your best efforts to eat right or exercise regularly.

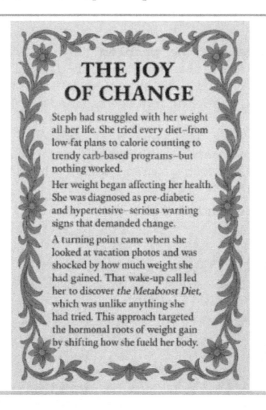

THE JOY OF CHANGE

Steph had struggled with her weight all her life. She tried every diet–from low-fat plans to calorie counting to trendy carb-based programs–but nothing worked.

Her weight began affecting her health. She was diagnosed as pre-diabetic and hypertensive–serious warning signs that demanded change.

A turning point came when she looked at vacation photos and was shocked by how much weight she had gained. That wake-up call led her to discover *the Metaboost Diet*, which was unlike anything she had tried. This approach targeted the hormonal roots of weight gain by shifting how she fueld her body.

Hormones and You

Hormones are the body's chemical messengers. They're produced by glands and organs like the ovaries, brain, adrenal glands, and gut. These hormones send signals to cells, regulating how your body functions and maintaining balance.

When it comes to weight and menopause symptoms, **hormones are in control**. They impact hunger, cravings, metabolism, fat storage, and more. When even one hormone is off, it can derail your efforts to lose weight.

As noted in Chapter 1, imbalanced hormone levels are linked to weight gain and increased risk of chronic conditions like inflammation, heart disease, stroke, and diabetes.

The good news? By using the nutrition strategies in the Metaboost Diet, **you can restore balance to your hormones** and prevent many of these issues.

Nine key hormones are involved in midlife weight gain—and nutrition plays a powerful role in managing them.

Estrogen: A Major Player

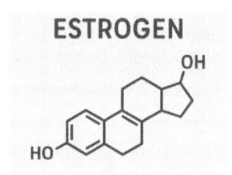

ESTROGEN

Estrogen is the female hormone and a key factor in both perimenopause and menopause. It's actually a group of three hormones: **estrone, estradiol**, and **estriol**. These regulate menstrual cycles and develop female characteristics, while also influencing how fat is stored in the hips, thighs, and abdomen—important for pregnancy and breastfeeding.

Estrogen also affects your body in many other ways:

- Maintains bone density
- Helps control cholesterol
- Increases skin blood flow and thickness
- Supports the health of vaginal, bladder, and pelvic floor tissues
- Helps regulate mood and may reduce anxiety and depression

During midlife, estrogen levels begin to fluctuate dramatically. As your ovaries reduce estrogen production in perimenopause, your body increases follicle-stimulating hormone (FSH) in an attempt to trigger more estrogen. This leads to those dramatic hormonal swings.

As estrogen declines during menopause, your liver produces less **sex hormone-binding globulin (SHBG),** a protein that normally binds hormones and keeps them in check. With less SHBG, hormone activity—especially androgens like testosterone—increases. This shift contributes to increased belly fat, higher cholesterol, and unwanted facial hair.

How the Metaboost Diet Supports Estrogen Balance

In Chapter 7, you'll learn how specific foods can help regulate estrogen. Some of the most powerful hormone-supporting foods include:

- **Cruciferous vegetables** (like broccoli, Brussels sprouts, cauliflower): These are closely tied to estrogen regulation. Research shows that women who consume these veggies regularly have lower risks of heart disease, stroke, cancer, and estrogen imbalance.
- **Leafy greens**: Contain compounds like **DIM, indole-3-carbinol (I3C),** and **calcium D-glucarate**, which assist the liver in removing estrogen by-products.
- **Avocados**: Full of healthy fats that promote hormone balance, especially between estrogen and progesterone.
- **Salmon** (and other fatty fish): Rich in omega-3 fatty acids that support estrogen production and overall hormone function.
- **Flax and pumpkin seeds**: High in **lignans**, plant-based nutrients that help regulate estrogen metabolism and serve as antioxidants. Pumpkin seeds also provide **zinc,** healthy fats, and protein—all essential for hormone health.

Sometimes, excess estrogen—not a deficiency—is the issue. This may happen when ovulation becomes irregular, leading to more estrogen and not enough progesterone. It can also be caused by poor estrogen breakdown or exposure to **xenoestrogens**—environmental chemicals that mimic estrogen inside the body. Too much alcohol, liver dysfunction, and excess body fat (which can convert androgens into estrogen) can also contribute to elevated estrogen levels. The Metaboost Diet helps address all of this—especially through foods like cruciferous veggies and leafy greens, which naturally assist with detoxification and hormone clearance.

Insulin

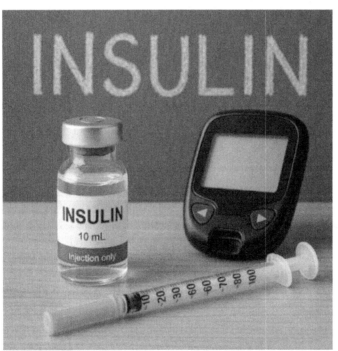

Insulin is a hormone made by the pancreas in response to the carbohydrates you eat. Its main job is to help your cells absorb sugar (glucose) from your bloodstream and either use it for energy or store it for later.

Insulin also plays a major role in fat storage. It prevents your body from breaking down fat and actually encourages fat accumulation. That's why, if you're overweight, diabetic, or at risk for diabetes, it's crucial to bring your insulin levels under control to avoid storing more fat and to better manage your weight. A key way to do this is by **reducing your intake of carbohydrates**, especially **refined carbs and added sugars**.

As we age and gain more belly fat, **insulin resistance** (IR) often develops. This means your body needs to release more insulin than normal to do the same job of moving sugar into your cells.

Diets high in sugar, refined carbs, and fast food are a major driver of insulin resistance and the resulting weight gain. One study found that people who regularly ate fast food (twice or more per week) gained more weight and were more likely to develop insulin resistance—raising their risk for obesity and type 2 diabetes.

Hot Flash: Possible Signs of Insulin Resistance

- Constant thirst or hunger
- Feeling hungry even after eating
- Recurring bladder or vaginal infections
- Increase in belly fat
- Frequent urination
- Tingling in hands and feet
- Skin tags
- Dark, velvety patches on the skin (acanthosis nigricans), especially on the neck or underarms

How the Metaboost Diet Supports Healthy Insulin Levels

The Metaboost Diet is designed to help regulate insulin and improve your body's sensitivity to it by making smarter food choices:

- **Cutting carbs**: Reducing carbs helps lower insulin levels and stabilizes blood sugar. You'll learn how to do this effectively in the Fuel Refocus phase.
- **Avoiding added sugars**: Especially those in the form of high-fructose corn syrup and sucrose, which promote insulin resistance.
- **Including protein in every meal**: While protein briefly increases insulin, in the long term it helps reduce belly fat and support insulin sensitivity.
- **Eating healthy fats**: Especially omega-3s, which are shown to lower fasting insulin levels.
- **Getting enough fiber**: Aim for at least 25 grams daily (ideally 35). Both soluble (found in oats, lentils, nuts, fruits, and certain veggies) and insoluble fiber (found in vegetables and whole grains) are essential for blood sugar balance and digestive health.
- **Supplementing with magnesium**: Many people with insulin resistance are low in magnesium, which helps improve insulin response. Chapter 7 goes into more detail.
- **Adding antioxidant-rich foods**: Vibrant fruits and vegetables help fight inflammation and support lower insulin levels.
- **Using herbs and spices**: Spices like fenugreek, turmeric, ginger, garlic, and cinnamon can improve insulin function and lower blood sugar.
- **Drinking green tea**: Rich in antioxidants that help reduce inflammation and improve insulin sensitivity.
- **Exercising regularly**: Both cardio and strength training boost insulin sensitivity over time.

Leptin

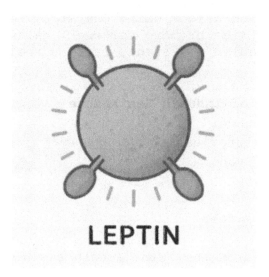

Leptin is a hormone made by fat cells that signals when you're full. It tells your brain you've had enough to eat and that your body has sufficient fat stores, helping to prevent overeating.

However, when you're overweight, you may have **excess leptin in your system**—so much that your brain stops responding to it. This is called **leptin resistance**. One study found that obese individuals had four times more leptin in their blood than people of normal weight.

With leptin resistance, your brain doesn't get the message that you're full, which leads to more eating, weight gain, and a cycle that's hard to break. As body fat increases, so does leptin and insulin, disrupting hunger signals even more. Your brain thinks you're starving—so you eat more and continue gaining fat.

Hot Flash: Six Foods That Contribute to Leptin Resistance

To avoid leptin resistance, eliminate or limit these processed, high-sugar foods:

- Soda and soft drinks
- Sweetened juices
- Canned fruits in syrup
- Boxed dessert mixes
- Flavored yogurts
- Sugary cereals

How the Metaboost Diet Helps Regulate Leptin

Managing leptin starts with changing what and how you eat:

- **Avoid ultra-processed foods**: These drive inflammation, which disrupts leptin signaling.
- **Increase your fiber intake**: Soluble fiber in particular helps with satiety, weight control, and gut health.
- **Lower your triglycerides**: High triglycerides block leptin from reaching the brain. Reducing your carb intake can help lower these fat levels in your blood.
- **Eat more protein**: This supports healthy leptin signaling and appetite regulation. Women should aim for 20-25 grams of protein per meal. A 3-ounce portion of animal protein provides around 21-24 grams. Vegetarian sources like beans or eggs also contribute valuable protein.

- **Exercise consistently**: Physical activity can help reset your leptin response.
- **Prioritize good sleep**: Poor sleep is linked to problems with leptin regulation.

Ghrelin

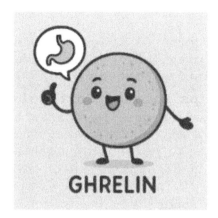

Ghrelin is often referred to as the "hunger hormone." It's produced in your stomach and travels through your bloodstream to your brain, signaling the need to eat.

When you drastically reduce calories, **ghrelin levels spike**, which makes you feel even hungrier. This is one of the main reasons restrictive calorie diets can be so difficult to maintain.

How the Metaboost Diet Supports Healthy Ghrelin Function

To keep ghrelin levels balanced and reduce hunger:
- **Reduce sugar intake**: Cut back on added sugars and high-fructose corn syrup, especially in beverages.
- **Include protein at every meal**: This is particularly important when breaking a fast. Women over 50 should aim for 20-25 grams of protein per meal.
- **Eat plenty of fiber**: High-fiber foods fill you up, improve satiety, and help stabilize blood sugar after meals.

Cortisol

CORTISOL

OH

OH

CH₃OH

As if midlife weren't already a challenge, add in the constant presence of stress—whether it's at home, work, or within family dynamics. When you're stressed, your body produces stress hormones, and one of the most important is **cortisol.**

In times of stress, cortisol prompts the release of fat and glucose into your bloodstream, giving you a burst of energy for the classic "fight or flight" response. This was useful in life-or-death scenarios, but today, cortisol can't distinguish between immediate danger and ongoing stressors like deadlines or financial concerns.

When stress becomes chronic, cortisol stays elevated. This can raise blood sugar, increase appetite and cravings, encourage fat storage—especially around the abdomen—and worsen insulin resistance.

How the Metaboost Diet Helps Balance Cortisol

If you've gone through a period of feeling constantly stressed, drained, and unlike yourself, high cortisol may be to blame. The Metaboost Diet includes foods and lifestyle strategies to help bring cortisol back to a healthy level:

- **Dark chocolate** (70% cocoa or higher): Rich in nutrients and shown in studies to reduce cortisol in response to stress.
- **Probiotic and prebiotic foods**: Yogurt, kimchi, sauerkraut, and other fermented foods increase good gut bacteria and may lower inflammation and cortisol. Prebiotics, found in soluble fiber, also support cortisol regulation.
- **Stay hydrated**: Dehydration increases physical stress on your body, raising cortisol. A pale yellow or clear urine color is a good sign of proper hydration.
- **Eat omega-3 fats**: Found in fish, omega-3s help reduce cortisol, while omega-6 fats (found in processed and fried foods) promote inflammation.

Lifestyle habits also play a major role in cortisol management:

- **Practice stress reduction**: Meditation, music, yoga, or relaxation programs are great options. Try apps like *Calm* or *Headspace* to get started.
- **Prioritize sleep**: Poor sleep raises cortisol, so good sleep hygiene is crucial.
- **Exercise moderately**: Regular movement helps lower cortisol levels.

Neuropeptide Y (NPY)

If you've ever felt hooked on carbs, you're not imagining things. That strong pull toward carbohydrate-heavy foods is often driven by a hormone called **neuropeptide Y (NPY).**

Produced in the brain and nervous system, NPY is one of the most powerful appetite triggers. It's responsible for those pantry raids and fridge searches for snacks. NPY levels rise when leptin is low, during calorie restriction, or

when you're stressed—all of which can lead to cravings and fat gain, especially around the belly.
It also shortens the time between meals and delays the signal to your brain that you're full.

How the Metaboost Diet Reduces NPY
By shifting your fuel sources and eating nutrient-dense meals, you can lower NPY levels and beat carb cravings. Here's how:
- **Eat enough protein**: Inadequate protein can raise NPY. Women over 50 should aim for 20-25 grams of high-quality protein, three times a day.
- **Boost prebiotic fiber**: Soluble fiber feeds healthy gut bacteria, supports digestion, and curbs unnecessary cravings.
- **Lower stress**: Like cortisol, NPY can be decreased by incorporating stress-relief strategies into your daily routine.

Glucagon-Like Peptide-1 (GLP-1)

GLP-1 is a gut hormone released when food enters your intestines. It reduces appetite, supports weight loss, slows digestion, and helps your pancreas release insulin. It also prevents your liver from sending out excess glucose—making it a key player in blood sugar control.

How the Metaboost Diet Increases GLP-1
On the Metaboost Diet, you'll notice feeling less hungry and having fewer cravings. That's partly due to higher GLP-1 levels from these foods:
- **Protein sources like fish, whey (cottage cheese, ricotta), and yogurt**: These enhance GLP-1 production and boost insulin sensitivity.
- **Antioxidant-rich fruits and vegetables**: These reduce inflammation and help raise GLP-1. Leafy greens like spinach and kale are particularly effective.
- **Probiotic foods**: Found in yogurt and other fermented items, these can also support GLP-1 levels and reduce appetite.

Cholecystokinin (CCK)

CHOLECYSTOKININI

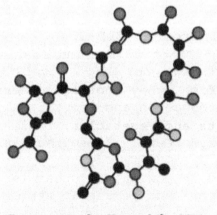

CCK is a digestive hormone that helps you feel full and promotes fat breakdown. It slows how quickly food moves through your gut, so you stay fuller longer, and it signals your body to burn fat more efficiently.
CCK is released when you eat meals that contain fat, and it also triggers digestive enzymes and bile for fat processing.

How the Metaboost Diet Boosts CCK
Foods that are rich in **protein, healthy fats, fiber,** and **omega-3s** all support CCK production. You'll be eating these regularly as part of your plan.

Pancreatic Peptide YY (PYY)

Pancreatic Peptide YY

PYY is another satiety hormone released after meals, especially meals with fat and protein. It slows the rate at which your stomach empties, helping you feel full and satisfied longer.

46

PYY levels peak about two hours after a meal and then taper off. Low levels are linked to increased hunger, and people with obesity or type 2 diabetes often have lower PYY levels.

How the Metaboost Diet Increases PYY

The meal structure in the Metaboost Diet is designed to support optimal PYY levels:

- **Lower carbohydrate intake**: Helps stabilize blood sugar and supports proper PYY function.
- **Get enough protein**: Both animal and plant sources will do the job.
- **Eat plenty of fiber**: A fiber-rich diet is essential for boosting fullness and supporting digestion.

Hot Flash: Is Hormone Replacement Therapy Right for You?

Hormone replacement therapy (HRT) has seen major advancements and continues to be a powerful option for many women going through menopause. For some, it can be truly transformative.

HRT offers a wide range of benefits, including:

- Trimming excess belly fat
- Redistributing body fat for a more balanced shape
- Lowering fasting blood sugar and insulin, which helps prevent insulin resistance and type 2 diabetes
- Improving cholesterol and triglyceride levels, which reduces the risk of heart disease
- Slowing bone loss, which helps prevent osteoporosis
- Enhancing memory and focus by reducing brain fog
- Boosting overall well-being

Deciding whether HRT is right for you is a personal decision to be made with your doctor. But the more informed you are, the better equipped you'll be to make a confident, evidence-based choice. Here are a few important considerations I often discuss with women exploring this option:

- The best time to begin HRT is typically during perimenopause or within a few years after menopause starts.
- Many of the symptoms you're experiencing—such as weight gain, hot flashes, and vaginal dryness—stem from declining estrogen levels. While HRT is only FDA-approved for treating hot flashes and vaginal symptoms (like thinning tissues and dryness), it may also help reduce belly fat and inflammation.
- If you still have your uterus, you should not take estrogen by itself, as this increases the risk of endometrial cancer. Adding progesterone balances this risk, and a combination of both hormones is the recommended approach. If you've had a hysterectomy, estrogen-only therapy is generally fine.

Always consult a knowledgeable provider who understands HRT and can tailor the treatment to your needs. For guidance, see the Resources section on my website, where you'll find a list of menopause-informed healthcare professionals.

CHAPTER 3

Get Ready to Transform Your Life

By now, you understand that following the Metaboost Diet can help you lose weight and ease many midlife symptoms. The great news is that once you're into the program, you can experience major improvements—such as reduced belly fat, fewer hot flashes, more energy, better mood, improved focus, and overall better health. In fact, many women start noticing these benefits within just two weeks. Every effort you make will pay off!

That said, I know you're excited to get started—but don't rush. I encourage you to take a few days, or even a week, to read through the entire book first. It's essential that you understand what's happening in your body during this stage of life, why the Metaboost Diet works the way it does, and how all the key components fit together. You'll want to be familiar with the meal plans and their purpose so you can get the most out of them.

Let the knowledge truly settle in. When you understand the "why" behind this program, you're more likely to stick with it and succeed. So take your time—this is a long-term lifestyle, not a quick fix. And when you're ready, here are a few important steps to set yourself up for success.

Track Your Starting Point

To measure your success, you need to know where you're beginning. That means tracking some key body measurements—and yes, stepping on the scale, but with the right mindset.

1. Record Your Weight

While the scale can be useful, it's not the only way—or even the best way—to measure health. In fact, I encourage women in the program to "break up" with their scale. Why? Because it's common to lose inches (especially around your waist) without seeing much movement on the scale. That's because you may be gaining lean muscle and losing fat. Muscle weighs more than fat but takes up less space—so even if your weight stays the same, your body is getting healthier.

Weigh yourself today, write it down along with the date, and keep that note in a small journal. Just remember: your weight is one data point—not the final verdict on your progress.

2. Take Body Measurements

Use a cloth tape measure to record the circumference of your waist, hips, and thighs. Keep these in the same notebook where you track your weight.

Measurement tips:

- Take measurements in the morning, before you've eaten, and without clothing to avoid bloating or distortion.
- Breathe normally—don't suck in your stomach to get better numbers.
- Use a mirror to make sure the tape measure is level.
- For **waist measurement**, exhale and measure around the smallest part of your torso—usually above your belly button.
- For **hip measurement**, wrap the tape around the widest part of your hips or buttocks—typically 7 inches below your waist.
- Keep the tape snug, but not too tight.

Note: Your waist size is one of the most important indicators of your health. A measurement over 35 inches can signal excess visceral fat, which carries serious health risks.

3. Calculate Your Waist-to-Hip Ratio (WHR)

This is a key health indicator in the Metaboost Diet. To calculate it, divide your waist circumference by your hip circumference. Write it down in your journal. A better WHR typically reflects improved health and lower disease risk.

4. Take Progress Photos

This might feel awkward now, but you'll be thankful later. Take full-body photos from the front, side, and back. These will help you visually track your transformation over time.

You'll repeat these measurements and take new photos after four weeks. Most women are inspired and encouraged by the results—visible proof that they're burning fat and becoming healthier.

What Your Waist-to-Hip Ratio Says About Your Health

Scientific studies have consistently linked a high WHR to increased risk of:

- Heart disease
- High blood pressure
- Diabetes
- Gallbladder issues
- Some cancers

After menopause, WHR often increases, which is associated with a higher risk of conditions like heart disease, fractures, and hormone-related cancers (such as breast and endometrial cancer).

But here's the good news: **lowering your WHR significantly improves your health outlook.**

Here's a general guide for women:

Health Risk	Waist-to-Hip Ratio
Low	0.80 or lower
Moderate	0.81-0.85
High	0.86 or higher

Use a Nutrition Tracker

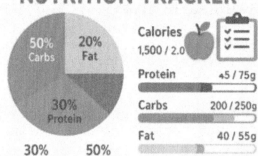

NUTRITION TRACKER

50% Carbs
20% Fat
30% Protein
30%   50%

Calories 1,500 / 2.0
Protein 45 / 75g
Carbs   200 / 250g
Fat   40 / 55g

Since creating the Metaboost Diet in 2017, I've seen that the women who have the most success are the ones who track their food intake—especially macronutrients and micronutrients.

- **Macronutrients** are carbs, fats, and proteins—the main sources of energy.
- **Micronutrients** include vitamins, minerals, fiber, antioxidants, and plant compounds.

You can track both with a smartphone app. My favorite is **Cronometer**, which has a large, detailed food database. Other great options include **Carb Manager, MyFitnessPal, Fitbit, Lose It!**, and **MyNetDiary**.

Once downloaded, use the app to begin monitoring your nutrition choices. Think of it like managing a budget—you can see exactly where your nutritional "spending" goes.

Be sure to choose an app that allows you to customize your **macro targets** and track **net carbs** (total carbs minus fiber). As an experiment, begin tracking your food intake this week—even before starting the full plan.

Important Note:

The Metaboost Diet does *not* involve counting calories. That approach doesn't reflect how food actually affects your body. Calories differ in how they influence your hormones, energy use, and hunger.

For example, eating processed foods full of empty calories leaves your body unsatisfied and craving more nutrients, leading to overeating.

On the flip side, when you choose **nutrient-dense, high-quality foods**—like the ones in this plan—your body feels nourished and satisfied. That's how you naturally reduce cravings, lose fat, and improve your health.

Begin a Daily Journaling Routine

I'm a big advocate for journaling every day. Taking a few minutes to write out your thoughts can help you stay focused on your goals—whether those are related to nutrition, exercise, mindset, or self-care. Journaling also encourages gratitude and helps you stay accountable.

Your journal can be a place to track your body measurements, waist-to-hip ratio, and set personal health goals.

The amount you write is totally up to you, and you can explore any topic that feels relevant. But for those following this program, here are some helpful daily prompts to guide your entries:

- **Today I am grateful for:** _____

- **Two self-care actions I'll take today:** _____

- **Victories or moments to celebrate today:** _____

- **My intentions today:** _____
   (Examples: "I'll try something new," "I will honor my body," "I'll stick to my meal plan," "I believe in myself.")

- **What I'm letting go of today:** _____
   (Examples: self-criticism, regrets, negativity, overwhelm.)

- **Exercise plan:** _____

- **Fasting window:** _____ (e.g., 8 p.m. to 12 p.m. the next day)

- **Macronutrient goals:** Carbs _____ Fats _____ Protein _____

You don't need a fancy journal—just a notebook or a digital document will do. If you'd like more structure, check out the *Daily Recharge Journal* available on my website. It's designed with prompts like these built in.

Think About Taking Supplements

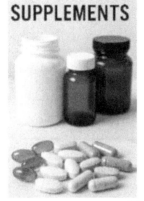

Many people ask if supplements are necessary. While I always stress that real, whole food should be your source of nutrients, I understand that it's not always easy to get everything your body needs through diet alone.

Fruits, vegetables, and nutrient-dense foods provide powerful health benefits that can't be duplicated in pill form. But because many of our diets fall short—especially in magnesium, vitamin D, and fiber—supplements can help fill in the gaps.

The Metaboost Diet is designed to be rich in essential nutrients like fiber, magnesium, omega-3 fats, and vitamin D. Still, if your diet is lacking in these areas, the following three supplements are worth considering.

1. Fiber Supplements

It can be tough to get 25-30 grams of fiber a day from food alone—I've struggled with it too! Supplementing is a great way to boost your fiber intake and support your health.

Personally, I prioritize fiber because of my family history with cancer. Several relatives, including my uncle and two brothers, died from different forms of the disease, so I do everything I can to support my body. Research strongly suggests that a high-fiber diet may help protect against colon, breast, ovarian, endometrial, and other gastrointestinal cancers.

If you're shopping for a fiber supplement, here's what to look for:

- **Choose products with both soluble and insoluble fiber.**

- **Opt for natural sources** over synthetic ones. I chose gluten-free, whole-food-based fibers like buckwheat, quinoa, chia, millet, and amaranth for the supplement I formulated. Other good sources include **pectin** (found in fruits) and **psyllium husk** (from the *Plantago* plant).

- **Avoid sugar-laden products**. Some popular fiber powders and gummies contain up to 16 grams of sugar per serving! Instead, look for unsweetened or naturally sweetened options (e.g., monk fruit or stevia).

Tip: If you're new to fiber supplements, **start slow**. Jumping in too fast can cause bloating or gas. Begin with half a dose for a week or two and gradually increase, always drinking plenty of water.

2. Vitamin D
We get vitamin D from sunlight, but many people don't get enough—especially if they spend most of their time indoors, wear sunscreen frequently, live in northern climates, or have darker skin.
Vitamin D is essential for bone health, immune support, and hormone function. The best form is **vitamin D3 (cholecalciferol)**, which your body absorbs more efficiently.

3. Omega-3 Fatty Acids
Omega-3s are incredibly important for your brain and body. They're found in foods like fatty fish, nuts, and seeds—but getting enough from diet alone can be challenging, which is why I recommend supplements.
When choosing an omega-3 supplement, **look for one that includes both EPA and DHA**—the two most beneficial types found in fish oil and marine algae.
While there's no universal dosage recommendation, most health organizations suggest at least **500 mg of combined EPA and DHA daily**, unless your doctor advises otherwise.

Hot Flash: Three Essential Actions to Take Right Now
If you're in perimenopause or menopause, here are **three things** you should start doing immediately to support your health and success on the Metaboost Diet:
1. **Commit to the right kind of exercise**
   Focus on a mix of **strength training** and **cardiovascular activity**. If you haven't started yet, now is the time! Join a gym, work with a trainer, or follow a home workout routine. Aim for at least **three 45- to 60-minute sessions per week**. Research shows that many age-related changes linked to menopause are actually due to **inactivity**—not aging itself.
2. **Mentally prepare to change your eating habits**
   Start learning which foods are high in protein, fiber, vitamins, minerals, and antioxidants. Add more whole foods like **fruits, vegetables, fish, and poultry** to your daily routine. Cut down on processed snacks, sugary drinks, and alcohol.

   Don't forget to stay hydrated—**aim for 64 ounces (2 quarts) of water daily**. Water helps transport nutrients, hormones, and oxygen through your body, removes waste, lubricates joints, and supports both physical and mental energy.
3. **Stop smoking**
   Smoking makes menopause symptoms worse. Women who smoke tend to experience more hot flashes and often enter menopause earlier. That's because **nicotine lowers estrogen levels**.

Smoking also increases your risk for **heart disease, stroke, osteoporosis, and cancer**—and most doctors won't prescribe HRT to smokers due to the heightened risks. If you smoke, look into a cessation program or ask your doctor for help in quitting.

When your body is going through major hormonal shifts, it makes sense to support it in every way possible. These three steps are a powerful place to start.

Create an Environment That Supports Your Success

Both your physical space and your social circle have a huge impact on your ability to stay consistent and succeed long-term. Your surroundings shape your daily habits, choices, and mindset more than you might realize.

Let's start with your **social environment.**

It's essential to let your family, friends, and coworkers know what lifestyle changes you're making. Their understanding and encouragement can make a big difference. I can say from experience that I wouldn't have been able to develop or stick with the Metaboost Diet without the full support of my family.

Research shows we tend to adopt the habits and attitudes of the people we spend time with. That's why having a supportive and uplifting group around you is so important. Stay away from people who undermine your goals or have negative energy.

Consider doing the Metaboost Diet alongside a friend or partner. Find a workout buddy. Surround yourself with people who are also prioritizing health and wellness. Many women find incredible support and motivation in the Metaboost Diet online community—come join us! (See Resources for details.)

Your **physical environment** matters just as much. A well-prepared kitchen and home can make it easier to stick with your goals. Here are a few simple but powerful strategies:

- **Keep your kitchen stocked** with the key ingredients and foods recommended in the Metaboost Diet.
- **Clear out tempting, unhelpful foods** and replace them with better options that align with your goals. Save indulgent treats for special occasions, and buy them in small portions.
- **Practice meal prepping** using the guides in Chapter 8. Prepping your meals and snacks ahead of time gives you easy access to healthy choices. Even buying pre-cut vegetables can save time and reduce the urge to reach for junk food.

Setting up a positive environment makes healthy choices more accessible and unhealthy habits harder to fall into. You're taking control of your surroundings before they take control of you.

Remember, achieving sustainable weight loss and better health is not about quick fixes or drastic diets—they rarely last and often do more harm than good. The only lasting results come from **slow, steady progress** supported by a nourishing, hormone-friendly eating plan like the Metaboost Diet.

So instead of cutting out all your favorite things, focus on balance. Yes, you can still enjoy pizza or a glass of wine occasionally. Adopting healthier habits shouldn't feel like punishment—it's actually about gaining freedom. You're creating a lifestyle you can happily maintain for years to come.

Part 2 Actions

CHAPTER 4

Action 1: Intermittent Fasting

Here's a paraphrased version of the section on **intermittent fasting**—from the author's initial skepticism to the wide range of health benefits—while keeping the meaning, structure, and tone consistent:

Embracing Intermittent Fasting

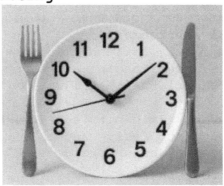

At first, I was reluctant to try intermittent fasting (IF). I assumed it was just another diet trend. I didn't want to give up my morning coffee the way I liked it, and I wasn't ready to skip breakfast.

But as I continued building the Metaboost Diet, I decided to dig into the research with an open mind. One of the most influential pieces I came across was a TED Talk by Dr. Mark Mattson, former chief of the Laboratory of Neurosciences at the National Institute on Aging. His research showed that intermittent fasting could significantly reduce inflammation. That one insight changed everything for me. Since the Metaboost Diet already focused on anti-inflammatory foods, adding IF as a complementary tool made perfect sense.

I've now experienced firsthand how powerful intermittent fasting can be. Let's take a closer look at how it works—and why it's such a transformative practice for long-term health and vitality.

What Is Intermittent Fasting?

Intermittent fasting is a style of eating that alternates between periods of eating and fasting (not eating). There are several ways to practice it:

- **5:2 Method:** Fast for two full days each week (non-consecutive), then eat normally the other five days.

- **Eat Stop Eat:** Do a full 24-hour fast once or twice a week—for example, from dinner one day to dinner the next.

- **OMAD (One Meal a Day):** Eat one large meal a day, choosing any time (morning, afternoon, or evening).

- **Alternate-Day Fasting:** Cycle between one day of fasting (or very low-calorie intake) and one day of normal eating.

- **Early Time-Restricted Feeding (eTRF):** Limit eating to morning and early afternoon, then fast for the rest of the day.

Why the Metaboost Diet Uses the 16:8 Method

For this program, I recommend the **16:8 approach**—a daily fasting cycle where you eat within an 8-hour window and fast for the remaining 16 hours, much of which occurs overnight while you sleep.

You can do this method every day or a few times a week, but the most consistent benefits come from daily practice. It's one of the simplest, most sustainable methods because it fits easily into a normal routine. Many participants in our online community say it's the easiest plan to stick with.

Most people follow this pattern by skipping breakfast, eating their first meal around noon, and finishing dinner by 8 p.m. That gives you a full 16-hour fasting window. But if you prefer an earlier eating schedule, that's fine too—as long as your eating window stays within 8 hours.

During your eating window, you'll enjoy **two Metaboost Diet-approved meals and two snacks**, without counting calories. But to be effective, your food choices matter—avoid processed foods, added sugars, and refined carbs.

During your fasting window, water, black coffee, and plain tea are allowed and encouraged to stay hydrated.

Science backs this up—a study published in *Cell Metabolism* found that 16:8 intermittent fasting led to **weight loss, reduced belly fat, lower blood pressure, and improved cholesterol**. It's also shown to reduce brain fog and enhance mental clarity.

Fasting Has Deep Roots

Fasting isn't new. It's been part of religious and cultural traditions for centuries. Muslims fast during Ramadan, and fasting is also practiced by Jews, Buddhists, Hindus, and Christians. In fact, fasting has long been viewed as a way to show spiritual devotion.

Even before organized religion, **our ancestors practiced fasting by necessity**. As hunter-gatherers, they would feast when food was plentiful and fast when it wasn't. Our bodies evolved to thrive under these "feast and fast" cycles, which makes intermittent fasting a return to how we're naturally built to function.

The Many Benefits of Intermittent Fasting

1. Blood Sugar & Insulin Control

Fasting improves insulin sensitivity, lowers insulin levels, and helps your body burn fat more efficiently. It can lower blood sugar by 3-6% and insulin levels by 20-31%, helping prevent and manage type 2 diabetes.

One study from 2018 found that nearly half of participants with type 2 diabetes **were able to stop taking medication** and achieve remission after a year of intermittent fasting. (Note: Always consult your doctor before changing any medication.)

2. Cellular Rejuvenation

Intermittent fasting creates mild stress at the cellular level, which triggers a repair response—similar to how exercise strengthens muscles.

One of the most powerful processes activated by fasting is **autophagy**, which clears away damaged or dysfunctional components in your cells. This cellular "clean-up" process may help protect against **Alzheimer's, Parkinson's,** and other age-related diseases.

Fasting also boosts **chaperone proteins**, which help other proteins fold properly, support cellular repair, and remove harmful free radicals.

3. Reduced Inflammation

Chronic inflammation is at the root of many diseases—from arthritis and MS to IBD and heart disease. Intermittent fasting reduces inflammatory markers in the body.

For example, **monocytes**—a type of white blood cell involved in inflammation—become less active during fasting, according to research in *Cell*.

Fasting also appears to reduce **galectin-3,** a protein linked to inflammation and disease progression.

In one study, **people with asthma** who practiced alternate-day fasting not only lost weight but also experienced fewer asthma symptoms and reduced inflammation.

4. Better Brain Health

Fasting enhances **neuroplasticity**, especially in the **hippocampus**, the brain region linked to memory and learning. It also promotes the production of **ketones**, which have neuroprotective effects.

Autophagy helps remove toxins and damaged cells from the brain, potentially lowering the risk of dementia.

Additionally, fasting increases levels of **brain-derived neurotrophic factor (BDNF)**, a molecule essential for brain function and mood regulation.

5. Cancer Prevention Potential

Among women, the most common cancers include **breast, colorectal, lung, cervical, and stomach cancers.** Intermittent fasting may help protect against these by:

- **Reducing inflammation** (a known risk factor for cancer)

- **Inhibiting angiogenesis** (the growth of new blood vessels that feed tumors)

- **Promoting fat loss,** which lowers cancer risk

- **Decreasing IGF-1,** a growth hormone linked to cancer and aging

High IGF-1 levels speed up cell growth but also increase the chance of cell damage. Fasting slows IGF-1 production, shifting the body from growth mode to **repair and maintenance**—a shift that may reduce cancer risk and support healthy aging.

Gene Expression and Slowing the Aging Process

Genes are tiny sections of DNA that carry instructions for nearly everything your body does—from how you metabolize food to how your immune system functions and how long you live. When a gene is "expressed," it acts as a guide for building proteins that direct the cells in your body.

Gene expression can be either turned up (upregulated) or turned down (downregulated) depending on different factors—and **intermittent fasting** is one of them. According to a 2020 study, just 30 days of moderate intermittent fasting (similar to the 16:8 plan) led to notable changes in gene expression that may enhance health and longevity.

Fasting has also been linked to **slower DNA breakdown** (which occurs with aging) and **faster DNA repair,** both of which help delay the aging process. In addition, fasting boosts antioxidant levels, helping protect your cells from damage caused by free radicals—unstable molecules that contribute to cellular aging and disease.

Intermittent Fasting and Weight Management

Research has shown that people who adopt intermittent fasting not only lose weight but also maintain it long-term. A 2014 review in *Translational Research* found that participants lost between 3-8% of their body weight over periods ranging from 3 to 24 weeks—an impressive result compared to many other approaches.

Even more notable, participants lost 4-7% of their **waist circumference,** signaling a reduction in **visceral fat,** the harmful fat that collects around your organs and is linked to serious health conditions.

This works because, after about 12 hours without food, your body switches from burning glucose to burning stored **fat.** The liver converts fatty acids into **ketone bodies,** which become a clean, efficient fuel source for both your body and brain.

Another key advantage? **Muscle preservation.** This is especially important for midlife women, who often experience muscle loss as they age. Intermittent fasting helps **maintain lean muscle mass** while reducing fat, which helps prevent a slower metabolism and accelerated aging.

Fasting also causes **growth hormone (GH)** levels to rise—by as much as five times. GH supports fat burning and helps build and maintain lean muscle tissue.

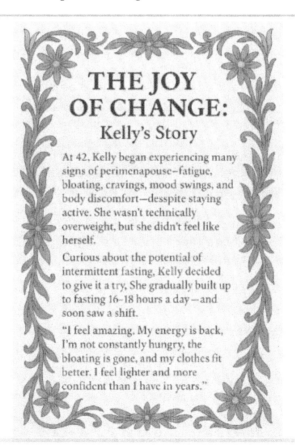

THE JOY OF CHANGE: Kelly's Story

At 42, Kelly began experiencing many signs of perimenapouse—fatigue, bloating, cravings, mood swings, and body discomfort—desspite staying active. She wasn't technically overweight, but she didn't feel like herself.

Curious about the potential of intermittent fasting, Kelly decided to give it a try, She gradually built up to fasting 16–18 hours a day—and soon saw a shift.

"I feel amazing. My energy is back, I'm not constantly hungry, the bloating is gone, and my clothes fit better. I feel lighter and more confident than I have in years."

How to Start Intermittent Fasting—and Stick With It
Start Slowly

If you're new to IF, take your time easing in. I started by delaying breakfast by just 30 minutes every few days. I gradually worked from eating at 6:30 a.m. to waiting until noon. It took about a month to fully adjust, but by moving slowly, I avoided the hunger and irritability that can come from jumping in too fast.

Pick Your Fasting Window

Once you're ready, choose an 8-hour time block for eating. Here are a few popular examples:

- **12 p.m. to 8 p.m.** → Eat

- **8 p.m. to 12 p.m. (next day)** → Fast

Or try:

- **10 a.m. to 6 p.m.**, or

- **9 a.m. to 5 p.m.**

Find the time frame that works best for your lifestyle.

Stay Adaptable

The 16:8 model works for many people, but you might find that a 14:10 or even an 18:6 routine feels better. What matters most is choosing a method you can stick with.

Follow the Meal Plans

Refer to the nutrition guidelines in Chapter 7 to make sure you're eating enough **protein** and nutrients during your eating window. Without sufficient protein, your body may begin breaking down muscle for energy during a fast. Balance your meals with **fiber-rich vegetables**, healthy fats, and **complex carbs**. The Metaboost Diet is built to complement intermittent fasting with high-quality, nutrient-dense foods that keep you full and energized.

Hydrate!

Staying well hydrated is key—especially during fasting hours. You're not getting water from food, so you'll need to drink more fluids. Hydration also helps curb hunger and cravings.

Remove Temptation

Keep trigger foods out of reach. If certain snacks or treats tempt you to break your fast or overeat, clear them out of your kitchen. The sight and smell alone can spark cravings, so create a supportive food environment.

Use Your Extra Time

One surprising bonus of fasting is gaining extra time. Without needing to prep or eat meals constantly, you free up time for things you enjoy—reading, journaling, taking a walk, or listening to music.

Get Enough Sleep

Restful sleep supports hunger regulation and helps control cravings. Aim for 6-8 hours per night. Bonus: the time you spend sleeping counts toward your fast, making it easier to reach your fasting goals.

Incorporate Exercise

Exercise enhances the benefits of IF. Light movement—like walking or stretching—can boost energy, mood, and circulation. Try different times of day to see what works best for you.

Make Time to Relax

Daily relaxation improves your mental clarity, lowers stress, and boosts emotional well-being. Whether it's meditation, deep breathing, or simply sitting quietly, these practices support both mind and body.

Celebrate Your Wins

As you hit your IF milestones—whether it's completing a day, a week, or a month—reward yourself. Treat yourself to something you enjoy: a relaxing bath, a walk in nature, journaling, calling a friend, or getting a manicure. Recognizing your efforts keeps motivation high and reinforces your commitment.

Hot Flash: 5 Common Misconceptions About Intermittent Fasting

Like any popular health trend, intermittent fasting (IF) comes with its fair share of myths. Let's clear up some of the most widespread misunderstandings:

Myth #1: Intermittent fasting just means skipping breakfast.

While many people do choose to skip their morning meal, IF is really about choosing a structured eating window. You can absolutely design your schedule to include a later breakfast—say, if you stop eating at 6 p.m., you could break your fast at 10 a.m. the next day and still follow the 16:8 approach. The goal is flexibility and finding what fits your natural rhythm.

Myth #2: Intermittent fasting is suitable for everyone.

Although IF offers numerous health benefits, it isn't for everyone. I don't recommend it for individuals with a history of eating disorders, those who are underweight, pregnant or nursing women, or anyone with type 1 diabetes. It's also not advised for children, teens, or those recovering from surgery or actively dealing with serious health issues. Always consult your doctor before starting.

Myth #3: You can eat anything you want during your eating hours.

The fasting window doesn't give you a free pass to load up on junk food. What you eat still matters. For best results, combine IF with nutritious, whole foods as recommended in the Metaboost Diet. Healthy eating and intermittent fasting work best as a team.

Myth #4: Intermittent fasting slows your metabolism.

Actually, research shows the opposite. Fasting can **enhance** your metabolic rate. It helps balance key hormones like norepinephrine and growth hormone, both of which support metabolic function. Fasting also improves metabolic flexibility—your body becomes more efficient at switching between burning carbs and fat for energy.

Myth #5: You'll feel constantly hungry while fasting.

It's common to worry that IF will leave you feeling ravenous. While a bit of hunger is normal at the start, easing into the routine helps your body adapt. Over time, hunger becomes manageable and less frequent. Fasting also influences hunger hormones—**ghrelin** (which signals hunger) tends to decrease, and **leptin** (which signals fullness) tends to increase—meaning you're more likely to feel satisfied and less prone to cravings.

Are You Ready?

Even though intermittent fasting is effective, flexible, and easy to follow once you get into the groove, starting can feel like a big step. The key is believing in your ability to make this change and being open to trying something new that can improve your health and wellbeing.

So—ask yourself:

- Are you ready to burn fat and feel more energized?
- Do you want to clear your mind and sharpen your focus?
- Are you ready to build strength and resilience?
- Do you want to prevent—or even reverse—health challenges that often appear during midlife?
- Are you ready to feel empowered in your body again?

If you said **yes** to even one of those questions, then you're more than ready to begin your intermittent fasting journey.

CHAPTER 5

Action Step 2: Focus on Anti-Inflammatory Nutrition

As a doctor, I've seen many patients who didn't realize they were dealing with something serious happening inside them—**chronic inflammation**. This hidden condition can increase the risk of many illnesses, including asthma, arthritis, cardiovascular disease, and stroke. If you're overweight or obese, there's a strong chance your body is already inflamed on a chronic level.

The good news? Numerous studies now confirm that a diet filled with **anti-inflammatory foods** can help reduce inflammation, manage weight, and boost your overall well-being. The key is staying consistent. Stick with this style of eating, and in time you'll begin to feel better—and likely notice weight loss as well.

Inflammation: Short-Term vs. Long-Term

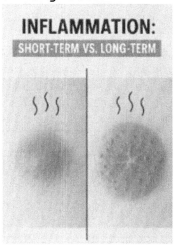

Inflammation is a natural response from your immune system when the body encounters something harmful—such as an infection, injury, or foreign substance. For instance, when you twist your ankle and it swells or a paper cut turns red and tender, that's **acute inflammation** at work. It allows white blood cells to flood the affected area, heal the damage, and then fade once the job is done.

This type of inflammation is vital—it protects us from daily threats and keeps the body running smoothly.

But **chronic inflammation** is a different story. It's a low-grade, long-lasting response that quietly damages tissue over time. Because it often happens without pain or noticeable symptoms, it can linger undetected for years, contributing to disease.

It plays a key role in **seven of the top ten causes of death** in the U.S., including:

- **Heart disease,** where LDL ("bad") cholesterol particles enter artery walls, triggering an inflammatory reaction that leads to plaque buildup and blockage.
- **Type 2 diabetes,** where inflammatory molecules interfere with insulin function, causing elevated blood sugar and potential organ damage.
- **Alzheimer's disease,** where overactive immune cells in the brain release inflammatory chemicals (cytokines) that damage healthy brain cells.

In women, **estrogen decline** during perimenopause and menopause can trigger inflammation in multiple areas, especially the **gut**. When the gut lining weakens, harmful substances can pass through into surrounding tissues, causing inflammation that may affect digestion, bones, and more.

This inflammation can also:

- **Interrupt bone remodeling**, contributing to **osteoporosis**
- **Affect brain function**, leading to cognitive issues like **brain fog**
- **Cause muscle loss** (sarcopenia)
- **Trigger joint pain**, as estrogen normally helps keep joint inflammation in check
- **Worsen weight gain**, particularly abdominal fat, which increases inflammatory markers like **cytokines** and **C-reactive protein**

Clearly, chronic inflammation is not just uncomfortable—it's a serious health threat. That's why reducing inflammation is at the heart of the Metaboost Diet and many modern approaches to disease prevention.

The Power of Eating to Fight Inflammation

The standard American diet is packed with processed, highly inflammatory foods that quietly contribute to serious health issues—harming the heart, brain, kidneys, and even increasing fat around your midsection.

That's why one of the most powerful tools to reduce or reverse chronic inflammation is **a nutrient-dense, anti-inflammatory diet**. Making smarter food choices can support your body in lowering inflammation, maintaining a healthy weight, and promoting long-term wellness. The key? Avoid or minimize foods that are known to fuel inflammation.

Understanding Omega-6 vs. Omega-3 Fatty Acids

I often remind my patients of the importance of **reducing the ratio of omega-6 to omega-3 fats** in their diets. But what makes these fats different?

Both omega-3 and omega-6 are considered polyunsaturated fatty acids (PUFAs), but their chemical structures vary. Omega-3s have their final double bond three carbons from the molecular tail, while omega-6s are six carbons away. While that might seem like a small difference, it has a big impact on how these fats behave in the body.

Historically, our ancestors likely consumed these fats in about a **1:1 ratio**, which helped the body function efficiently. Today, thanks to processed foods and seed oils, the average Western diet has a **20:1 ratio**—a heavy tilt toward omega-6s. This imbalance promotes inflammation.

Where are all these omega-6 fats coming from? Mostly from:

- Refined seed and vegetable oils like **corn, soybean, sunflower, and cottonseed**
- Ultra-processed snacks like chips, crackers, salad dressings, and fried fast foods

When omega-6 fats are metabolized, they create **pro-inflammatory by-products**. And when these oils are hydrogenated to make margarine or shortening, they become **trans fats**—which are even more harmful. Trans fats harden cell membranes, increase inflammation (especially in overweight individuals), lower good cholesterol (HDL), raise bad cholesterol (LDL), and impair immune function.

To push back against this inflammatory cascade, **increase your intake of omega-3s.** You can get them from:

- Fatty fish like **salmon, sardines, and mackerel**
- Plant sources like **flaxseeds and walnuts**
- **Grass-fed meat**

- **Omega-3 supplements**, like fish oil, if fish isn't a regular part of your diet

Also, reduce omega-6 sources by cutting back on refined vegetable oils and avoiding trans fats.

Added Sugar and Its Inflammatory Impact

"Added sugar" refers to sugar that's not naturally occurring in whole foods but added during processing—like table sugar, high-fructose corn syrup, honey, syrups, and concentrated fruit juices. Natural sugars in fruits, vegetables, and dairy are not included in this category.

According to the **World Health Organization**, added sugars should make up less than 10% of your daily calories—ideally under 5%. For a person on a 2,000-calorie diet, that's no more than **25 grams (6 teaspoons)** of added sugar per day.

But the average American consumes nearly **80 grams of added sugar daily**—over three times the recommended amount.

Why is this a problem? Excess sugar:

- Causes **blood glucose spikes**, which trigger inflammatory chemicals throughout your body
- Stimulates **insulin production**, which is itself pro-inflammatory
- Disrupts **phagocytosis**, the immune system's process of clearing out harmful invaders

To help consumers, the **FDA now requires "added sugars" to be listed** on food labels. But be aware—sugar has many names. Look out for ingredients ending in **"-ose"** (like dextrose or maltose), **syrups**, or **nectars**.

Cutting back on processed foods and sweetened drinks can dramatically reduce your sugar intake and lower inflammation.

Hot Flash: The Truth About Artificial Sweeteners

Artificial sweeteners—like those found in diet sodas or "sugar-free" snacks—may seem like a healthier option, but research suggests they can **trigger inflammation** by damaging your gut health.

These sweeteners alter your gut microbiome, turning beneficial bacteria into harmful forms. This can weaken the gut wall, making it more permeable or "leaky," which increases the risk for chronic diseases.

Common artificial sweeteners include:

- **Aspartame**
- **Sucralose**
- **Acesulfame-K (Ace-K)**

You'll often find them on ingredient lists—even in foods labeled "healthy." Always check your labels carefully.

Here's the encouraging part: as you cut back on artificial sweeteners, your **taste buds will reset**. Over time, your body will start to appreciate the natural sweetness of whole foods, and you'll rely less on overly sweetened, processed items.

Nitrites, Nitrates, and Inflammation from Processed Foods

Nitrites and nitrates are nitrogen-based compounds that differ slightly in structure: nitrates have three oxygen atoms, nitrites have two. These compounds naturally exist in certain vegetables like celery, leafy greens, and cabbage and may provide health benefits in their natural form.

However, the **synthetic versions** used in processed foods—particularly in cured meats like bacon, deli meats, and hot dogs—can pose health risks. When consumed, these additives may convert into **nitrosamines,** harmful compounds linked to inflammation and an increased risk of various cancers.

Another concern with processed meats is their ability to generate **advanced glycation end products (AGEs),** which can also fuel inflammation in the body. To lower these risks, try to reduce your intake of processed meats—or opt for **uncured, nitrate-free alternatives** when available.

Artificial Colors, Flavors, and Preservatives

Many packaged foods contain additives meant to improve flavor, appearance, shelf life, or texture. But the body does not recognize these artificial ingredients as food. Instead, it sees them as **foreign substances,** often triggering an **inflammatory immune response.**

To cut down on exposure to these additives:

- Cook more meals at home
- Choose minimally processed or **organic options** whenever possible
- Limit prepackaged and ultra-processed items

Fried Foods and Inflammation

While fried foods may be tasty, they're often cooked in oils high in omega-6 fats. These oils disrupt the **omega-3 to omega-6 ratio,** leading to increased inflammation.

Additionally, frying foods at high heat (like making French fries or potato chips) produces **acrylamide,** a chemical associated with inflammation and possibly cancer. The National Toxicology Program lists acrylamide as a potential carcinogen.

Healthier cooking alternatives:

- Use the **oven** to bake foods instead of frying
- Try an **air fryer,** which has been shown to reduce acrylamide by up to 90%

Saturated Fats and Gut Inflammation

Years ago, when working in the oil industry, I saw firsthand how early versions of low-carb diets encouraged people to eat large amounts of meat, cheese, and bacon—while skipping vegetables. While weight loss may have occurred, the high intake of **saturated fat** came at a cost.

Foods like **fatty beef, cheese, and butter** contain high levels of saturated fat, which triggers inflammation through various biological pathways:

- **Toll-like receptors (TLRs)** in the gut are normally used to identify harmful invaders. But when TLR4 is exposed to excess saturated fat, it misfires, recognizing fat as a threat and triggering inflammation—potentially leading to **leaky gut syndrome.**
- Saturated fats also encourage the production of inflammatory agents such as **leukotrienes and prostaglandins,** which contribute to **joint damage** and **cardiovascular issues.**

Additionally, **excess saturated fat** can affect **hormone levels** in women, elevating **estradiol,** which may increase the risk of breast cancer.

You don't need to eliminate saturated fats completely on the Metaboost Diet. Just aim for **balance** and incorporate more **healthy fats,** such as those found in:

- **Olive oil**
- **Avocados**
- **Coconut oil**

- Nuts and seeds

Tips to reduce saturated fat:
- Choose **leaner cuts of red meat** and trim excess fat
- Opt for **ground turkey or chicken** instead of beef
- Remove **chicken skin** before cooking
- Substitute **plain full-fat yogurt** for sour cream
- Use cheeses lower in saturated fat like **feta, ricotta,** or **cottage cheese**
- Always check food labels to avoid hidden sugars in "low-fat" products

The Inflammatory Impact of Excessive Alcohol

Drinking too much alcohol—more than 5-7 drinks per day—damages the gut's balance of good and bad bacteria, weakening your **immune system** and increasing inflammation. Over time, excessive alcohol promotes **gut permeability,** allowing harmful toxins and bacteria to enter the bloodstream and damage organs. Limit alcohol intake to **one drink per day,** which equals:

- 5 oz of wine

- 12 oz of beer

- 1.5 oz of spirits

Is Your Body Inflamed?

Take this **inflammation quiz** based on your eating habits over the past 24 hours. Tally your score to assess your current inflammatory load.

Scoring Instructions:

- Option (a): 0 points

- Option (b): 1 point

- Option (c): 2 points

Total Score:

- **0-15:** Very low inflammation

- **16-30:** Moderate inflammation

- **31-50:** High inflammation

Prioritize Foods That Heal

While we've already discussed the foods that can contribute to chronic inflammation, it's now time to focus on the ones that can *heal*. These inflammation-fighting foods are central to the **Metaboost Diet** and play a powerful role in improving your overall health.

Instead of reaching for medications, many of the best tools to combat chronic inflammation can be found in your local **grocery store**. Studies continue to show that certain nutrients and components in foods and drinks offer potent **anti-inflammatory** effects—and these are the very foods highlighted in the Metaboost Diet.

At the forefront of this defense are **antioxidants**—compounds that protect cells from damage caused by **free radicals**. Free radicals are unstable molecules missing an electron. To stabilize, they steal electrons from other cells, which can damage or destroy those cells, contributing to chronic inflammation and disease.

But antioxidants come to the rescue. These nutrients can neutralize free radicals by donating an electron, *without* becoming unstable themselves. As a result, they stop the damaging chain reactions that lead to inflammation.

Key **antioxidant vitamins** include A, C, and E, while **mineral-based antioxidants** include selenium, zinc, copper, and manganese. Here's a list of foods rich in these protective nutrients:

- **Berries** - Blueberries, raspberries, strawberries, blackberries, and cranberries are standout antioxidant-rich fruits.
- **Vegetables** - Kale, bell peppers, artichokes, broccoli, beets, red cabbage, asparagus, and tomatoes are excellent veggie sources.
- **Nuts and seeds** - Almonds, walnuts, pistachios, hazelnuts, and pecans deliver antioxidants and healthy fats.
- **Legumes** - Foods like lentils, edamame, and kidney beans are both anti-inflammatory and high in fiber.
- **Herbs and spices** - Garlic, turmeric, ginger, cloves, and fresh herbs boast strong anti-inflammatory powers.
- **Beverages** - Moderate amounts of coffee, tea, and red wine are also known for their antioxidant content.
- **Omega-3 fatty acid sources** - Salmon, mackerel, and other fatty fish help fight inflammation. If fish isn't part of your diet, consider an omega-3 supplement like fish oil.

To maximize the health benefits, aim for **diversity** in your food choices. No single item can do it all, so vary your intake across **fruits, vegetables, nuts, seeds, legumes,** and **anti-inflammatory spices**.

The **Metaboost Diet meal plans** (outlined in Chapter 8) are specifically designed to give you this variety and can serve as both a framework and inspiration for building nutrient-dense meals.

Hot Flash: My Go-To Anti-Inflammatory Foods

Here's a list of favorites that are consistently featured in anti-inflammatory eating:

- Asparagus
- Avocados
- Beans and legumes
- Beets
- Berries
- Broccoli
- Carrots
- Celery
- Kale
- Olive oil
- Oranges
- Pineapple
- Salmon
- Shiitake mushrooms
- Spinach
- Sweet potatoes
- Swiss chard
- Tomatoes

- Walnuts

Whether your goal is to reduce symptoms of **perimenopause or menopause, shed weight,** or **lower your risk of chronic illness** like cancer, heart disease, diabetes, or cognitive decline, adopting **anti-inflammatory nutrition** as early as possible is one of the best choices you can make for your health.

CHAPTER 6

CHAPTER 6

Action 3: Fuel Refocus

Fuel Refocus

I've worked with countless women who felt completely dependent on processed carbs—especially foods loaded with added sugars, Some started their mornings with sugary cereal and still added sugar on top, snacked on chocolate throughout the day, and ended with ice cream at night. Their cravings for sweets felt never-ending.

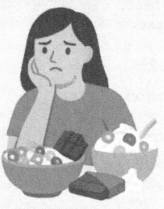

And that's no surprise, Sugar is practically everywhere, and its appeal is strong. Food companies make matters worse—more than 600,000 processed food products line grocery store shelves, and around 80% of them contain hidden sugars.

HIDDEN SUGARS

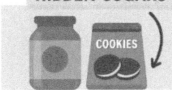

More and more research suggests that those who are overweight, pre-diabetic, or struggling with sugar addiction may thrive on a diet that's higher in healthy fats and lower in carbs.

That's where the Fuel Refocus phase of the Metaboost Diet comes in

More and more research suggests that those who are overweight, pre-diabetic, nr struggling with sugar addiction

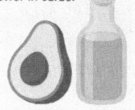

What Does Fuel Refocus Mean?

Your body is naturally programmed to burn glucose—produced from carbs—for energy. This occurs through a process called **gluconeogenesis** in the liver. Once glucose runs out, your body can switch to **fat** as its fuel source.

But with the average American diet being so carb-heavy (think: bread, pasta, rice, baked goods, and sugary drinks), your body is rarely forced to burn fat. Instead, glucose keeps flooding the system, insulin is repeatedly triggered, and fat gets stored—not burned.

Fuel Refocus changes that pattern. By shifting your intake of **macronutrients** (carbs, protein, and fat), your body enters a fat-burning state, producing **ketone bodies**—a more efficient energy source derived from fat. This shift is key to helping your body use stored fat for fuel rather than constantly relying on sugar.

Fuel Refocus Macro Breakdown

Here's how the standard American diet breaks down:

- **50% carbohydrates**

- **15% protein**

- **35% fat**

On the **Metaboost Diet**, you'll change those ratios to trigger fat-burning:

- **70% healthy fats**

- **20% lean protein**

- **10% carbohydrates**

You'll find these macros reflected in the Metaboost Diet meal plans. Once you start crafting your own meals, use a **nutrition tracking app** (like Cronometer or MyFitnessPal) to help you hit your daily targets.

Approved Macro Sources

70% Healthy Fats

- Avocados & avocado oil
- Olive oil & olives
- Coconut oil
- Nuts (almonds, walnuts, macadamia, pecans)
- Nut butters (unsweetened)
- Seeds (chia, flax)
- Butter and full-fat mayonnaise (preferably avocado or olive oil based)

20% Lean Protein

- Grass-fed meats (beef, bison, pork, lamb)
- Poultry (chicken, turkey)
- Wild-caught seafood
- Sardines, anchovies, eggs
- Low-carb, low-sugar protein powders
- Nitrate-free jerky

10% Carbohydrates

Focus on **complex carbs**—they're rich in fiber, stabilize blood sugar, and keep you full longer. These include:

- **Vegetables**: broccoli, spinach, Brussels sprouts, cauliflower, leafy greens
- **Fruits**: apples, berries
- **Legumes and whole grains** (in moderation)
- **Nuts and seeds**

Avoid **simple carbs**—these spike insulin and are often stored as fat. Common examples:

- Candy, baked goods, sodas
- White bread, pasta, and most processed foods

The Maintenance Transition (Metaboost Diet for Life)

Once you've reached your health goals, you'll slowly transition to a more balanced macro ratio:
1. **Week 1+:** 60% fat, 20% protein, 20% carbs
2. **Following weeks:** 50% fat, 20% protein, 30% carbs
3. **Long-term maintenance:** 40% fat, 20% protein, 40% carbs

Hot Flash: Hit Your Carb Goals with Non-Starchy Veggies

When managing your carb intake, understand the difference between **starchy** and **non-starchy** vegetables.

- **Starchy Veggies:** Sweet potatoes, corn, peas, legumes.

  o ½ cup = ~15g carbs, 80 calories

  o Raise blood sugar faster

- **Non-Starchy Veggies:** Broccoli, cauliflower, zucchini, spinach

  o ½ cup = ~5g carbs, 25 calories

  o Lower glycemic impact

If your goal is **weight loss**, limit your starchy veggie intake to stay within your daily carb macros and support fat burning.

Vegetable Comparison Chart.

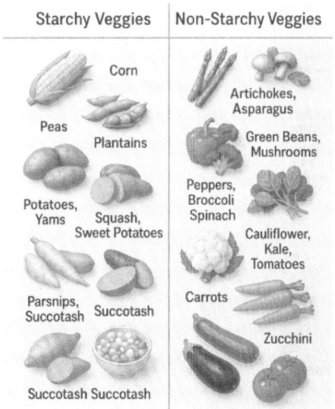

By shifting your fuel source from carbs to healthy fats, you empower your body to burn fat more efficiently, reduce inflammation, and support hormonal balance during midlife and beyond.

Understanding the Difference Between Net Carbs and Total Carbs

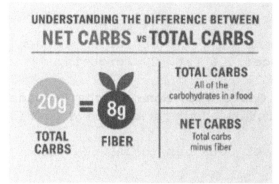

On the **Metaboost Diet,** you'll focus on tracking **net carbs** rather than total carbs. Net carbs represent the amount of carbohydrates your body actually absorbs and uses for energy, and they're calculated by subtracting the fiber content from the total carbohydrates in a food.

The formula is straightforward:

Total Carbohydrates - Fiber = Net Carbohydrates

When you check a food label, you'll find the **total carbohydrates** listed per serving. Directly beneath that, you'll see **fiber** and **sugar** amounts (including added sugars). Although fiber is part of the total carbohydrate number, it isn't digested or absorbed by the body—so we subtract it to find the net carbs. Why is this important? Because **net carbs** are the ones that influence your blood sugar. Since **fiber doesn't spike blood sugar levels,** foods that are **low in net carbs** tend to support **weight loss** and better **blood sugar control.**

Nutrition Facts

8 servings per container
Serving size   2/3 cup (55g)

Amount per serving
Calories   230

	% Daily Value*
Total Fat 8g	**10%**
Saturated Fat 1g	**5%**
Trans Fat 0g	
Cholesterol 0mg	**0%**
Sodium 160mg	**7%**
Total Carbohydrate 37g	**13%**
Dietary Fiber 4g	**14%**
Total Sugars 12g	
Includes 10g Added Sugars	**20%**
Protein 3g	
Vitamin D 2mcg	10%
Calcium 260mg	20%
Iron 8mg	45%
Potassium 235mg	6%

* The % Daily Value (DV) tells you how much a nutrient in a serving of food contributes to a daily diet. 2,000 calories a day is used for general nutrition advice.

Calculating Net Carbs
To figure out net carbs, simply subtract the fiber content from the total carbohydrates. For example, if a nutritional label shows 37 grams of total carbs and 4 grams of dietary fiber, then the net carbs would be 33 grams (37 - 4 = 33 grams).

Common Challenges During Fuel Refocus
As you adjust your macronutrients, you might worry about missing bread, pasta, or potatoes—or fear that your sweet tooth will get the best of you. But don't worry! Many women have shared that cravings fade (along with unwanted pounds and inches), and they feel more energized, satisfied, and healthier on the Metaboost Diet.

  Keep in mind, though, that your body has relied on carbs for energy for most of your life. Now, you're asking it to burn stored fat instead. That shift takes time and may come with some challenges. But you're not alone—many experience similar symptoms when starting the Metaboost Diet.

Impatience with Fat Adaptation
When you begin the program, you're training your body to use fat instead of carbohydrates for fuel. But this transformation doesn't happen overnight. Research shows that fat adaptation takes weeks—usually three to four—for most people to fully transition. That means noticeable changes might take time, so be patient! Once your body adapts, the results can come quickly.

Carbohydrate Withdrawal
If your diet has included a lot of complex carbs, shifting to just 10% of calories from carbs might affect your mood and energy. This early phase can come with withdrawal symptoms such as:
- Fatigue
- Headaches
- Cough
- Sniffles
- Irritability
- Nausea

Ironically, these symptoms are a good sign—they indicate that your body is moving away from burning glucose and starting to use fat for energy. This transition, though uncomfortable at first, is a key step in becoming fat-adapted.

  To ease the symptoms, focus on replenishing your electrolytes. These vital minerals—magnesium, potassium, sodium, calcium, phosphorus, and chloride—are crucial for energy production, cell stability, and overall bodily function.

  Stay well-hydrated and eat electrolyte-rich foods. For potassium, load up on leafy greens and avocados (aim for one a day). Nuts and seeds—like almonds, walnuts, pistachios, pumpkin, and sunflower seeds—are excellent magnesium sources. Green veggies supply calcium, lightly salting your meals can provide sodium and chloride, and foods like chicken and tuna are great for phosphorus.

Not Eating Enough Fat
You might have been taught to avoid fat, but on this plan, fat becomes your priMeredithenergy source—and it's essential. Without enough fat, your energy will dip, and the program may feel harder than it needs to be.

Think of the Metaboost Diet not just as a low-carb plan, but as a high-healthy-fat diet. Rather than focusing on cutting carbs, shift your mindset to include enough fat.

Aim for 70% of your daily calories to come from fat. This includes foods like eggs, nuts, seeds, avocados, butter, uncured bacon, and oils such as olive, avocado, and coconut oil.

Steering Clear of Hidden Carbs

Carbohydrates and added sugars often sneak into foods in unexpected ways, making them tough to avoid. Many products contain more sugar and refined carbs than you'd guess, so it's crucial to not only check nutrition labels but also consider how the food was made and calculate your actual carb intake.

Carbs don't just appear in the usual suspects—they're also present in foods that seem harmless. Here's a quick list of common culprits where hidden carbs and added sugars often appear:

- Reduced-fat products
- Liquid egg substitutes
- Sauces
- Condiments
- Peanut butter
- Salad dressings
- Protein and energy bars

Hot Flash: Smart Carb Substitutions

Try these tasty, low-carb alternatives to your favorite high-carb foods to help you stay within your 10% carbohydrate target:

HIGH-CARB FOOD | LOW-CARB SWAP

HIGH-CARB FOOD	LOW-CARB SWAP
Bread	Lettuce wraps or shredded
Breading	Almond flour or shredded che
Chips	Mashed cauliflowar
Mashed potatoes	Zooblies or spiralizeα
Pasta	Sparkling water
Soda	Almond flour

Getting Enough Protein

One common challenge is figuring out the best timing for your protein intake. Many people concentrate protein at a single meal, often dinner. However, to help preserve muscle mass—especially as you approach or enter midlife—it's ideal to spread your protein evenly across your meals during your 8-hour eating window.

 This strategy also supports hormone balance, particularly leptin and ghrelin, which regulate hunger and fullness.

You might've heard that it's necessary to consume protein within 30 to 60 minutes after a workout. That advice came from research involving 25-year-old male athletes, who showed increased muscle gains when consuming protein shortly after exercising. But for most women, especially those not aiming for maximum muscle growth, this guideline doesn't really apply.

As a rule of thumb, aim for 25 to 30 grams of protein (about 3 ounces) per meal, and 10 to 20 grams (roughly 1.5 ounces) for snacks. Always pair protein with healthy fats and carbs to help you stay full and satisfied.

Be careful not to go overboard, though. Consuming too much protein can backfire. Extra amino acids can be converted into glucose by your body, which may interfere with fat burning.

Kick Sugar in 10 Days—My Sugar Detox Plan

Our bodies adapt to the level of sugar we regularly consume—the more we eat, the more we crave. This is especially true for *added sugars*, which include sugars introduced during food processing, as well as table sugar, honey, syrups, and sugars we add ourselves. The good news? You *can* retrain your taste buds and overcome your sweet tooth.

A study published in the *American Journal of Clinical Nutrition* proves this point. Researchers studied 29 people who regularly drank two or more sugar-sweetened beverages each day. Participants rated the sweetness of various drinks and puddings at the beginning of the study. Then, half of the group cut their sugar intake by 40%, while the other half continued with their usual habits.

Three months later, all participants resumed eating whatever they liked for a month. When they re-rated the same sweetened foods, those who had reduced sugar intake found the items too sweet and liked them less. Their cravings had actually diminished!

If you have a sweet tooth, this is promising news. Once you cut back on sugar, your desire for it starts to fade. Here's a 10-day sugar detox to get you started—feel free to repeat as needed.

Day 1: Set Your Intentions

Write your sugar detox goals in a journal. Some examples:

- Reduce my intake of added sugars.
- Learn more about the health risks of too much sugar.
- Take small daily steps, like:
  - Eating more whole, unprocessed foods.
  - Replacing sugary drinks with water or unsweetened seltzer.
  - Drinking black coffee while intermittent fasting.
  - Flavoring plain Greek yogurt with berries instead of buying sweetened varieties.
  - Eating whole fruit instead of sugary snacks.
  - Swapping candy for homemade trail mix with dried fruit and nuts.

Day 2: Track Your Added Sugar

Start logging your sugar intake using an app. You might be shocked by the numbers. For women, the American Heart Association recommends no more than **25 grams of added sugar per day**. Seeing how much you're actually consuming can be a powerful motivator.

Day 3: Ditch Sugary Drinks

Replace sodas, sweetened teas, sugary cocktails, and commercial juices with flavored sparkling water. Infuse it with cucumber, lemon, or lime. Clear your kitchen of sweetened beverages.

Day 4: Manage Stress

Stress can fuel sugar cravings. Incorporate calming activities like yoga or meditation into your day. Eat magnesium-rich foods such as apples, avocados, and almonds, paired with eggs or fatty fish for additional mood-boosting nutrients.

Day 5: Create Balanced Snacks

Highly processed foods with added sugars—especially those with high-fructose corn syrup—keep you craving more. Today, focus on satisfying combinations of healthy carbs, fats, and proteins. For example, pair an apple with almonds or squash with hummus instead of grabbing chips or cookies.

Day 6: Read Labels Religiously

Make label reading a daily habit. Many condiments, sauces, and packaged foods contain hidden sugars. Always scan for added sugars and refined carbs.

Day 7: Rethink Dessert

Still craving something sweet after dinner? Ask yourself if it's true hunger or just habit. If you're hungry, opt for a protein-and-fat combo like walnuts or unsweetened Greek yogurt with berries and shredded coconut. It's a satisfying replacement for dessert.

Day 8: Stay Hydrated

Drinking enough water helps curb sugar cravings. Aim for **64 ounces** (about 8 cups) per day. Add lemon, lime, or herbs to boost flavor and encourage consistency.

Day 9: Cut Back on Artificial Sweeteners

While they may seem helpful, artificial sweeteners can actually increase cravings and promote weight gain. Start weaning off them by halving your current use and reducing further every couple of days. If you need a sweet touch, opt for natural alternatives like **stevia** or **erythritol**.

Day 10: Celebrate Your Progress

By now, you've likely noticed a big reduction in cravings—maybe you've eliminated added sugar altogether. Keep tapering off artificial sweeteners and stay hydrated. Revisit your journal to reflect on your original goals, and note how you feel after these 10 days.

Sugar is not essential in your diet. Your body requires protein, healthy fats, and quality carbs—but not added sugar. The **Metaboost Diet** is designed around this principle and can help you break free from sugar addiction. You *can* do this—and once you do, you'll leave that sugar habit in the past for good.

Part 3-The Plan

CHAPTER 7: The Metaboost Diet Nutritional Foundation

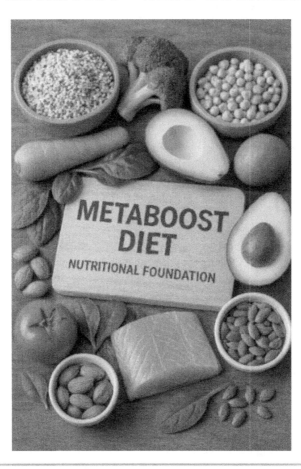

The body you're caring for in your 40s, 50s, 60s, and beyond is very different from the one you fueled in your 20s. As you move through perimenopause, menopause, and postmenopause, many aspects of your body undergo change—your shape, metabolism, muscle mass, bone density, energy levels, appearance, and overall health are all affected. These shifts call for specific nutrients and foods that support not only weight management but also long-term wellness.

Often, we turn to medications for relief from these changes, rather than considering food as a first line of support. But the truth is, the right foods can balance hormones, nourish the body, and even reduce or eliminate symptoms. Having guided tens of thousands of women through this journey, I've seen firsthand that the Metaboost Diet is one of the most effective ways to improve midlife health, reduce symptoms, and achieve lasting weight loss. You might be surprised at how powerful this approach to eating can be.

What so many women have realized is that consuming the right types of food in the right balance is a potent form of medicine. The benefits extend beyond weight—they also impact hormone balance, reduce chronic inflammation, and boost overall health.

With that in mind, let's explore what you get to eat—and why it matters.

Healthy Fats

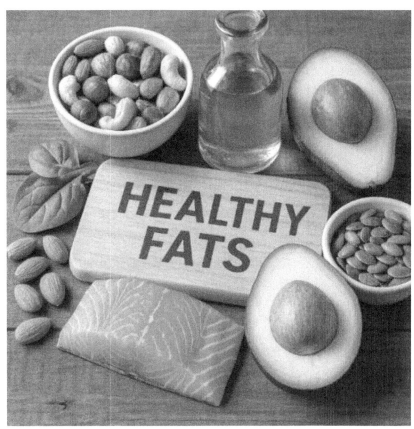

For decades, dietary fat was unfairly blamed for a range of health issues—from heart disease to obesity and diabetes. The low-fat trend of the late 1970s led to the widespread introduction of fat-free products. Unfortunately, these processed foods were stripped of important nutrients and often loaded with added sugar to enhance taste, which contributed to declining health.

Now, it's time to welcome fats back. On the Metaboost Diet, healthy fats play a central role. These "good" fats help lower the risk of heart disease and stroke, support cognitive function, promote hormonal balance, improve skin health, aid in recovery, and contribute to an overall sense of well-being.

Fats also help keep you full by triggering satiety hormones—another reason why you won't feel deprived on this plan. Additionally, fats can improve insulin sensitivity, reduce the occurrence of hot flashes, and ease night sweats.

Sources like olive oil, nuts, and seeds are excellent options. Flax seeds, for instance, are rich in lignans (plant-based estrogens) that help regulate hormones, as well as omega-3s, fiber, and antioxidants. Chia and hemp seeds also offer valuable omega-3 fats.

Nuts support blood vessel and hormone health, help manage cholesterol, and regulate blood sugar and insulin levels.

Here's a complete list of healthy fats approved for the Metaboost Diet:

Metaboost Diet-Approved Fats

- Avocados
- Avocado oil
- Butter (preferably grass-fed)
- Coconut flakes (in moderation)
- Coconut flour (used in recipes)
- Coconut oil (in moderation)
- Creamy dressings (used in recipes)
- Dairy fats (heavy cream, full-fat milk, if tolerated)

- Flaxseed oil
- Ghee (clarified butter)
- Hummus
- Mayonnaise (ideally made with olive or avocado oil)
- MCT oil (in moderation)
- Nuts (especially walnuts, almonds, pecans, macadamias); almond flour
- Nut butters (no sugar or added oils)
- Olive oil
- Olives
- Seed butters (no sugar or added oils)
- Seeds (especially chia, flax, hemp, pumpkin, sunflower)
- Sesame oil (in moderation)
- Tahini (sesame seed butter)

Quality Proteins

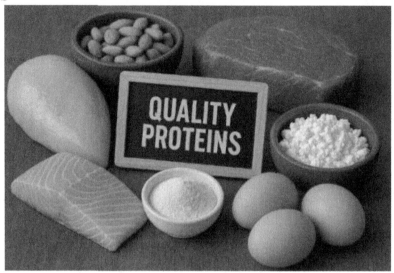

Protein serves as the structural foundation of your body, much like wood for a house or steel for a skyscraper. It's essential for maintaining and repairing tissues, which is why the Metaboost Diet includes a slightly higher protein intake than many traditional eating plans.

You may have heard conflicting opinions about protein in recent years, but let's clear things up: higher-protein diets have often been wrongly criticized. As women age, their need for protein increases due to a natural loss of lean muscle and a reduced ability to repair tissue—changes closely tied to declining estrogen levels, which also affect muscle mass and bone strength. Put simply, protein becomes crucial at this stage of life. One influential study, the Women's Health Initiative, showed that women who consumed more protein had a 32% lower risk of becoming frail and maintained better physical function.

Protein is also key in stabilizing blood sugar—helpful if you're experiencing mood swings—and in regulating appetite through its influence on leptin and ghrelin, two hormones that control hunger and fullness.

It's important to include a variety of protein sources: poultry, fish, lean red meats, legumes, dairy-based proteins, and more. Eggs, once wrongly maligned, are actually an affordable, nutrient-dense source of protein. They help regulate hunger and fat-storage hormones, supporting insulin balance and ghrelin response. Eggs also offer vitamin D, iron, and B vitamins—all critical for bone strength and overall wellness.

Fatty fish like wild salmon, trout, herring, and sardines are also excellent choices. Rich in omega-3 fats, these fish help fight inflammation and regulate hunger hormones, keeping you satisfied longer. They're also high in vitamin D, which supports healthy testosterone levels in women—something that can help with energy, mood, and weight management. These fish also support cardiovascular health and keep skin and hair looking healthy.

Poultry and lean beef are also great protein options. They stimulate leptin production, helping you feel full, and they're excellent sources of iron and vitamin B12.

Here's a list of the protein-rich foods you can enjoy on the Metaboost Diet:

Metaboost Diet-Approved Proteins

- Anchovies
- Bacon (uncured, nitrate-free)
- Lean cuts of beef
- Nitrate-free beef jerky
- Bison
- Buffalo
- Chicken
- Collagen protein powder
- Cornish hens
- Duck
- Eggs
- Wild-caught fish (especially salmon, trout, and tuna)
- Game meats like venison
- Legumes
- Nitrate/nitrite-free deli meats
- Ostrich
- Lean cuts of pork
- Protein powder (low sugar, low carbohydrate, minimal ingredients)
- Shellfish
- Tofu
- Turkey
- Turkey bacon

Dairy Proteins

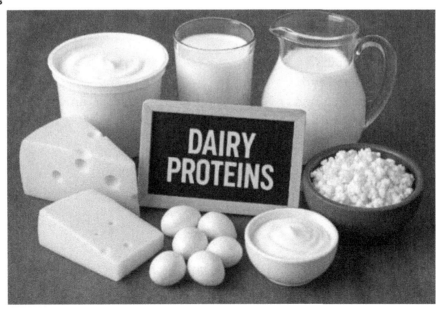

If you're not lactose intolerant or sensitive to dairy, the Metaboost Diet includes dairy as a beneficial option. As estrogen declines during menopause, the risk of bone fractures increases—making calcium-rich dairy an important part of bone health.

Bone strength relies not just on calcium, but also vitamin D—both found in dairy products. Without these nutrients, bones may become weak and more prone to fractures, so prevention is key.

One study of nearly 750 postmenopausal women found that those who consumed more dairy and animal protein had higher bone density than those who ate less.

Dairy may also promote better sleep. Foods rich in the amino acid glycine—like milk and cheese—have been shown to help perimenopausal and postmenopausal women experience deeper sleep.

Additionally, some dairy products like yogurt contain probiotics—beneficial bacteria that help balance the microbiome in the gut and vaginal area. Probiotics can reduce vaginal discharge and odor, making them useful for both prevention and treatment of infections.

Metaboost Diet-Approved Vegetable Proteins

- Almond milk/cheese/flour
- Cashew milk/cheese
- Chia seeds
- Chickpeas/chickpea flour
- Dried or canned beans
- Edamame
- Hemp hearts/milk
- Lentils
- Lupin beans
- Nutritional yeast
- Seitan
- Tempeh
- Tofu

Hot Flash: 10 Surprising Benefits of Probiotics

When you think of probiotics, you probably think of gut health—and rightfully so. These beneficial microbes help prevent and treat digestive issues like constipation, diarrhea, and inflammatory bowel diseases by keeping your gut's microbiome balanced. But their benefits extend far beyond digestion. Probiotics can also:

- Promote weight and belly fat loss
- Improve mental health conditions like depression, anxiety, and memory
- Support cardiovascular health
- Improve cholesterol and triglyceride levels
- Boost immune function
- Enhance urogenital health
- Help regulate blood sugar
- Strengthen bones and joints
- Protect liver function
- Improve outcomes in cancer care

Dairy Has a Lot to Offer!

Dairy provides a range of benefits, and if you tolerate it well, there are many delicious options you can include in your diet.

Metaboost Diet-Approved Dairy Proteins
- Cheddar
- Full-fat cottage cheese
- Cream cheese
- Feta
- Goat cheese
- Full-fat Greek yogurt
- Havarti
- Heavy cream
- Full-fat kefir
- Monterey Jack
- Mozzarella and other soft cheeses
- Parmesan and other hard cheeses
- Sour cream
- Swiss

Carbohydrates

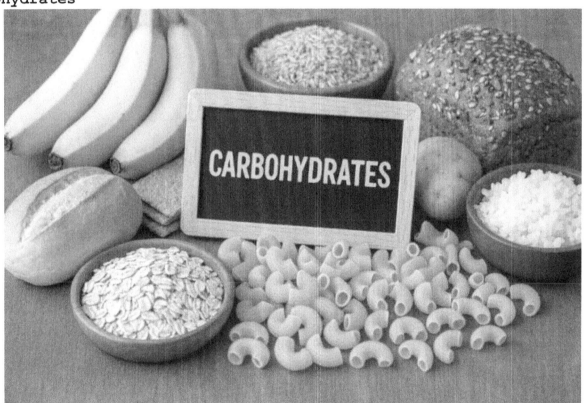

Carbs aren't the enemy—in fact, the right kinds of carbohydrates are essential for your health. Focus on nutrient-dense options like non-starchy vegetables, certain fruits, and some whole grains and starchy vegetables. These foods are loaded with fiber, vitamins, minerals, and antioxidants.

Leafy greens are especially important. Veggies like spinach, kale, collards, and chard are high in antioxidants, help fight inflammation, and support estrogen metabolism thanks to their fiber and nutrient content.

Cruciferous vegetables—such as broccoli, cauliflower, Brussels sprouts, cabbage, and kale—are also key players. They help your body eliminate excess estrogen. One study even found that eating broccoli reduced a potentially harmful form of estrogen linked to breast cancer and increased a protective form.

Many of these carbs also contain natural phytoestrogens—plant compounds that mimic estrogen in the body. Though once debated, recent studies suggest they can benefit menopausal women. You'll find these in soybeans, flaxseeds, chickpeas, peanuts, berries, and green or black tea.

Fruits are a fantastic, natural way to satisfy sweet cravings. They offer hydration, fiber, and antioxidants that help reduce inflammation while supporting satiety.

Metaboost Diet-Approved Non-Starchy Vegetables

- Leafy greens (all kinds)
- Artichokes
- Asparagus
- Bamboo shoots
- Bean sprouts
- Green and yellow beans
- Beets
- Bok choy
- Broccoli
- Broccolini
- Brussels sprouts
- Cabbage (any variety)
- Carrots
- Cauliflower
- Celery
- Cucumbers
- Eggplant
- Endive
- Kimchi
- Kohlrabi
- Jicama
- Mushrooms
- Okra
- Onions
- Parsley
- Peppers (all kinds)
- Pickles
- Radishes
- Rutabaga
- Sauerkraut
- Scallions
- Summer squash
- Tomatoes
- Watercress
- Zucchini

Metaboost Diet-Approved Starchy Vegetables

- Edamame (soybeans)
- Lentils and other legumes
- Parsnips
- Peas

- Plantains
- Potatoes
- Turnips
- Succotash (corn and lima beans)
- Sweet potatoes (yams)
- Winter squash

Metaboost Diet-Approved Whole Grains
- Amaranth (use like rice or as flour)
- Barley
- Brown rice
- Buckwheat (available as groats, flour, or noodles)
- Bulgur
- Corn
- Farro
- Millet
- Oats
- Quinoa
- Spelt (as whole berries or flakes)
- Wheat berries

Metaboost Diet-Approved Fruits
- Apples
- Bananas
- Blackberries
- Blueberries
- Cherries
- Fresh cranberries
- Citrus fruits (like grapefruit)
- Pears
- Plums
- Raspberries
- Strawberries

Hot Flash: My Top Foods to Help Cool Down Hot Flashes
Up to 85% of women going through menopause experience hot flashes, and around 55% of perimenopausal women also report them. As menopause approaches, both the frequency and intensity of hot flashes often increase.

If you're dealing with this frustrating symptom, the numbers might seem discouraging—but don't worry! What you eat can make a significant difference. The Metaboost Diet, in particular, can help ease hot flashes. Here are some key nutrients and foods that can help reduce those sudden heat surges:

- **Omega-3 Fatty Acids:** Found in salmon, tuna, walnuts, and flax seeds, these healthy fats can reduce both the frequency and intensity of hot flashes.

- **Vitamin E:** Leafy greens, pumpkin seeds, sunflower seeds, almonds, and red bell peppers are all excellent sources. Vitamin E not only helps ease hot flashes but also acts as a powerful antioxidant, helping to repair cell damage.

- **Soy-Based Foods:** Tofu and edamame are rich in phytoestrogens, plant compounds that mimic estrogen and may help manage hot flashes. They also deliver protein, fiber, and healthy fats.

- **Fruits and Vegetables:** Studies show that women who eat a diet rich in produce and avoid processed foods and sugar experience fewer menopausal symptoms, including hot flashes, weight gain, and abdominal fat.

Fiber Up! Why More Fiber Equals Better Health

As a physician, I've always emphasized the importance of fiber. In my experience, people who consume more fiber tend to enjoy better overall health. Fortunately, the Metaboost Diet makes it easy to increase your fiber intake, and the long-term benefits are well worth the effort. Here's how fiber supports your health:

- **Keeps Appetite in Check:** Fiber slows down how quickly food is digested, helping you feel full longer and naturally reducing appetite. It also helps lower ghrelin, the hormone responsible for hunger.

- **Helps Slim the Waistline:** Soluble fiber, in particular, is effective in targeting belly fat. And since high-fiber foods take longer to chew, they slow down your eating, giving your brain more time to recognize fullness—helping prevent overeating.

- **Supports Weight Loss in Multiple Ways:** Fiber may reduce how many calories your body absorbs from other foods. Eating fiber-rich meals can make losing weight feel almost effortless.

- **Balances Blood Sugar and Insulin:** One of fiber's most well-documented effects is its ability to regulate blood sugar. Research shows that when fiber is eaten alongside carbs, it helps prevent sharp spikes in blood sugar and insulin.

- **Lowers Breast Cancer Risk:** A meta-analysis found that women who follow fiber-rich diets reduce their breast cancer risk by about 12%. Fiber achieves this by:

  - Lowering excess estrogen levels in the bloodstream
  - Binding with and removing harmful substances from the gut
  - Supporting the growth of beneficial gut bacteria while suppressing bad bacteria
  - Enhancing the activity of immune-supporting white blood cells (macrophages)
  - Promoting short-chain fatty acids (SCFAs), which help prevent tumor development

Aim for at least **25 grams of fiber per day**—or more if you can. It's easier than you might think when you fill your plate with plenty of vegetables and a variety of fruits.

Metaboost Diet: Top Fiber-Rich Foods

Looking to boost your fiber intake? These Metaboost Diet-approved foods are some of the richest sources of fiber—helping you stay full longer, manage weight, and support overall health.

Food Source	Serving Size	Grams of Fiber
Artichoce	1 medium, cooked	10
Avocado	1 cup, diced	10
Peas	1 cup, cooked	9
Winter squash	1 cup, cooked	9
Lentils	½ cup, cooked	7.5
Black beans	½ cup, cooked	6
Parsnips	1 cup, cooked	6,5
Broccoli	1 cup, cooked	5
Collard greens	1 cup, cooked	5
Apple (white)	1 medium	4,3
Brussels sprouts	1 cup, cooked	4
Green beans	1 cup, cooked	4
Okra	1 cup, cooked	4
Cherries (fresh)	1 medium, cooked	3
Kale	½ cup, cooked	3
Barley	½ cup, cooked	3

Why Magnesium Matters (Especially During Menopause)

Magnesium is one of the most important minerals for women's health, yet about half of all women don't get enough of it. On the Metaboost Diet, you'll naturally increase your magnesium intake—and the benefits are impressive, especially during and after menopause. Here's why magnesium should be on your radar:

- **Supports Bone Health:** Around 60% of your body's magnesium is stored in your bones. It helps prevent osteoporosis by supporting bone structure and promoting calcium absorption. It also reduces inflammation, which can weaken bones over time.

- **Helps Prevent Diabetes and Insulin Resistance:** Magnesium deficiency is strongly linked to insulin resistance and type 2 diabetes. It plays a role in managing blood sugar and may reduce complications related to diabetes.

- **Promotes Heart Health:** Magnesium helps keep the heart rhythm steady, prevents clots, and supports healthy blood pressure. It's also found in foods that are high in antioxidants, healthy fats, fiber, and protein—all great for cardiovascular function. One study of nearly 4,000 postmenopausal women linked higher magnesium levels to reduced inflammation and better heart health.

- **Improves Sleep:** Trouble sleeping is common during menopause. Magnesium helps regulate the body's internal clock (circadian rhythm), promotes muscle relaxation, and increases melatonin production. In one small study, adults who took 500 mg of magnesium daily experienced better sleep quality and longer sleep duration.

- **Lifts Mood:** Magnesium supports brain function, emotional balance, and your ability to handle stress—all of which impact mood and may help reduce symptoms of depression.

- **Boosts Fat Burning:** Though often overlooked in weight loss, magnesium helps improve insulin sensitivity, allowing your body to burn fat more efficiently—especially stubborn belly fat. It can also reduce water retention and bloating while curbing cravings for carbs.

- **Supports Overall Wellness:** Adequate magnesium intake can help prevent or manage a variety of chronic conditions, including Alzheimer's, high blood pressure, heart disease, insulin resistance, migraines, and type 2 diabetes.

Daily Goal: Women should aim for 310-320 mg of magnesium per day. The Metaboost Diet helps you meet this target through whole, nutrient-dense foods. (A list of top magnesium-rich foods is often included alongside this section in the program.)

Metaboost Diet: Top Magnesium-Rich Foods

Magnesium is vital for women's health—especially during and after menopause. Luckily, the Metaboost Diet includes many foods that are naturally high in this essential mineral. Here's a list of the best magnesium sources you can enjoy on the plan:

Magnesium

Food Source		Serving Size	Magnessium
	Leafy greens	1 cup cooked	156
	Pumpkin seeds	1 cooked fillet	150
	Salmon	1 small cooked fillet	97
	Almonds	1 oz (about 2 tablespoons)	80
	Cashews	1 oz	72
	Dark choco-	½ cup cooked	60
	Avocado	1 medium	58
	Avocado	3½ oz cooked square	58
	Flax seeds	½ cup cooked	40
	Flax seeds	1 oz couoked	40
	Black beans	½ cup cooked	40
	Lima beans	½ cup cooked	40

Omega-3 Fatty Acids: Why They Matter in Menopause

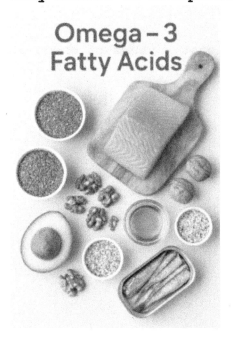

Omega-3 fats offer powerful support for women during midlife—and they're a cornerstone of the Metaboost Diet. These healthy fats come with a long list of benefits:

- **Tackle Belly Fat:** EPA and DHA—two key omega-3 fatty acids found in fatty fish—have been shown to reduce abdominal fat. One analysis of seven studies found omega-3 supplements significantly reduced waist size in overweight adults.

- **Manage Hunger:** In a study involving 232 overweight participants, those given higher doses of omega-3s during a weight-loss program reported feeling fuller and less hungry after meals than those receiving lower doses.

- **Lower Triglycerides:** As you approach or go through menopause, triglyceride levels can rise, while good HDL cholesterol drops—raising the risk of heart disease. Omega-3s help counteract this by reducing triglycerides, especially when paired with a low-sugar, low-refined-carb diet.

- **Relieve Joint Pain:** Omega-3 fats reduce the production of inflammatory compounds like prostaglandins, which can cause joint pain. They act much like anti-inflammatory medications, easing discomfort and stiffness.

- **Boost Mood:** Women are twice as likely as men to experience depression, and the risk increases after menopause. Omega-3s support brain cell health and can help reduce symptoms of sadness, irritability, and cognitive decline.

- **Protect Bone Health:** These fats are linked to increased bone mineral density and may help prevent osteoporosis.

- **Improve Vaginal Dryness:** Omega-3s promote natural lubrication in the body, including the vaginal tissues—helping to relieve dryness associated with hormonal changes.

Most women benefit from **at least 2 grams of omega-3s per day**. Here's a list of Metaboost Diet-approved foods that are especially rich in these essential fats:

Metaboost Diet: Highest Omega-3 Foods

Food	Serving Size	Omega-3 (mg)
Flaxseed oil	1 tablespoon	7.260
Chia seeds	3½ oz. cooked	5.060
Salmon	3½ oz. cooked	4.123
Walnuts, chopped	1 tablespoon	2.570
Flax seeds	1 tablespoon	2.350
Sardines	3½ oz can	1.480
Hemp seeds	2 oz. can	1.000
Anchovies	2 oz. can	951
Herring	3 oysters	946
Soybeans	½ cup sookad	670
Tofu	3½ oz square	495
Oysters	6 oysters	370
Omega-3 enriched eggs	1 cup cooked	332

Ease Menopause Symptoms with Vitamin D

Vitamin D is one of the most essential nutrients for women—especially during menopause. Technically a hormone, not just a vitamin, it plays a crucial role in supporting your immune system, heart, lungs, and blood vessels. When it comes to menopause, here's how vitamin D can make a big impact:

- **Aids in Weight Loss**: Vitamin D supports fat loss in several ways. First, it boosts leptin production, the hormone that tells your brain you're full. Second, it helps reduce fat production and storage in fat cells. Third, it works with calcium to regulate cortisol—the stress hormone responsible for storing belly fat when chronically elevated.

- **Improves Muscle Strength**: Muscle loss is a natural part of aging, but vitamin D can help preserve and even enhance strength. One study on Brazilian postmenopausal women showed that those taking 1,000 IUs of vitamin D daily for nine months experienced a 25% increase in muscle strength. In contrast, the placebo group lost an average of 6.8% of muscle mass and were nearly twice as likely to fall.

- **Supports Mental Health**: Research shows vitamin D plays a role in mood regulation. A 2020 review of over 7,500 people found that those with negative emotions who supplemented with vitamin D saw improvements in their symptoms, particularly if they had low levels to begin with.

- **Fights Fatigue**: Feeling constantly tired? It may be due to low vitamin D levels. A 2015 study of female nurses revealed that 89% of those reporting fatigue were deficient in vitamin D.

- **Strengthens Bones**: As estrogen drops, bone mineral density declines, raising the risk of fractures. Vitamin D works with calcium to help your body absorb and retain this vital mineral, making your bones stronger and more resilient.

- **May Lower Breast Cancer Risk**: Lab studies have shown that vitamin D can stop the growth and spread of breast cancer cells and even trigger cell death.

Recommended Intake:
- Women aged 19-50: **600 IUs daily**

- Women over 50: **800 IUs daily**

Although food sources are helpful, supplementation is often necessary to meet daily needs.

Metaboost Diet Foods Highest in Vitamin D

Food	Serving Size	Vitamin D (IUs)
Mushrooms	3½ oz cooked	2.300
Salmon, wild-caught	3½ oz cooked	1.300
Sardines	3½ oz can	270
Tuna	3½ oz o⁻	268
Oatmeal	½ cup cooked	150
Milk	1 cup	100
Yogurt	¾ cup	100
Almond milk (fortified)	1 cup	100
Cheese, hard	1 oz or 1 slice	40
Egg yolk	1 large	37

Stay Hydrated

Aim to drink **at least 64 ounces (8 cups) of water per day**. Water is often overlooked but is crucial for nearly every body function—from flushing out toxins to supporting brain and heart health.

In menopause, hydration becomes even more important. Drinking enough water helps prevent dryness (skin and vaginal), reduces bloating, and supports overall body lubrication.

Tip: Avoid store-bought flavored waters, which often contain added sugars and artificial ingredients. Instead, try infusing plain water with fresh fruits, herbs, or cucumber slices for a naturally refreshing twist.

Smart Sugar Alternatives

The best sugar substitutes on the Metaboost Diet are **stevia** and **erythritol**, either alone or combined with **monk fruit**. These do not spike blood sugar or insulin levels.

A common question is whether these can be used during fasting. While the scientific consensus isn't final, some experts believe sweet tastes may trigger insulin release—even without calories—which could reduce the benefits of fasting. Personally, I avoid anything sweet during fasting periods.

Suggested Brand: *Swerve*, a popular erythritol-based sweetener, comes in both granular and confectioners' forms.

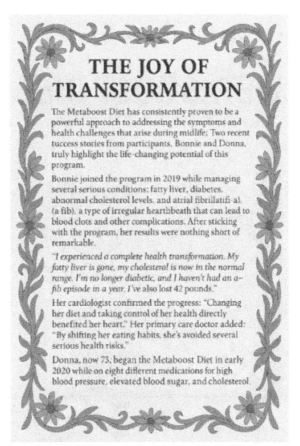

THE JOY OF TRANSFORMATION

The Metaboost Diet has consistently proven to be a powerful approach to addressing the symptoms and health challenges that arise during midlife. Two recent success stories from participants, Bonnie and Donna, truly highlight the life-changing potential of this program.

Bonnie joined the program in 2019 while managing several serious conditions: fatty liver, diabetes, abnormal cholesterol levels, and atrial fibrillatifi-a), (a-fib), a type of irregular heartbeath that can lead to blood clots and other complications. After sticking with the program, her results were nothing short of remarkable.

"I experienced a complete health transformation. My fatty liver is gone, my cholesterol is now in the normal range. I'm no longer diabetic, and I haven't had an a-fib episode in a year. I've also lost 42 pounds."

Her cardiologist confirmed the progress: "Changing her diet and taking conttol of her health directly benefited her heart." Her primary care doctor added: "By shifting her eating habits, she's avoided several serious health risks."

Donna, now 73, began the Metaboost Diet in early 2020 while on eight different medications for high blood pressure, elevated blood sugar, and cholesterol.

Stories like Bonnie's and Donna's are not rare—they're typical among those who follow the Metaboost Diet. The foods you eat on this plan do far more than help you shed inches; they actively promote healing and vitality, leading to truly life-changing outcomes.

As I often emphasize, your daily food choices on the Metaboost Diet have a lasting impact on your health, weight, and overall lifespan. Food is made up of powerful nutrients that enter your cells and enhance their function. With the right nourishment, your body becomes stronger and more resilient, increasing your chances of living a long, vibrant, and healthy life.

CHAPTER 8- Putting It All Together: The Meal Plans and Shopping Lists

Welcome to the Metaboost Diet Meal Plans

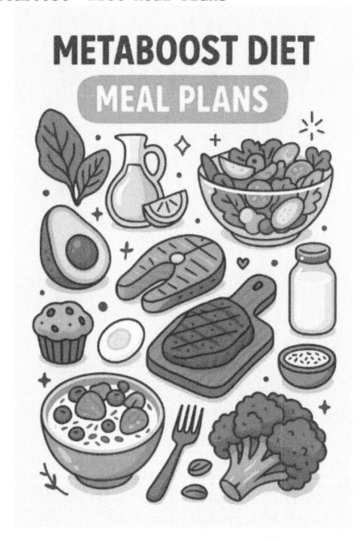

To help you ease into this new way of eating, I've created **four weeks of standard meal plans** along with **two weeks of vegetarian options**—no need to do any math! Each meal is thoughtfully balanced with healthy fats, lean proteins, and smart carbohydrates in optimal proportions. These meals also offer key nutrients like fiber, magnesium, omega-3s, vitamin D, and more—all crucial for supporting midlife wellness. Plus, the portion sizes are designed to keep you satisfied and energized.

You'll find **two meals and two snacks** in each daily plan, all intended to be eaten within your eating window. Every day includes a breakdown of the **macronutrient ratios** so you can see how closely you're hitting the recommended **70/20/10** ratio. No calorie counting here—just focus on keeping those macronutrients in balance.

At the end of each week's plan, you'll find a **shopping list** tailored to that week's meals. These lists are designed to simplify your planning and grocery trips. Feel free to adjust them to suit your preferences, favorite recipes, or the number of people you're cooking for.

Being prepared is key—especially in the early stages. Having your meals and ingredients ready means less guesswork, fewer temptations, and a smoother transition into this lifestyle.

Why Meal Prep Matters
Spending a little time prepping your meals each week can lead to big rewards:
- **Better nutrition**: You stay in control of your ingredients, portions, and nutrients—no more last-minute choices that work against your health goals.
- **A faster metabolism**: Planned snacks keep you nourished and satisfied, reduce inflammation, and support fat-burning.
- **Smart spending**: Ditch the pricey daily takeout and save serious money. That $15 salad five days a week adds up to $75—money you could put toward something more enjoyable, like a massage or self-care treat.

Tips for Smarter Meal Prep
- **Plan ahead**: Map out your weekly meals and take stock of what's already in your kitchen. Track what staples you're running low on.
- **Make a grocery list before shopping**: Stick to it once you're at the store. Focus on the store's outer aisles for fresh produce and whole foods. Stock your pantry with essentials like olive oil, nuts, seeds, spices, and condiments. And consider visiting local farmers' markets for fresh, seasonal produce. If time is tight, use grocery store pickup or delivery services to simplify the process and skip the lines.
- **Review your recipes in advance**: If you're new to cooking, start with familiar or simple dishes. As your confidence builds, experiment with new techniques and ingredients. If you're unsure about grilling, start with stovetop alternatives until you're more comfortable.
- **Mix things up**: Start with a protein base, then switch up the veggies, fruits, and healthy fats throughout the week to create colorful, nutrient-dense meals.
- **Use proper food storage**: Glass containers are ideal for reheating, while plastic containers are great for on-the-go meals. Zip-top bags are perfect for portioning out snacks like nuts and seeds.
- **Be efficient**: Stock up on frozen vegetables when they're on sale, buy pre-chopped veggies or pre-cooked proteins to save time, and always check the ingredient list on any pre-prepared foods.
- **Make it enjoyable**: Turn on a favorite podcast, playlist, or show to make meal prep time something you look forward to.

Meal Prep Styles to Explore
- **Make-ahead meals**: Cook complete meals in advance and store them in the fridge to heat and serve later—perfect for busy evenings.
- **Batch cooking**: Prepare a large quantity of a dish, like chili or soup, divide it into single portions, refrigerate what you'll eat soon, and freeze the rest for later.
- **Individual portions**: Prepare grab-and-go meals in small containers—great for breakfasts or quick lunches, hot or cold.

The Metaboost Diet – Week 1: Conventional Meal Plan
Get ready to jumpstart your journey with a full week of delicious, nutrient-rich meals! Each day includes two satisfying meals and two balanced snacks—designed to fit within your eating window and aligned with the recommended 70/20/10 macronutrient ratio (Fat/Protein/Net Carbs). You'll also benefit from

plenty of fiber and nutrients to support midlife health. Here's how Week 1 looks:

Day 1
Meal 1: MeredithShirk's Parfait
 Snack 1: Celery Sticks with Almond Butter
 Meal 2: Meatloaf with Cauliflower Mash
 Snack 2: Pecans and Dark Chocolate
 Macros: Fat: 70% | Protein: 20% | Net Carbs: 10% | Fiber: 23g

---

Day 2
Meal 1: Egg Scramble
 Snack 1: Caprese Bites
 Meal 2: Grilled Chicken Salad
 Snack 2: Chia Pudding
 Macros: Fat: 71% | Protein: 21% | Net Carbs: 8% | Fiber: 29g

---

Day 3
Meal 1: Meatloaf with Cauliflower Mash *(leftover from Day 1)*
 Snack 1: Avocado Crisps
 Meal 2: Baked Salmon with Grilled Summer Squash
 Snack 2: Chia Pudding
 Macros: Fat: 70% | Protein: 23% | Net Carbs: 7% | Fiber: 24g

---

Day 4
Meal 1: MeredithShirk's Parfait
 Snack 1: Easy Guacamole with Bell Pepper Strips
 Meal 2: Grilled Chicken Salad *(from Day 2)*
 Snack 2: Raspberries with Pecans
 Macros: Fat: 70% | Protein: 21% | Net Carbs: 9% | Fiber: 31g

---

Day 5
Meal 1: Tuna Salad with Snacky Side Salad
 Snack 1: Easy Guacamole *(leftover from Day 4)* with Baby Carrots
 Meal 2: Baked Salmon with Grilled Summer Squash *(from Day 3)*
 Snack 2: Raspberry-Flax Muffin
 Macros: Fat: 74% | Protein: 18% | Net Carbs: 8% | Fiber: 32g

---

Day 6
Meal 1: Tuna Salad with Snacky Side Salad
 Snack 1: Carrots and Celery with Flaxseed and Almond Butter
 Meal 2: Chicken Taco Salad
 Snack 2: Raspberry-Flax Muffin
 Macros: Fat: 73% | Protein: 19% | Net Carbs: 8% | Fiber: 25g

---

Day 7
Meal 1: Egg Scramble
 Snack 1: Caprese Bites
 Meal 2: Meatloaf with Cauliflower Mash *(from Day 1)*
 Snack 2: Pecans with Berries and Coconut
 Macros: Fat: 66% | Protein: 17% | Net Carbs: 15% | Fiber: 25g

---

Each recipe for these meals and snacks can be found in **Chapter 9**, so refer there for preparation steps. Remember: no calorie counting needed—just follow the macronutrient guidance and enjoy the variety, flavor, and health benefits!

Shopping List Guidelines for the Metaboost Diet

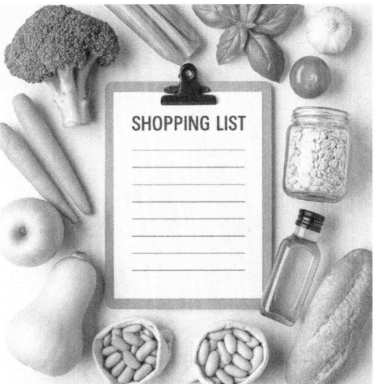

As you begin your first week of eating the Metaboost Diet way, it's helpful to stock up on essential pantry staples and frequently used items that will support you throughout the program. Below, you'll find a list of those staples. Then, each week you'll refer to the specific shopping lists to gather fresh ingredients and any additional items needed for that week's meals.

The quantities listed in the weekly shopping guides are as close as possible to the actual amounts needed for the recipes. When appropriate, amounts are rounded to common package sizes, but many reflect exact recipe quantities to ensure accuracy.

These weekly shopping lists are based on the assumption that you'll mostly be cooking for yourself. Recipes that serve more than one meal reflect this and are intended to be eaten more than once during the week. If you're preparing meals for multiple people, you'll need to adjust quantities accordingly—either by purchasing more or by doubling up on meal prep.

Be sure to review each recipe's yield and adjust your grocery list based on how many servings you'll need. Also, keep in mind that these lists are meant to serve as flexible guides—you may already have certain ingredients in your pantry, or you might choose to skip or swap out some meals.

Pantry Staples for the Metaboost Diet

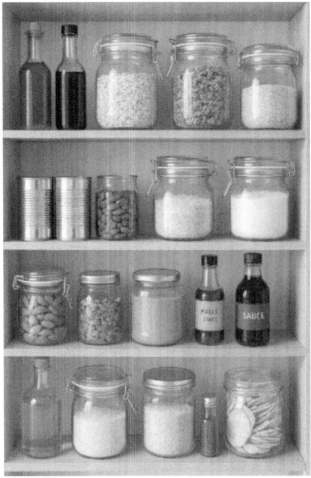

Spices, Seasonings & Flavor Enhancers

- Almond extract
- Black pepper (ground)
- Cayenne pepper
- Chili powder
- Cinnamon (ground)
- Cumin (ground)
- Curry powder
- "Everything bagel" seasoning
- Garlic powder
- Garlic salt
- Italian seasoning
- Mustard (stone-ground)
- Nutmeg (ground)
- Onion powder
- Oregano (dried)
- Paprika (smoked and sweet)
- Pumpkin pie spice
- Red pepper flakes
- Salt (kosher, sea, and table varieties)
- Turmeric (ground)
- Vanilla bean paste
- Vanilla extract

- White pepper (ground)

Oils and Healthy Fats
- Avocado oil
- Butter (salted & unsalted)
- Coconut oil
- Ghee (clarified butter)
- Mayonnaise (no added sugar, avocado oil, or olive oil-based)
- Olive oil
- Ranch dressing
- Toasted sesame oil

Nuts and Seeds
- Almonds (slivered and whole)
- Chia seeds
- Coconut flakes (unsweetened)
- Flaxseed (ground)
- Hemp hearts
- Macadamia nuts (whole and halved)
- Mixed nuts
- Peanuts (roasted and salted)
- Pecans
- Pumpkin seeds
- Sesame seeds (black and white)
- Sunflower seeds
- Walnuts

Condiments
- Primal Kitchen BBQ sauce
- Spicy brown mustard
- Sriracha or other hot sauce
- Tamari or soy sauce

Miscellaneous Essentials
- Almond butter (unsweetened)
- Almond flour
- Apple butter
- Baking powder
- Cacao powder
- Coconut flour
- Coconut milk (unsweetened)
- Cocoa powder (unsweetened)
- Collagen powder
- Honey
- Maple syrup
- MCT powder
- Oat flour
- Peanut butter (no sugar added)
- Vinegars: red wine, rice wine, balsamic, apple cider

- Sweeteners: stevia, monk fruit (with or without erythritol), Swerve

---

This base list will support most of your cooking throughout the Metaboost Diet. Review it as you begin, and check off what you already have. Then, refer to your weekly list for the fresh ingredients and additional items you'll need for your meals.

Metaboost Diet: Week 1 Shopping List

Note: Quantities reflect what's needed for that week's recipes, not necessarily how items are sold.

Proteins
- Ground beef (lean, grass-fed): 1½ lbs
- Chicken breasts (boneless, skinless): 1 lb
- Pre-cooked chicken breast: 1 (approx. 8 oz)
- Salmon fillet: 3 lbs
- Eggs: 7 large
- Whole-milk mozzarella balls: 1 (8 oz) package
- Plain full-fat Greek yogurt (e.g., Fage): 1 (16 oz) container
- Tuna (canned in water): 2 (2 oz) cans

Vegetables
- Baby carrots: 10 oz package
- Carrots: 2 medium
- Cauliflower: 1 large head
- Celery: 1 stalk
- Cherry tomatoes: 2 pints
- Garlic: 1 bulb
- Onion (white or yellow): 1 medium
- Onion (red): 1 medium
- Romaine lettuce: 1 head
- Roma tomato: 1 large
- Round tomatoes: 1-2 ripe
- Spinach: 1 (10 oz) bag
- Yellow summer squash: 1 medium
- Zucchini: 1 medium
- Assorted raw vegetables (for dipping)
- Mixed salad greens: 1 bag

Fresh Herbs
- Basil
- Cilantro
- Parsley

Fruits
- Avocados: 4 medium
- Blueberries: ½ pint
- Lemons: 6 medium
- Raspberries: ½ pint
- Strawberries: 1 pint

Miscellaneous
(Small packages/containers recommended)
- Unsweetened coconut milk
- Pre-grated Parmesan cheese
- Heavy cream

- Sour cream
- Sugar-free dark chocolate chips
- No-sugar-added tomato sauce

Metaboost Diet: Week 2 Meal Plan Overview

Each day includes two meals and two snacks, supporting the Metaboost Diet's macronutrient goals. Recipes are referenced by their page in the meal plan guide.

Day 1
- **Meal 1:** Roasted Tomato Bisque
- **Snack 1:** Everything-Bagel Cucumber Bites
- **Meal 2:** Portobello Pizzas
- **Snack 2:** Blueberry Pie Smoothie
- **Macros:** Fat 72% | Protein 16% | Net Carbs 12% | Fiber 28g

Day 2
- **Meal 1:** TGD Cobb Salad
- **Snack 1:** Fresh blueberries
- **Meal 2:** Cheeseburger Lettuce Sliders
- **Snack 2:** Chocolate-Cinnamon Apple Bites
- **Macros:** Fat 66% | Protein 24% | Net Carbs 10% | Fiber 21g

Day 3
- **Meal 1:** Roasted Tomato Bisque (leftover from Day 1)
- **Snack 1:** Chocolate-Cinnamon Apple Bites (from Day 2)
- **Meal 2:** TGD Cobb Salad (from Day 2)
- **Snack 2:** Tropical Berries
- **Macros:** Fat 70% | Protein 23% | Net Carbs 7% | Fiber 24g

Day 4
- **Meal 1:** Chicken and BLT Wrap
- **Snack 1:** Herbed White Bean Dip with cucumber slices
- **Meal 2:** Cheeseburger Lettuce Sliders (from Day 2)
- **Snack 2:** Chocolate-Cinnamon Apple Bites
- **Macros:** Fat 70% | Protein 19% | Net Carbs 11% | Fiber 21g

Day 5
- **Meal 1:** Portobello Pizzas
- **Snack 1:** Chocolate Peanut Butter Yogurt
- **Meal 2:** Chicken and BLT Wrap (from Day 4)
- **Snack 2:** Apple and Mixed Nuts
- **Macros:** Fat 67% | Protein 20% | Net Carbs 13% | Fiber 25g

Day 6
- **Meal 1:** Avocado "For Life" Toast
- **Snack 1:** Herbed White Bean Dip (leftover from Day 4)
- **Meal 2:** Sesame Ginger Pork with Green Beans
- **Snack 2:** Coconut and Walnut Chia Pudding
- **Macros:** Fat 68% | Protein 18% | Net Carbs 14% | Fiber 34g

Day 7
- **Meal 1:** Sesame Ginger Pork with Green Beans (from Day 6)
- **Snack 1:** Cheese and Walnuts
- **Meal 2:** Grilled Shrimp with Broiled Tomato Bites
- **Snack 2:** Chocolate-Peanut Butter Mug Cake
- **Macros:** Fat 74% | Protein 20% | Net Carbs 6% | Fiber 27g

---

Shopping List for Week 2
Proteins
- Ground beef (90% lean, grass-fed): 6 oz
- Chicken breast (boneless, skinless): 6 oz
- Rotisserie-cooked chicken: 1-2 breasts (12 oz total)
- Eggs: 1 dozen large
- Pork loin (boneless): 1 (8 oz) piece
- Turkey bacon: 1 lb
- Large shrimp: 1 lb
- Plain full-fat Greek yogurt: 1 (5.3 oz) container

Vegetables
- Cucumbers: 2 medium
- Garlic: 10 cloves (1 bulb)
- Fresh green beans: 8 oz
- Portobello mushrooms (caps): 8
- Onion (red): 1 medium
- Onion (white or yellow): 1 medium
- Romaine lettuce: 1 large head
- Cherry tomatoes: 1 pint
- Grape tomatoes: 1 pint
- Roma (plum) tomatoes: 8 medium
- Round tomatoes: 1-2 ripe
- Spinach: 1 (10 oz) bag
- Cannellini beans: 2 (15 oz) cans
- Dill pickles: 1 (18 oz) jar

Fresh Herbs
- Basil
- Dill
- Ginger
- Parsley

Fruits
- Apple: 1
- Avocados: 3 medium
- Blueberries: ½ pint
- Lemons: 2 medium
- Raspberries: ½ pint

Miscellaneous Items (Additional for Weeks 2-3)
- Cheddar cheese (pre-shredded): 9 oz
- Cheese sticks: small pack
- Chicken broth (canned): 16 oz
- Dark chocolate chips (sugar-free): 1 oz
- Unsweetened full-fat coconut milk: 15 oz can
- Cream cheese: 4 oz package
- Mozzarella (pre-shredded): 2 oz (about ½ cup)
- Parmesan (pre-grated): 1 oz (about ¼ cup)
- Sprouted-grain bread (e.g., Food For Life)

Week 3 Meal Plan Overview

Each day includes two meals and two snacks, designed to support fat-burning, nutrient balance, and satiety with minimal prep repetition.

Day 1
- **Meal 1:** Stuffed Bell Peppers (Turkey + Cauliflower Rice)
- **Snack 1:** Marinated Olives, Chickpeas & Veggies w/ Herbs
- **Meal 2:** Shrimp & Asparagus
- **Snack 2:** Aloha Avocado
  Macros: Fat 69% | Protein 20% | Net Carbs 11% | Fiber 25g

Day 2
- Repeat Shrimp & Aloha Avocado
- **Meal 2:** Sirloin, Spinach & Blue Cheese Salad
- **Snack 2:** Marinated Olives & Veggies
  Macros: Fat 71% | Protein 19% | Net Carbs 10% | Fiber 26g

Day 3
- Repeat Stuffed Peppers
- **Snack 1:** Apple Clusters
- **Meal 2:** Grilled Steak with Creamed Spinach & Mushrooms
- **Snack 2:** Veggie Slices w/ Italian Mayo Dip
  Macros: Fat 65% | Protein 22% | Net Carbs 13% | Fiber 22g

Day 4-7
Rotation of previous meals plus:
- **Broccoli & Cheese Chicken Bake**
- **Cottage Cheese Omelet**
- **Poached Eggs with Cabbage Hash & Avocado**
- **Tuna Salad over Mixed Greens**
- **Herbed Cottage Cheese Dip**
- **Meredith Shirk's Parfait (blended)**
  Macros Range: Fat 65-70% | Protein 20-24% | Net Carbs 7-13% | Fiber 22-27g

---

Shopping List - Week 3
Proteins
- Sirloin steak: 12 oz + 4 mini steaks (3 oz each)
- Pre-cooked chicken: 2 breasts (1 lb)
- Ground turkey (lean): 1½ lbs
- Shrimp: 1 lb
- Eggs: 2 medium, 2 large
- Cottage cheese (full-fat): 4 oz
- Greek yogurt (plain, full-fat): 5.3 oz
- Tuna (canned): 1 (2 oz) can

Vegetables
- Asparagus: 1½ lbs
- Broccoli (crown): 4 cups
- Pre-shredded cabbage: 12 oz (about 2 cups)
- Carrots: 5 medium
- Cauliflower rice: 1 lb (about 2 cups)
- Celery: 1-2 stalks
- Cucumbers: 4 large, 1 small

- Garlic: 6 cloves
- Mushrooms (portobello or button): 1 lb
- Onions (white/yellow): 1 medium
- Radishes: 8
- Red bell peppers: 4
- Spinach: 10 oz + 16 oz baby (combined ~7½ cups)
- Tomato: 1 ripe
- Mixed salad greens: 10 oz
- Chickpeas: 1 (15 oz) can

Fresh Herbs
- Basil
- Cilantro
- Dill
- Thyme

Fruits
- Apple: 1 small
- Avocados: 2 medium
- Blackberries: ½ pint
- Blueberries: ½ pint
- Lemons: 2-3
- Raspberries: ½ pint
- Strawberries: 1 pint

Miscellaneous
- Blue cheese (crumbled): 1½ oz
- Cheddar cheese (shredded): 24 oz
- Parmesan (grated): about ¼ cup
- Whole milk: 1 pint
- Heavy cream: ½ pint
- Sour cream: 8 oz
- Olives: 1 lb (approx. 2 cups)

Week 4 Meal Plan Overview
This week builds on familiar favorites like pumpkin pancakes and turkey-spaghetti squash bowls, with new savory and sweet options.

Day 1
- **Meal 1:** Pumpkin Pancakes
- **Snack 1:** Cucumber, Tomato & Feta Salad
- **Meal 2:** Spaghetti Squash with Turkey, Bacon, Spinach & Goat Cheese
- **Snack 2:** Turkey Mayo Lettuce Wraps
  Macros: Fat 66% | Protein 22% | Net Carbs 12% | Fiber 25g

Day 2
- Repeat Spaghetti Squash meal
- **Snack 1:** Deviled Eggs
- **Meal 2:** BLT Salmon Burgers
- **Snack 2:** Kale Chips & Pecans
  Macros: Fat 67% | Protein 25% | Net Carbs 8% | Fiber 28g

Day 3-7
- Rotation of:

- o Pumpkin Pancakes
- o Raspberry Almond Smoothie
- o Egg & Veggie Salad
- o Chicken Curry with Cauliflower Rice
- o Lemon Chicken with Capers
- o Peanut Butter Cup Smoothie
- o Naked Turkey Roll-Ups
- o Creamy Avocado Dip with veggie sticks or green beans
  - **Macros Range:** Fat 66-69% | Protein 20-22% | Net Carbs 10-13% | Fiber 25-31g

---

Metaboost Diet: Week 4 Shopping List
Proteins
- Uncured bacon: 6 slices
- Boneless, skinless chicken breast: 4 oz
- Pre-cooked chicken breasts: 1 lb
- Eggs: 6 large
- Lean ground turkey: 1 lb
- Turkey deli slices: approx. 2 oz
- Turkey bacon: 12 slices
- Salmon fillet: 8 oz
- Greek yogurt (plain, full-fat): 5.3 oz container

Vegetables
- Broccoli crown: enough for ~4 cups florets
- Cauliflower rice: 1 pack (approx. 1 cup)
- Cucumbers: 2 medium
- Garlic: 2 cloves
- Green beans: ¼ lb (approx. 10 beans)
- Green bell pepper: 1
- Kale: 1 large bunch
- Lettuce (butter or similar): 1 small head
- Red onion: 1 medium
- Red bell pepper: 1
- Spaghetti squash: 2 medium
- Baby spinach: 1 (16 oz) package (~4 cups)
- Round tomatoes: 2 ripe
- Cherry tomatoes: 1 pint
- Pumpkin purée: 15 oz can (~2 cups)

Fresh Herbs
- Chives
- Cilantro
- Basil
- Thai basil

Fruits
- Avocados: 3 medium
- Lemons: 2 medium
- Raspberries: ½ pint

- Strawberries: 1 pint

Miscellaneous
- Cheese sticks: small package
- Cheddar (pre-shredded): ~1 cup
- Feta (pre-crumbled): ~1 oz
- Goat cheese: 4 oz
- Swiss cheese: 2 oz piece
- Heavy cream: ½ pint
- Sour cream: 8 oz container
- Assorted olives: 8 oz (~¼ cup)

Metaboost Diet: Vegetarian Meal Plan – Week 1

This 7-day plant-based plan focuses on healthy fats, fiber, and moderate protein with satisfying, delicious meals and snacks.

Sample Meals & Highlights
- **Flaxseed Pancakes**
- **Tofu in Peanut Sauce**
- **BBQ Tempeh with Greens & Cauliflower Rice**
- **Mushroom Stroganoff with Creamy Garlic Cauliflower Rice**
- **Chia Puddings, Vegan Yogurt Parfaits, Nut-Based Snacks, and Smoothies**

Macros (daily ranges):
- Fat: 65-71%
- Protein: 14-20%
- Net Carbs: 10-17%
- Fiber: 25-49g

Shopping List – Vegetarian Week 1

Proteins
- Eggs: 4 large
- Tempeh: 1 lb
- Firm tofu: 14 oz (~1⅜ cups)
- Greek yogurt (plain, full-fat): 5.3 oz
- Unsweetened almond milk yogurt: 5.3 oz

Vegetables
- Broccolini: 12 oz (~2¼ cups)
- Cauliflower (whole): 1 small head
- Garlic: 9 cloves
- Chopped kale: 1 lb (~6 cups)
- Button mushrooms: 2 (10 oz) packages (~5 cups)
- Yellow onions: 2 medium

Fresh Herbs
- Flat-leaf parsley
- Fresh ginger

Fruits
- Fresh blueberries: ½ pint

- Lemons: 2 medium

Miscellaneous
- Frozen blueberries: 10 oz (~2 cups)
- Babybel cheese round: 1
- Orange juice: 4 oz
- Parmesan cheese (pre-grated): ~½ cup
- Vanilla protein powder (plant-based, e.g., KOS): 1 jar
- Vegetable broth (canned/jarred): 15 oz (~2 cups)

Metaboost Diet: Vegetarian Week 2 Meal Plan

Enjoy a full week of plant-based meals packed with fiber, healthy fats, and clean protein sources. Meals are rotated throughout the week to simplify prep while still offering plenty of variety.

Day-by-Day Breakdown

Day 1
- **Meal 1:** Breakfast Salad
- **Snack 1:** Pear Slices with Ricotta Cheese
- **Meal 2:** Blackened Tofu with Sesame Broccoli Slaw
- **Snack 2:** Herbed White Bean Dip with snap peas, radishes, broccoli & cauliflower
   Macros: Fat 68% | Protein 16% | Net Carbs 16% | Fiber 27g

Day 2
- **Meal 1:** Grape Tomato & Pea Salad on Ricotta + 1 tbsp Ground Flaxseed
- **Snack 1:** Hard-Boiled Egg with Avocado
- **Meal 2:** Blackened Tofu with Sesame Broccoli Slaw *(repeat)*
- **Snack 2:** Peanut Butter-Mocha Smoothie
   Macros: Fat 74% | Protein 14% | Net Carbs 12% | Fiber 30g

Day 3
- **Meal 1:** Blackened Tofu with Sesame Broccoli Slaw *(repeat)*
- **Snack 1:** Herbed White Bean Dip with raw veggie medley *(repeat)*
- **Meal 2:** Spicy Edamame Bowl with Creamy Chili Sauce
- **Snack 2:** Green Almond Butter Smoothie
   Macros: Fat 63% | Protein 20% | Net Carbs 17% | Fiber 35g

Day 4
- **Meal 1:** Breakfast Salad *(repeat)*
- **Snack 1:** Blackened Tofu with Sesame Broccoli Slaw
- **Meal 2:** Spicy Edamame Bowl *(repeat)*
- **Snack 2:** Chocolate Banana "Nice" Cream
   Macros: Fat 71% | Protein 15% | Net Carbs 14% | Fiber 32g

Day 5
- **Meal 1:** Spicy Edamame Bowl *(repeat)*
- **Snack 1:** Grape Tomato & Pea Salad on Ricotta *(repeat)*

- **Meal 2**: Veggie Cheese Enchiladas with Grain-Free Tortillas
- **Snack 2**: Edamame Mash Salad
  Macros: Fat 72% | Protein 15% | Net Carbs 13% | Fiber 25g

Day 6

- **Meal 1**: Vegan Protein Salad
- **Snack 1**: Hard-Boiled Egg with Avocado *(repeat)*
- **Meal 2**: Spicy Edamame Bowl *(repeat)*
- **Snack 2**: Strawberries with Almond Milk Greek Yogurt
  Macros: Fat 67% | Protein 18% | Net Carbs 15% | Fiber 30g

Day 7

- **Meal 1**: Veggie Cheese Enchiladas *(repeat)*
- **Snack 1**: Edamame Mash Salad *(repeat)*
- **Meal 2**: Vegan Protein Salad *(repeat)*
- **Snack 2**: Chocolate Banana "Nice" Cream *(repeat)*
  Macros: Fat 65% | Protein 17% | Net Carbs 19% | Fiber 38g

Shopping List – Vegetarian Week 2
Proteins

- Eggs: 10
- Tempeh: 16 oz package
- Tofu:
  - Medium or firm: 10 oz
  - Extra firm: 12 oz
- Greek yogurt (plain, full-fat): 5.3 oz
- Almond milk yogurt (unsweetened, Greek-style): 5.3 oz

Vegetables

- Arugula: 1 oz (~1 cup)
- Bell pepper: 1 (any color)
- Broccoli slaw: 14 oz bag
- Coleslaw mix: 14 oz bag
- Garlic: 7 cloves
- Romaine lettuce: 1 head
- Onion:
  - Red: 1 medium
  - White/yellow: 1-2 medium
- Red cabbage (pre-shredded): ~1 cup
- Scallions: 6
- Spinach:
  - Chopped: 10 oz (~6 cups)
  - Baby: 1 small pack (~1 cup)
- Tomatoes:
  - Cherry: 1 pint
  - Grape: 1 pint
- Zucchini: 1 medium
- Mixed raw veggies: sugar snap peas, radishes, broccoli & cauliflower florets

Fresh Herbs

- Cilantro
- Dill
- Ginger
- Mint

Fruits
- Avocados: 4 medium
- Bananas: 2 ripe
- Blueberries: ½ pint
- Lemons: 2 medium
- Limes: 2 medium
- Pear: 1 firm
- Strawberries: 1 pint

Miscellaneous
- Cacao nibs: small pack (~3 tbsp)
- Cheddar cheese (pre-shredded): ~1½ cups
- Cannellini beans: 1 (15 oz) can (~½ cup)
- Frozen edamame: 10 oz package
- Ricotta: 15 oz container (~1½ cups)
- Tomato sauce (no sugar added): 15 oz (about 1½ cups)
- Vegetable broth: 8 oz (about 1 cup)

If You Prefer to Create Your Own Meals

Not interested in sticking strictly to the meal plans? That's totally fine—you can easily design your own menus. Here are a few ideas to get you started:

Meal 1

Midday Salad

Around lunchtime, a large mixed green salad makes a great first meal. Add a high-quality protein like salmon, chicken, or eggs. If you're vegetarian or vegan, swap in chickpeas or other legumes. Top it off with nuts or seeds and slices of avocado. Dress it with lemon juice or a blend of vinegar, olive or avocado oil, and herbs. Salads are an easy and delicious way to include your healthy fats—like olive oil, nuts, seeds, and avocado—right at lunch.

Lettuce Wrap Option

You can also go for a lettuce wrap filled with egg salad, tuna, or hummus and veggies. Or try stuffing a tomato with these same fillings. Another great option for Meal 1 is a brunch-style plate with scrambled eggs, nitrate-free bacon, and sautéed vegetables. The key is to fuel your body with a balanced mix that includes plenty of healthy fats.

Drink Choices

Stick to water, herbal tea, or coffee for beverages during meals and snacks. Just be cautious with caffeine, as it might worsen hot flashes.

Meal 2

Protein + Veggies + Starch

Choose a protein, pair it with non-starchy vegetables like broccoli, Brussels sprouts, or cauliflower, and optionally include a starchy vegetable such as sweet potato, winter squash, or a regular potato for a complete meal.

Stir-Fry Combo

Make a stir-fry using chicken tenders and veggies, served over cauliflower rice and cooked in a healthy fat like avocado oil. Want to keep it simple? Use a 4-ounce portion of lean steak (or another protein), a side salad with vinaigrette, and a small baked potato with butter and sour cream.

Vegetarian Option

  If you want a meat-free meal, sauté zucchini noodles with pesto or olive oil and herbs, then sprinkle with grated Parmesan.

  Each meal focuses on combining protein, vegetables, fats, and salads to deliver a balanced intake that supports hormonal health and metabolic function.

You can also enjoy two daily snacks. Prioritize whole, minimally processed foods. Great snack choices include hard-boiled eggs, yogurt, cheese sticks, nuts, raw vegetables, fresh berries, dill pickles, olives, or uncured beef jerky to help manage hunger between meals.

You've likely noticed these meals are centered around healthy fats, moderate-quality protein, ample non-starchy carbs, and some starchy vegetables. This combination supports fat loss, reduces inflammation, balances hormones, boosts metabolism, and contributes to overall wellness.

Also, you'll see there's no mention of calorie counting or portion control. The Metaboost Diet is designed so you can eat freely without stressing over those numbers. Because your meals are rich in protein, healthy fats, and fiber-filled carbs, you'll feel full and satisfied—no cravings for sugar or processed carbs. Over time, you'll naturally learn which foods work best for you and how to assemble meals that keep you feeling your best. And don't forget—tracking your macronutrients can give you an added edge for success!

CHAPTER 9 - The Metaboost Diet Recipes

Since launching the Metaboost Diet as an online program, I've teamed up with coaches, nutritionists, and chefs to craft even more mouthwatering recipes you'll want to make again and again—keeping you both satisfied and on track. As someone who loves to cook and play around with flavors in my own kitchen, I've also contributed some of my personal creations.

While developing these recipes, we focused not just on taste, but also on simplicity and speed. Let's be honest—life is busy, and we all need meals that are both delicious and easy to prepare.

These are all brand-new recipes you won't find online. They've been created with both versions of the Metaboost Diet in mind—the traditional plan that includes animal-based foods, as well as the vegan/vegetarian variation for those who steer clear of animal products.

Enjoy every bite!

MEALS AND SNACKS

Meredith Shirk's Parfait or Smoothie

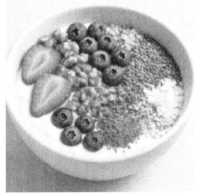

Serves 1

Ingredients:

- ¾ cup plain full-fat Greek yogurt (e.g., Fage)
- ¼ cup sliced strawberries
- ¼ cup fresh blueberries
- ¼ cup chopped walnuts
- 1 tbsp ground flaxseed
- 1 tbsp chia seeds
- 1 tbsp hemp hearts
- 1 tbsp unsweetened coconut flakes
- 2-3 ice cubes (for smoothie)
- Water, as needed (for smoothie)

Parfait Instructions:

Combine all ingredients in a bowl, stir well, and enjoy immediately.

Smoothie Instructions:

Add all ingredients except water to a blender. Blend until smooth, adding water gradually to reach the desired texture.

Chocolate Strawberry Smoothie

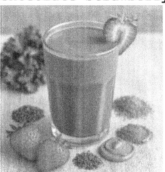

Serves 1

Ingredients:

- 1 scoop protein powder
- 1 cup chopped kale
- ½ cup sliced strawberries
- 1 tbsp ground flaxseed
- 1 tbsp unsweetened almond butter
- 1 tbsp unsweetened cocoa powder
- ½ cup coconut milk
- 2 tbsp chia seeds
- Ice cubes (optional)

Instructions:

Blend all ingredients until smooth.

Note: Choose a vegetarian or vegan protein powder to suit your dietary preference.

Egg Scramble

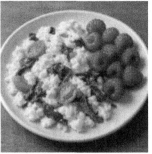

Serves 1
Ingredients:

- 2 large eggs
- Salt and black pepper, to taste
- 1 tbsp butter
- 1 cup spinach
- ½ cup chopped tomatoes
- 1 cup fresh raspberries (optional)

Instructions:

1. Crack eggs into a bowl, season with salt and pepper, and whisk well.
2. Heat butter in a skillet over low heat.
3. Pour in eggs and cook until edges start to set. Gently fold and continue to cook for about a minute.
4. Stir in spinach and tomatoes, folding until just set but slightly runny on top.
5. Serve with raspberries on the side, if desired.

Cottage Cheese Omelet

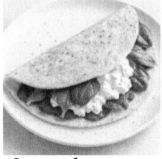

Serves 1
Ingredients:

- 2 large eggs
- 1 tbsp milk
- Salt and black pepper, to taste
- 1 tbsp olive oil
- ½ cup spinach
- 3 tbsp full-fat cottage cheese

Instructions:

1. In a bowl, whisk eggs with milk, salt, and pepper.
2. Heat olive oil in a skillet over medium heat. Pour in egg mixture and cook 1-2 minutes, until mostly set.
3. Flip, then place spinach and cottage cheese on one side. Cook another 1-2 minutes, fold, and serve.

Poached Eggs with Cabbage Hash Browns

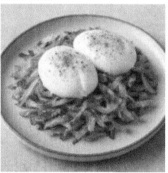

Serves 1
Ingredients:

- 1 tsp olive oil
- 2 cups shredded green cabbage
- ½ cup sliced onion
- 2 medium eggs
- Salt and pepper, to taste
- Smoked paprika (optional)

Instructions:

1. Heat olive oil in a skillet over medium heat. Add cabbage and onion; cook 8-10 minutes until browned and softened.
2. Transfer to a plate and cover to keep warm.
3. Simmer water in a medium pan. Crack eggs into water and poach for 4-5 minutes, flipping once.
4. Remove eggs with a slotted spoon and place on top of the cabbage. Season with salt, pepper, and paprika if using.

Avocado "For Life" Toast

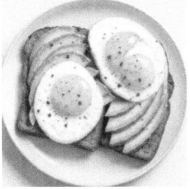

Serves 1
Ingredients:
- 1 tbsp olive oil
- 2 large eggs
- 2 slices sprouted grain bread (e.g., Food For Life)
- 1 avocado, halved, pitted, and sliced
- Salt and pepper, to taste
- Red pepper flakes (optional)

Instructions:
1. Heat olive oil in a skillet over medium-high heat. Cook eggs to your liking.
2. Toast bread slices.
3. Place toast on a plate, layer with avocado and eggs, and season. Sprinkle with red pepper flakes, if desired.

Flaxseed Pancakes

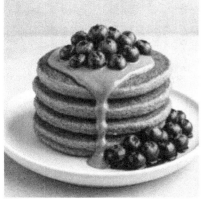

Makes 4 servings
Ingredients:
- 1 cup ground flaxseed
- 4 large eggs, beaten
- ⅓ cup unsweetened almond milk (or more as needed)
- 2 tsp fresh lemon juice

- 1 tsp baking soda
- 1 tsp vanilla extract
- 1 tsp ground cinnamon
- ⅛ tsp salt
- ½ tbsp coconut oil
- 4 tbsp unsweetened almond butter
- 2 cups frozen blueberries

Instructions:
1. Mix flaxseed, eggs, milk, lemon juice, baking soda, vanilla, cinnamon, and salt in a large bowl. Add more liquid if needed to get a pourable batter.
2. Heat coconut oil in a skillet over medium heat. Pour ¼ cup of batter per pancake and cook 2-3 minutes per side. Keep warm while making the rest.
3. Warm almond butter in the microwave. Heat blueberries until soft and juicy.
4. Serve pancakes topped with almond butter and berries.

Pumpkin Pancakes

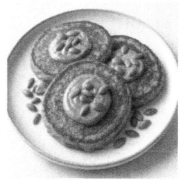

Serves 3
Ingredients:
- 2 tbsp ground flaxseed
- ¾ cup almond flour
- 1 tbsp coconut flour
- 1 tsp stevia
- ½ tsp baking powder
- ½ tsp pumpkin pie spice
- ½ cup canned pumpkin puree
- 2 large eggs, beaten
- 1 tbsp avocado oil
- 6 tbsp unsweetened almond butter
- 3 tbsp pumpkin seeds

Instructions:

1. In a mixing bowl, stir together the flaxseed, flours, stevia, baking powder, and pumpkin spice. Add the pumpkin and eggs and mix until fully combined.
2. Preheat a skillet or griddle over medium heat. Add ½ tbsp avocado oil, then spoon in 2-3 portions of batter, spreading each into a 3- to 4-inch pancake.
3. Cook about 3 minutes per side until golden. Transfer to a plate, cover to keep warm. Repeat with remaining oil and batter.
4. Serve pancakes topped with almond butter and pumpkin seeds.

Breakfast Salad

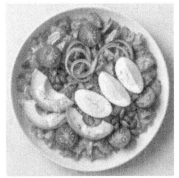

Serves 2

Ingredients:

- 3 tbsp avocado oil mayo
- 1 clove garlic, crushed
- 2 tsp fresh lemon juice
- 4 cups torn romaine lettuce
- 1 cup cherry tomatoes, halved
- 1 medium avocado, sliced
- ¼ small onion, thinly sliced
- Salt and pepper
- ½ cup pumpkin seeds
- 4 hard-boiled eggs, peeled and quartered

Instructions:

1. Mix mayo, garlic, and lemon juice to make the dressing.
2. Divide lettuce between two plates and top with tomatoes, avocado, onion, and seasoning.

3. Add pumpkin seeds and egg wedges, drizzle with dressing, and serve.

Chicken and BLT Wrap

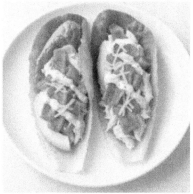

Serves 2

Ingredients:

- 2 large romaine or Bibb lettuce leaves
- 1 avocado, sliced
- 1 cup shredded rotisserie chicken
- ½ cup chopped tomato
- 2 slices turkey bacon
- 4 tbsp ranch dressing (homemade or Primal Kitchen)
- ⅛ tsp black pepper
- ¼ cup shredded cheddar cheese

Instructions:

1. Lay lettuce flat and layer each with avocado, chicken, tomato, bacon, dressing, pepper, and cheese.
2. Fold sides inward and serve immediately.

Tuna Salad with Snacky Side Salad

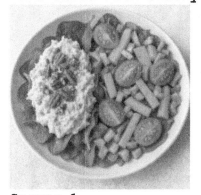

Serves 1

Tuna Salad:

- 1 (2 oz) can tuna, drained

- 1 tbsp chopped red onion
- 2 tbsp avocado oil mayo
- 2 tbsp chopped pecans

Side Salad:
- 1 cup mixed greens
- ½ cup chopped tomato
- 1 medium chopped carrot
- 1 chopped celery stalk
- 1 tbsp olive oil
- Juice of 1 lemon

Instructions:
1. In a bowl, combine tuna, onion, mayo, and pecans.
2. In a separate bowl, mix greens, tomato, carrot, and celery, then drizzle with olive oil and lemon juice.
3. Serve the tuna salad over the greens.

TGD Cobb Salad

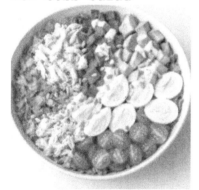

Serves 4
Ingredients:
- 8 cups chopped romaine
- 2 cups shredded rotisserie chicken
- 12 slices turkey bacon
- 2 chopped avocados
- 8 hard-boiled eggs
- 1½ cups halved cherry tomatoes
- ½ cup ranch dressing
- 4 tbsp sunflower seeds

Instructions:
Toss all ingredients in a large bowl with the dressing, then sprinkle with sunflower seeds before serving.

Grape Tomato and Pea Salad on Ricotta Spread

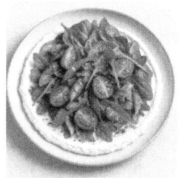

Serves 1
Ricotta Base:
- 1 cup full-fat ricotta
- 1 tbsp olive oil
- ½ tsp salt

Salad:
- 1 cup arugula
- 1 cup spinach
- ½ cup halved sugar snap peas
- ½ cup halved grape tomatoes

Dressing:
- 2 tbsp white balsamic vinegar
- 1 cup chopped basil
- 2 tbsp olive oil
- Pinch of red pepper flakes
- Salt and black pepper

Instructions:
1. Blend ricotta, oil, and salt until smooth; spread on a plate.
2. In a bowl, toss arugula, spinach, peas, and tomatoes.
3. Blend dressing ingredients until smooth.
4. Drizzle dressing over greens, toss, and layer over the ricotta base.

Vegan Protein Salad

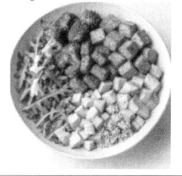

Serves 2
Marinated Tempeh:

- 2 tbsp balsamic vinegar
- 1 tbsp tamari or soy sauce
- 1 tbsp maple syrup
- ½ tsp garlic powder
- Salt and pepper
- 4 oz tempeh, cubed

Baked Tofu:

- 5 oz firm tofu, cubed
- ½ tsp garlic powder
- 1 tbsp tamari
- Salt and pepper

Salad Base:

- 1 cup steamed chopped broccoli
- 2 cups arugula
- 1 cup diced cucumber
- 1 chopped avocado
- 4 tbsp hemp seeds
- 1 tbsp tahini
- 1 tbsp olive oil
- Fresh lemon juice

Instructions:

1. Marinate tempeh for 2+ hours.
2. Preheat oven to 400°F. Bake tempeh 20 minutes and tofu 30 minutes.
3. In a bowl, combine greens, broccoli, cucumber, avocado, tofu, and tempeh.
4. Drizzle with tahini, olive oil, and lemon juice. Toss well before serving.

Roasted Tomato Bisque

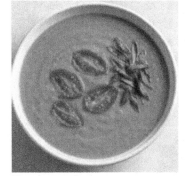

Serves 4
Ingredients:

- 4 tbsp olive oil
- 8 Roma tomatoes, halved

- 4 garlic cloves, minced
- 1 (15 oz) can cannellini beans
- 2 cups chicken broth
- Salt and pepper
- 1 cup heavy cream
- Julienned fresh basil (optional)

Instructions:

1. Preheat oven to 400°F. Coat a baking sheet with olive oil.
2. Arrange tomatoes cut side up, sprinkle with garlic, and roast 20-25 minutes.
3. Blend tomatoes, garlic, and beans until smooth.
4. Transfer to a pot, add broth, season, and warm through. Stir in cream and garnish with basil, if desired.

Chicken Taco Salad

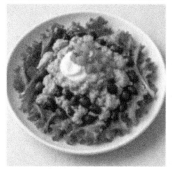

Serves 1
Ingredients:

- ¾ cup chopped cooked chicken
- Pinch of chili powder, cumin, oregano (or other spices)
- ½ tsp garlic salt
- 2 tbsp guacamole
- 2 tbsp sour cream
- 2 tbsp fresh salsa
- ½ cup black beans, rinsed and drained
- 2 cups mixed salad greens

Instructions:

1. Season chicken with spices and garlic salt.
2. Stir in guacamole, sour cream, salsa, and black beans.
3. Place greens on a plate, top with the chicken mixture, and serve.

Tuna Salad over Mixed Greens

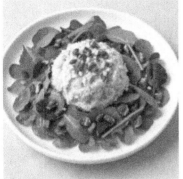

Serves 1
Ingredients:

- 2 cups torn mixed greens
- 1 (3 oz) can tuna in water, drained
- 1 tbsp minced onion
- 2 tbsp olive oil or avocado oil mayonnaise
- 2 tbsp chopped pecans

Instructions:

1. Place the salad greens in a medium bowl.
2. In a small bowl, mix the tuna, onion, and mayo, then spoon over the greens. Top with pecans and serve.

Sesame Ginger Pork with Green Beans

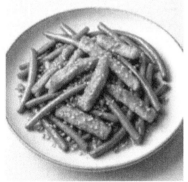

Serves 4
Ingredients:

- ¼ cup sesame seeds
- Nonstick spray
- 8 oz pork loin, cut into ½-inch strips
- Salt and pepper
- 2 tbsp coconut oil
- 4 garlic cloves, minced
- 2 tsp grated ginger
- 2 cups trimmed green beans
- 2 tsp tamari
- 1 tbsp toasted sesame oil

Instructions:

1. Toast sesame seeds in a dry skillet until fragrant and lightly golden.
2. Spray another skillet and cook pork for 6-8 minutes or until browned. Season with salt and pepper and set aside.
3. In the same pan, heat coconut oil, then sauté garlic, ginger, and green beans for 6-8 minutes.
4. Return pork to the pan, add tamari, and stir everything together.
5. Serve garnished with toasted sesame seeds and a drizzle of sesame oil.

Stuffed Bell Peppers with Turkey and Cauliflower Rice

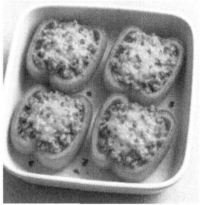

Serves 4
Ingredients:

- Nonstick spray
- 4 tbsp coconut oil
- 12 oz lean ground turkey
- 1 cup cauliflower rice
- 2 garlic cloves, minced
- Ground cumin, paprika, black pepper
- Fresh cilantro, minced
- 2 large red bell peppers, halved and cored
- 2 cups shredded cheddar cheese

Instructions:

1. Preheat oven to 300°F and grease a baking dish.

2. Sauté turkey in coconut oil over medium heat until no longer pink.
3. Transfer to a bowl and mix in cauliflower rice, garlic, spices, and cilantro.
4. Stuff pepper halves with the mixture and top with cheese.
5. Bake for 10 minutes or until cheese is melted and golden.

Shrimp and Asparagus Sauté

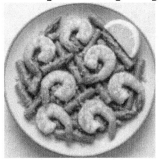

Serves 4
Ingredients:

- 2 tbsp butter
- 2 tbsp olive oil
- 1 lb shrimp, peeled and deveined
- 1 lb asparagus, trimmed and sliced
- 1 tbsp minced garlic
- Salt, pepper, smoked paprika (optional)
- Zest and juice of ½ lemon
- ¼ cup grated Parmesan
- 2 tbsp ground flaxseed

Instructions:

1. Heat butter and olive oil in a skillet over medium heat. Add shrimp and asparagus and cook 3-4 minutes.
2. Add garlic, seasonings, lemon zest, and juice. Cook until shrimp is pink and asparagus tender.
3. Combine Parmesan and flaxseed, sprinkle over the dish, stir, and serve.

Pumpkin Chicken Curry with Cauliflower Rice

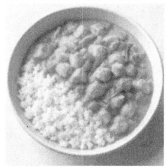

Serves 2
Ingredients:

- 2 tbsp coconut oil
- 1 (4 oz) boneless, skinless chicken breast or thigh, cubed
- ½ cup chopped red bell pepper
- ⅔ cup canned pumpkin
- Curry powder and optional spices
- 1 cup unsweetened coconut milk
- Thai basil, julienned
- 1 cup cooked cauliflower rice

Instructions:

1. Heat coconut oil in a skillet over medium heat, add chicken, and cook 3-4 minutes.
2. Stir in bell pepper, pumpkin, and spices to coat evenly.
3. Pour in coconut milk, bring to a boil, then reduce to a simmer and cook for 10 minutes.
4. Adjust seasoning, garnish with basil, and serve over cauliflower rice.

Tofu in Spicy Peanut Sauce

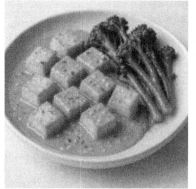

Serves 4
Ingredients:

- 1 (14 oz) block firm tofu
- ¼ cup natural peanut butter

- 2 tbsp tamari
- 2 tbsp water
- 3 tbsp turmeric
- 1 tsp toasted sesame oil
- ½ tsp red pepper flakes
- 1 tbsp grated ginger
- 2¼ cups chopped broccolini
- 1 tbsp coconut oil

Instructions:
1. Press tofu between paper towels for 30 minutes, then cube.
2. Whisk peanut butter, tamari, water, turmeric, sesame oil, pepper flakes, and ginger.
3. Steam or boil broccolini until tender.
4. Sauté tofu in coconut oil for 10-15 minutes until browned.
5. Add sauce, mix well, and serve with broccolini or cauliflower rice.

Egg and Veggie Salad

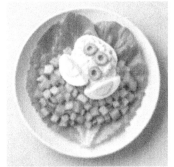

Serves 1
Ingredients:
- 2 hard-boiled eggs, quartered
- 2 tbsp olive or avocado oil mayo
- 1 tsp spicy brown mustard
- 1 tbsp apple cider vinegar
- ¼ cup sliced olives
- 1 small cucumber, chopped
- 1 tbsp diced red onion
- 1 diced celery stalk
- 1 medium diced carrot
- 2 large lettuce leaves

Instructions:
1. Mash eggs with mayo, mustard, and vinegar. Stir in olives.
2. Mix cucumber, onion, celery, and carrot in a separate bowl.

3. Layer lettuce on a plate, add veggie mix, then top with egg salad.

Grilled Chicken Salad

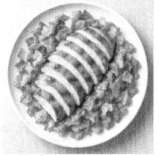

Serves 4
Ingredients:
- 4 cups water
- ¼ cup kosher salt
- 2 large chicken breasts (1 lb), quartered
- 3 tbsp olive oil
- 1½ tsp paprika
- 1 head romaine lettuce, chopped
- Juice of 1 lemon

Instructions:
1. Dissolve salt in water and brine chicken for 30 minutes.
2. Preheat grill or grill pan.
3. Pat chicken dry, toss with olive oil and paprika.
4. Grill over high heat until browned, then move to medium heat and cook to 155°F.
5. Let rest 10 minutes under foil.
6. Arrange romaine on a platter, add chicken, and drizzle with lemon juice.

Portobello Mushroom Pizzas

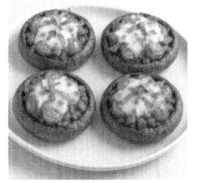

Serves 2
Ingredients:

- 2 tbsp olive oil
- ½ chopped red onion
- 4 portobello mushroom caps; stems chopped
- ½ cup halved grape tomatoes
- Salt and pepper
- ½ cup shredded mozzarella
- ¼ cup shredded Parmesan
- ¼ cup fresh basil, sliced

Instructions:
1. Sauté onion in olive oil, add mushroom stems and tomatoes, simmer 5 minutes. Season.
2. Cook mushroom caps 3-4 minutes per side.
3. Fill caps with tomato mixture, top with cheese, cover, and heat until melted.
4. Plate and garnish with basil.

Cheeseburger Lettuce Sliders

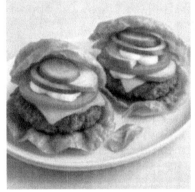

Serves 2
Ingredients:
- 6 oz 90% lean ground beef
- Salt and pepper
- 1 tbsp olive oil
- 4 large lettuce leaves
- 2 slices cheddar cheese
- 2 tbsp olive oil mayo
- 2 tomato slices
- 1 avocado, sliced
- 2 onion rings
- 2 dill pickle slices

Instructions:
1. Form beef into 4 mini patties; season.
2. Heat oil in skillet and cook patties 4-5 minutes per side.

3. Assemble sliders in lettuce leaves with cheese, mayo, tomato, avocado, onion, and pickle. Top with another lettuce leaf and serve.

BLT Salmon Burgers

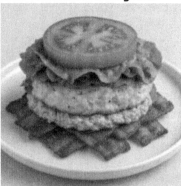

Serves 4
Ingredients:
- 16 slices turkey bacon, halved
- 8 oz poached salmon, flaked
- 2-3 tbsp mayo
- Salt and pepper
- 2 tbsp olive oil
- 2 mashed avocados
- 4 tbsp ground flaxseed
- Juice of ½ lemon
- 3 tbsp chopped chives
- 4 lettuce leaves
- 2 tomatoes, sliced

Instructions:
1. Preheat oven to 400°F. Make 4 bacon weaves using halved strips. Bake until crisp, 25 mins.
2. Mash salmon with mayo, season, and form into 4 patties.
3. Cook patties in olive oil until browned on both sides.
4. Mix avocado, flaxseed, lemon juice, and chives.
5. Layer bacon weave, avocado spread, salmon patty, lettuce, and tomato. Serve.

Baked Salmon with Grilled Summer Squash

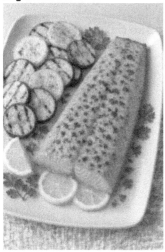

Serves 4
For the Squash:
- Oil for grilling
- 1 yellow squash, sliced
- 1 zucchini, sliced
- 1 tbsp melted unsalted butter
- Zest and juice of 1 lemon
- Salt and pepper
- 1 tsp cayenne (or to taste)

For the Salmon:
- Nonstick spray
- 1 lemon, thinly sliced
- 1 large salmon fillet (approx. 3 lbs)
- Salt and pepper
- 6 tbsp melted butter
- 1 tbsp honey
- 3 garlic cloves, minced
- 1 tsp chopped fresh thyme
- 1 tsp dried oregano
- Fresh parsley for garnish

Instructions:
1. **Grill the squash:** Preheat grill to medium and lightly oil the grates. Place sliced squash and zucchini on foil squares. Drizzle with butter, lemon zest, and juice. Season with salt, pepper, and cayenne. Wrap tightly in foil and grill for about 30 minutes until tender.
2. **Bake the salmon:** While squash is cooking, preheat oven to 350°F. Line a baking sheet with

foil and spray with cooking spray.
3. Lay lemon slices in the center, place seasoned salmon on top.
4. Mix butter, honey, garlic, thyme, and oregano. Pour over salmon and fold foil around it.
5. Bake for 15-20 minutes until salmon flakes. Broil for 2 minutes to brown the top slightly.
6. Serve with grilled squash and garnish salmon with parsley.

Grilled Shrimp with Broiled Parmesan Tomatoes

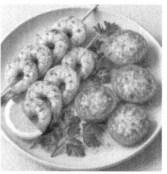

Serves 4
For the Shrimp:
- ⅓ cup olive oil
- 2 tbsp lemon juice
- 1 tsp salt
- ¼ tsp pepper
- 1 tsp Italian herbs
- 2 tsp minced garlic
- 1 lb large shrimp, peeled/deveined
- 4 soaked bamboo skewers
- Parsley and lemon wedges for serving

For the Tomatoes:
- Cooking spray
- 8 small tomatoes
- 2 tbsp olive oil
- ¼ cup grated Parmesan

Instructions:
1. **Marinate shrimp:** Combine oil, lemon juice, salt, pepper, herbs, and garlic in a bag. Add shrimp to a dish, pour marinade over, and chill for 15 minutes to 2 hours.

2. **Prep tomatoes**: Spray a baking dish. Halve tomatoes, trim bottoms to stand flat, brush with oil, and top with Parmesan.
3. Preheat grill and broiler. Skewer shrimp and grill 2-3 minutes per side until opaque.
4. Broil tomatoes for 3 minutes until cheese is golden.
5. Serve shrimp with broiled tomatoes, garnish with parsley and lemon wedges.

Lemon Chicken with Capers

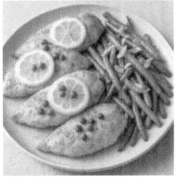

Serves 4
Ingredients:
- 4 boneless, skinless chicken breasts (about 1 lb)
- Salt and pepper
- 4 tbsp ghee or olive oil
- 2 lemons (1 juiced, 1 sliced)
- 1 garlic clove, sliced
- 2 tbsp capers, drained
- 1 sliced onion
- 4 cups trimmed green beans
- ¼ cup toasted slivered almonds

Instructions:
1. Season chicken with salt and pepper. In a skillet, heat 1 tbsp ghee and cook chicken 8-10 minutes, turning once. Remove and keep warm.
2. Add lemon juice, 1 tbsp ghee, garlic, capers, and lemon slices to the pan. Simmer, then return chicken and cook 5 more minutes.
3. In another pan, sauté onions and green beans in remaining ghee until beans are tender.

4. Toss in almonds and serve with the chicken.

Chicken Broccoli Casserole with Cheese

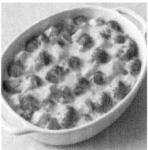

Serves 4
Ingredients:
- 3 cups cooked, chopped chicken
- 4 cups cooked broccoli florets
- 2 tbsp olive oil
- ½ cup sour cream
- ½ cup heavy cream
- 1 minced garlic clove
- 1 tsp fresh basil, minced
- Salt and pepper
- 1 cup shredded cheddar cheese

Instructions:
1. Preheat oven to 375°F.
2. In a casserole dish, mix chicken, broccoli, and olive oil.
3. In a bowl, combine sour cream, cream, garlic, basil, salt, and pepper. Pour over the casserole and stir.
4. Top with cheese and bake 7-10 minutes until bubbly and warm.

Sirloin Spinach Salad with Blue Cheese and Pecans

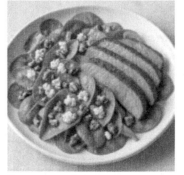

Serves 4
Ingredients:
- 2 cups baby spinach

- 3 tbsp crumbled blue cheese
- 2 tbsp chopped pecans
- 2 tbsp olive oil
- Juice of ½ lemon
- Salt and pepper
- 12 oz grilled sirloin steak, thinly sliced

Instructions:

1. Toss spinach, blue cheese, and pecans in a large bowl. Add olive oil and lemon juice, mix, and season.
2. Serve on plates topped with warm steak slices.

Spaghetti Squash with Turkey, Bacon, and Spinach Goat Cheese

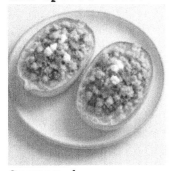

Serves 4

Ingredients:

- 2 medium spaghetti squash
- 2 tbsp olive oil
- Salt and pepper
- 6 slices bacon
- 1 lb lean ground turkey
- ¼ cup white wine
- 4 cups baby spinach
- 4 oz goat cheese

Instructions:

1. Preheat oven to 400°F. Cut squash in half, remove seeds, oil and season. Place face-down on foil-lined baking sheet and bake 40-60 mins.
2. Cook bacon until crispy; set aside. Brown turkey, then transfer to bowl.
3. In the same pan, deglaze with wine, cook for 1 minute, then add spinach. Once wilted, stir in goat cheese until creamy.
4. Crumble bacon into turkey, mix with spinach-goat cheese mixture.

5. Scrape squash into strands and place in bowls. Top with turkey-spinach mixture and serve.

Meatloaf with Cauliflower Mash

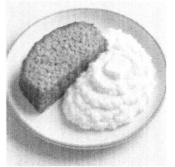

Servings: 6

- 2 tbsp olive oil
- ¼ cup diced onion
- 1½ lbs lean, grass-fed ground beef
- 1 cup almond flour
- 2 large eggs
- ⅓ cup tomato sauce (unsweetened)
- ½ cup grated Parmesan (approx. 2 oz)
- ½ tsp salt
- ½ tsp black pepper
- ½ tsp garlic powder
- 3 cups prepared mashed cauliflower (frozen or homemade), heated
- 6 tbsp butter (optional)

Instructions:

1. Preheat oven to 350°F.
2. In a small skillet, heat olive oil and sauté onion for about 3 minutes, or until translucent.
3. Mix ground beef, sautéed onion, almond flour, eggs, tomato sauce, Parmesan, and seasonings in a large bowl. Shape the mixture into a loaf.
4. Transfer loaf to a baking dish and bake for 1 hour.
5. Remove from oven, drain excess fat, and let the loaf rest for 10 minutes before slicing.
6. Serve slices with warmed mashed cauliflower. Add butter on top of the cauliflower if preferred.

Grilled Steak with Creamed Spinach and Mushrooms

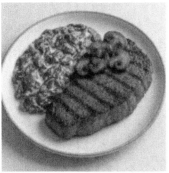

Servings: 4

- Four 3-ounce boneless sirloin steaks (or divide a 12-ounce steak)
- Salt and pepper
- 2 tbsp olive oil
- 2 cups chopped mushrooms (button or portobello)
- 4 cup baby spinach
- ½ cup heavy cream
- Dash of ground nutmeg

Instructions:

1. Heat a grill pan on medium-high. Season steaks with salt and pepper, then grill for 2-4 minutes per side for medium-rare. Remove to a platter and keep warm.
2. In a skillet, heat olive oil over medium-high. Sauté mushrooms for 3-4 minutes, until browned, then transfer to the platter with the steaks.
3. Lower heat to medium, add spinach and cream to the skillet, and stir until spinach wilts and the cream thickens. Add salt and nutmeg to taste.
4. Serve the steaks with mushrooms on top and spinach on the side.

Cauliflower Rice

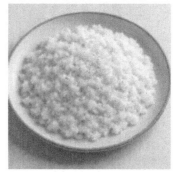

Ingredients:

- 1 medium cauliflower, cut into florets
- 3 tbsp olive oil
- 2 cloves garlic, minced
- 1½ tsp salt
- 1 tsp pepper
- ½ cup vegetable broth
- 4 tbsp ghee or unsalted butter
- ¼ cup heavy cream

Instructions:

1. For the stroganoff, add mushrooms, garlic, onion, broth, and paprika to a slow cooker. Cook on high for 4 hours.
2. Stir in yogurt, season with salt and pepper, and keep warm.
3. For the rice, pulse cauliflower in a food processor until it resembles rice.
4. Heat olive oil in a saucepan over medium, then add cauliflower rice, garlic, salt, and pepper. Cook for 3 minutes.
5. Add broth, cover, lower heat, and simmer for 12 minutes, stirring occasionally.
6. Mix in ghee and cream and simmer for 5 more minutes until creamy.
7. Serve stroganoff over the cauliflower rice.

Blackened Tofu with Sesame Broccoli Slaw

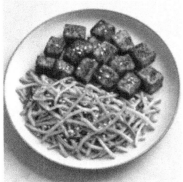

Servings: 4

- 12 oz extra-firm tofu, cubed
- Seasonings of choice
- 4 tbsp coconut oil
- 4 cups broccoli slaw
- 4 tbsp sesame seeds

Instructions:

1. Toss tofu with your selected herbs and spices in a bowl.
2. Heat 2 tbsp coconut oil in a large skillet over high heat. Sear tofu for 3-4 minutes on each side until blackened. Transfer to a bowl and keep warm.
3. Wipe out the skillet, then add the rest of the coconut oil over medium-high heat. Stir-fry broccoli slaw for about 2 minutes or until desired doneness.
4. Plate the slaw, top with tofu, sprinkle with sesame seeds, and serve.

BBQ Tempeh, Greens, and Cauliflower Rice

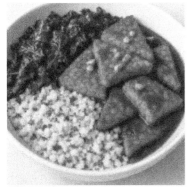

Servings: 4

- ½ cup Primal Kitchen BBQ sauc
- ½ cup fresh orange juice
- 2½ tbsp tamari
- 2 tbsp apple cider vinegar
- Two 8-oz packages of tempeh
- 1 small cauliflower head (approx. 1 lb)
- 2 tbsp ghee or unsalted butter
- ½ medium yellow onion, finely chopped
- 1-2 tsp garlic powder
- ¼ tsp freshly grated nutmeg
- Salt and black pepper to taste
- 2 tbsp olive oil
- 3 garlic cloves, minced
- 6 cups chopped kale
- 1 tbsp lemon juice
- 2 tbsp coconut oil
- ½ cup chopped flat-leaf parsley
- ½ cup (2 oz) grated Parmesan
- Chopped roasted salted peanuts (optional)

Instructions:

1. In a small bowl, whisk together the BBQ sauce, orange juice, tamari, and vinegar. Pour into a shallow pan. Slice the tempeh into thin triangles—16 total, each ¼ inch thick—and arrange in the marinade. Spoon sauce over the top and marinate for at least 1 hour (or overnight), flipping occasionally.
2. Cut the cauliflower into florets and pulse in a food processor until it resembles rice.
3. In a large skillet, melt the ghee over medium heat. Add the onion and cook until soft, about 4 minutes. Add the cauliflower, garlic powder, and nutmeg. Season with salt and pepper and cook for 5-7 minutes. Cover to keep warm.
4. Heat olive oil in another skillet over medium heat. Add garlic and cook for 1 minute until fragrant. Add kale and cook 2-3 minutes until wilted. Mix in lemon juice and a pinch of salt and pepper.
5. Preheat a grill, grill pan, or cast-iron skillet over medium-high. Lightly oil the surface with coconut oil. Remove tempeh

from marinade (reserve remaining marinade). Grill for 5 minutes on each side, brushing with the sauce as it cooks.

6. Stir parsley and Parmesan into the cauliflower rice, adjusting seasoning if needed.

7. To serve, layer cauliflower rice in bowls, top with grilled tempeh, drizzle with extra marinade, sprinkle with peanuts (optional), and serve the kale on the side.

Veggie Cheese Enchiladas with Grain-Free Tortillas

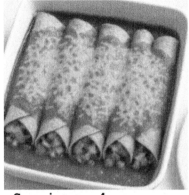

Servings: 4

Tortilla Dough:
- 1 cup almond flour
- ¼ cup coconut flour
- 2 tsp xanthan gum
- 1 tsp baking powder
- ½ tsp kosher salt
- 2 tsp lime juice
- 1 large egg, lightly beaten
- 1 tbsp water

Enchilada Sauce:
- 1½ cups no-sugar-added tomato sauce
- 1 cup vegetable broth
- 1 tsp apple cider vinegar
- 1½ tsp chili powder
- 1½ tsp smoked paprika
- 1½ tsp ground cumin
- ½ tsp onion powder
- ½ tsp garlic powder
- 1 tsp salt

Filling:
- 2 tbsp avocado oil
- ⅓ small onion, diced

- 1 small bell pepper, diced
- ½ small zucchini, diced
- 3 large eggs, lightly beaten
- 2 cups spinach
- 1 tbsp chili powder
- 1½ tsp garlic salt
- 1 tsp onion powder
- ½ tsp ground cumin
- 1½ cups (6 oz) shredded cheddar cheese

Instructions:

1. **Tortillas:** In a food processor, mix almond flour, coconut flour, xanthan gum, baking powder, and salt. With the machine running, add lime juice, then the egg, and water last. Once a dough forms, transfer to plastic wrap, knead briefly, wrap, and chill for 10 minutes.

2. **Sauce:** Combine all sauce ingredients in a saucepan. Simmer over low heat until reduced and thickened, about 15-30 minutes.

3. **Form tortillas:** Divide dough into 8 balls. Roll each between parchment to 5-6 inches wide and ⅛ inch thick. Cook on a hot skillet for about 20 seconds per side. Stack cooked tortillas with parchment in between.

4. **Filling:** Sauté onion and bell pepper in avocado oil for about 3 minutes. Add zucchini, then eggs. Stir in spinach and seasonings. Simmer until well combined and cooked through.

5. **Assembly:** Fill each tortilla with ½ cup filling and 1½ tbsp cheese. Roll and place seam-side down in a 9x13-inch baking dish.

6. Preheat oven to 350°F. Pour sauce over enchiladas and top with remaining cheese. Bake for 30 minutes or until hot and bubbling with golden cheese. Serve warm.

Spicy Edamame Bowl with Creamy Chili Sauce

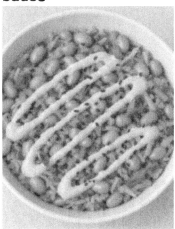

Servings: 4
Edamame Mixture:

- 2½ tbsp toasted sesame oil
- 6 scallions, sliced (white and green parts separated)
- ⅓ cup diced red onion
- 5 garlic cloves minced
- 2 cups frozen edamame
- 1 tsp grated fresh ginger
- 1 tbsp Sriracha or similar hot sauce
- 1 (14-oz) bag coleslaw mix
- 3 tbsp tamari or soy sauce
- 1 tbsp rice vinegar
- ⅛ to ¼ tsp ground white pepper
- Salt to taste
- Black sesame seeds, for garnish

Chili Sauce:

- ¼ cup olive oil mayo
- 1 tbsp Sriracha or hot sauce
- Salt to taste

Instructions:

1. Heat sesame oil in a skillet over medium. Add the white scallions, red onion, and garlic. Sauté for 3 minutes until soft.
2. Mix in edamame, ginger, and hot sauce. Cook for 3 minutes until warmed.
3. Add coleslaw mix, tamari, vinegar, white pepper, and salt. Stir and cook for 5 minutes until cabbage softens.
4. Mix chili sauce by whisking together mayo, hot sauce, and salt in a small bowl.
5. Spoon edamame mixture into bowls, drizzle with chili sauce, garnish with green scallions and sesame seeds.

Celery Sticks with Almond Butter

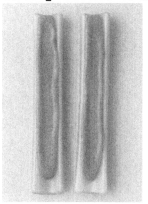

Servings: 1

- 2 tbsp unsweetened almond butter
- 2 celery stalks, trimmed

Spread 1 tbsp almond butter on each celery stalk and enjoy.

Carrots and Celery with Flaxseed and Almond Butter

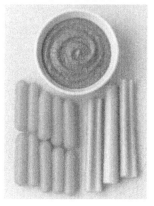

Servings: 1

- 2 tbsp ground flaxseed
- 2 tbsp unsweetened almond butter
- 10 baby carrots
- 2 celery stalks, halved

Mix flaxseed and almond butter in a bowl until smooth. Use as a dip for carrots and celery.

Caprese Bites

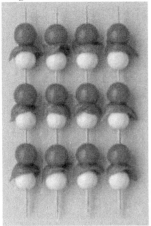

Yields: 24 skewers

- 24 cherry tomatoes
- 24 fresh basil leaves
- 1 (8 oz) package of whole-milk mozzarella balls
- 24 small skewers
- Olive oil

Thread each skewer with one tomato, a folded basil leaf, and one mozzarella ball. Arrange on a platter and drizzle lightly with olive oil. Plan for about 3 skewers per person.

Apple Clusters

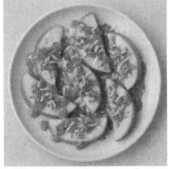

Yields: 1 serving

- 1 small apple, cored and sliced
- 2 tbsp unsweetened almond butter
- 1 tbsp chia seeds
- 1 tbsp ground flaxseed
- 2 tbsp unsweetened coconut flakes

Place the apple slices on a plate. In a small microwave-safe bowl, mix the almond butter, chia seeds, and flaxseed. Microwave for 15 to 30 seconds until slightly melted. Drizzle the mixture over the apples and sprinkle with coconut flakes.

Aloha Avocado

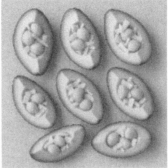

Yields: 4 servings

- 2 ripe avocados
- 1 cup macadamia nuts, halved
- ½ cup unsweetened coconut flakes

Slice the avocados in half, remove pits, then quarter each half. Fill the center of each piece with macadamia nuts and coconut flakes.

Pumpkin-Spiced Walnuts

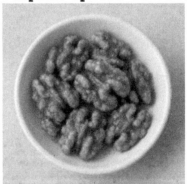

Yields: 1 serving

- ¼ cup whole walnuts
- 1 tsp avocado oil
- ½ tsp pumpkin pie spice

Place walnuts in a small dish. Drizzle with avocado oil and sprinkle with the pumpkin spice. Toss until evenly coated and serve.

Avocado Crisps

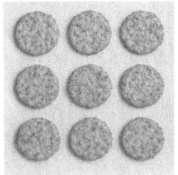

Yields: 1 serving

- 1 avocado, peeled, pitted, and chopped
- ¼ cup grated Parmesan
- 1 tsp lemon juice
- ½ tsp garlic powder
- ½ tsp Italian seasoning

Preheat oven to 325°F and line a baking sheet with parchment. In a medium bowl, mash the avocado. Stir in Parmesan, lemon juice, garlic powder, and Italian seasoning. Drop teaspoon-sized portions onto the sheet, flatten slightly, and bake for 15-18 minutes, until the edges are golden brown.

Cheese and Walnuts

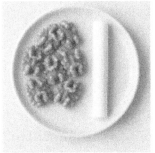

Yields: 1 serving

- ¼ cup walnut halves
- 1 cheese stick

Place the walnuts on a plate and add the cheese stick. Enjoy as a simple snack.

Cheesy Nuts

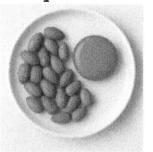

Yields: 1 serving

- 1 Babybel mini cheese wheel, unwrapped
- ½ cup almonds

Serve the cheese alongside almonds for a quick and easy snack plate.

Everything-Bagel Cucumber Bites

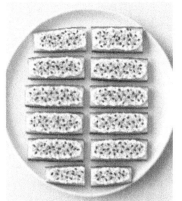

Yields: 4 servings

- 1 medium cucumber
- 1 (4 oz) package cream cheese
- 2 tbsp salted butter
- 2 tbsp plain full-fat Greek yogurt
- 4 tsp everything bagel seasoning

Slice the cucumber lengthwise. In a small bowl, blend cream cheese, butter, and yogurt until smooth. Spread the mixture over the cut sides of the cucumber, sprinkle with seasoning, and slice each half again for 4 total servings.

Crunchy Kale Chips with Pecans

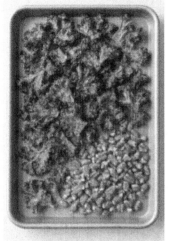

Yields: 3 servings
- Nonstick cooking spray
- 1 large bunch fresh kale, stems removed and leaves trimmed
- 2 tbsp olive oil
- 1 tbsp sea salt
- ¾ cup chopped pecans

Instructions:
1. Preheat oven to 350°F. Lightly coat a baking sheet with spray or line with a silicone mat.
2. Add kale to a large zip-top bag, drizzle with olive oil, seal, and massage until the leaves are evenly coated.
3. Spread kale in a single layer on the baking sheet. Bake for 12 minutes, or until crispy. Remove from oven and sprinkle with sea salt. Serve with chopped pecans.

Creamy Avocado Dip

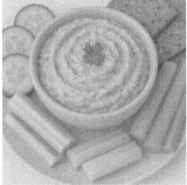

Yields: ½ cup (1 serving)
- 1 ripe avocado, peeled and pitted
- 1 tbsp avocado oil or olive oil mayo
- Juice of 1 lemon (approx. 3 tbsp)
- 1 tbsp chopped fresh cilantro

Mash the avocado in a bowl with the oil or mayo, lemon juice, and cilantro until creamy. Serve with veggies or crackers of your choice.

Easy Guacamole

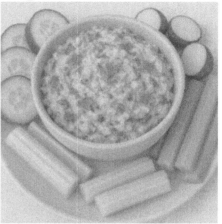

Yields: About 2 cups (8 servings)
- ¼ cup finely chopped onion
- 3 ripe avocados
- 2 tbsp lime or lemon juice
- 1 Roma tomato, seeded and diced
- ¼ cup chopped fresh cilantro
- ½ tsp ground cumin
- ½ tsp salt

Instructions:
1. Soak onion in warm water for 10 minutes to mellow the flavor.
2. Cut avocados in half, remove pits, and scoop the flesh into a bowl.
3. Add lime juice and mash until mostly smooth with some chunks.
4. Stir in tomato, cilantro, cumin, and drained onion. Season with salt.
5. Taste and adjust seasoning. Serve with fresh veggies for dipping.

Herbed White Bean Dip

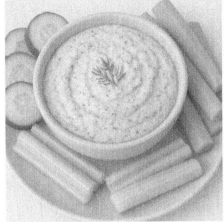

Yields: About ¾ cup (2 servings)

- ½ cup cooked cannellini beans
- Juice of ½ lemon (approx. 1½ tbsp)
- 1 tsp lemon zest
- 2 tbsp tahini or soy sauce
- 1 tbsp olive oil
- 1 tbsp chopped dill
- 1 garlic clove

Blend all ingredients in a food processor until smooth. Serve with sliced vegetables for dipping.

Herbed Cottage Cheese Dip with Cucumber

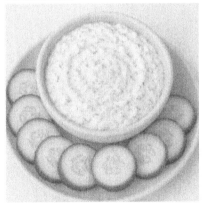

Yields: 2 servings

- ½ cup full-fat cottage cheese
- 1 tbsp lemon juice
- ½ tsp garlic powder
- ½ tsp onion powder
- ¼ tsp black pepper
- 1 tbsp chopped dill
- 1 small cucumber, sliced

Blend cottage cheese, lemon juice, seasonings, and dill until smooth. Transfer to a bowl and enjoy with cucumber slices.

Veggie Slices with Italian Mayo Dip

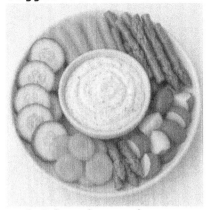

Yields: 4 servings

- 1 cup olive oil mayonnaise
- 1 tbsp Italian seasoning
- 2 large cucumbers, sliced
- 2 large carrots, sliced
- 8 asparagus spears, cut into bite-size pieces
- 8 radishes, halved or quartered

In a small bowl, mix mayonnaise with seasoning. Arrange the vegetables on a platter and serve with the dip.

Marinated Olives, Chickpeas, and Veggies with Thyme and Dill

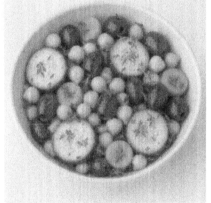

Yields: 4 servings

- 2 large cucumbers, sliced
- 2 medium carrots, sliced
- 1 (15 oz) can chickpeas, drained and rinsed
- 2 cups olives (any kind)
- ½ cup red wine vinegar
- ¼ cup fresh thyme leaves
- ¼ cup fresh dill

In a large bowl, mix together cucumbers, carrots, chickpeas, and olives. Add vinegar and herbs, stir well, and refrigerate for 15 minutes before serving.

Cucumber, Tomato, and Feta Salad

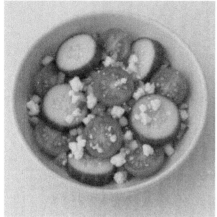

Yields: 1 serving

- 1 medium cucumber, sliced
- 1 cup halved cherry tomatoes
- ¼ small red onion, diced
- 1 garlic clove, minced
- 1 tbsp olive oil
- 1 tbsp red wine vinegar
- 2 tbsp crumbled feta

In a small bowl, combine cucumber, tomatoes, onion, and garlic. Drizzle with oil and vinegar, toss to coat, and top with crumbled feta.

Turkey and Mayo Lettuce Wraps

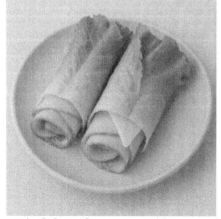

Yields: 2 wraps (1 serving)

- 1 tbsp olive oil mayo
- 1 tbsp red wine vinegar
- 1 tbsp ground flaxseed
- 2 large lettuce leaves
- 2 oz deli-sliced turkey
- 1 slice Swiss cheese

Mix mayo, vinegar, and flaxseed in a small bowl. Lay lettuce flat, spread with mayo mixture, add turkey and cheese, then roll up and serve.

Hard-Boiled Egg with Avocado

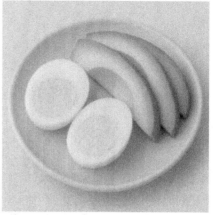

Serves: 1

- 1 large hard-boiled egg, peeled and halved
- ½ avocado, sliced

Arrange the egg halves and avocado slices on a plate and serve.

Deviled Eggs

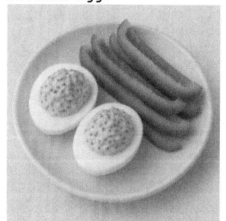

Serves: 1

- 2 large hard-boiled eggs
- 1 tbsp avocado oil mayo
- 1 tbsp chia seeds
- ¼ tsp ground turmeric
- 1 green bell pepper, sliced

Peel and halve the eggs. Remove yolks and mash them with mayo, chia seeds, and turmeric. Fill the egg whites with the mixture and serve alongside bell pepper slices.

Naked Turkey Roll-Ups

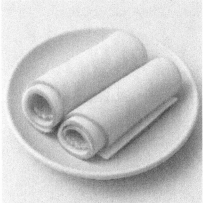

Serves: 1

- 2 oz deli turkey
- 2 oz Swiss cheese
- 1 tbsp spicy brown mustard

Layer turkey and cheese slices. Spread with mustard, roll tightly, and serve.

Edamame Mash Salad

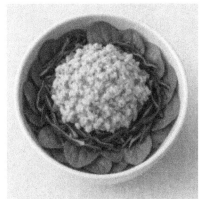

Serves: 4

- 1½ cups frozen edamame
- 2 cups boiling water
- 2 garlic cloves
- 1 tbsp lime juice
- 2½ tbsp avocado oil mayo
- 2 tbsp chopped cilantro
- 1 tbsp chopped mint
- 1 tbsp chopped dill
- ¼ tsp stone-ground mustard
- ¼ tsp salt
- ¼ tsp black pepper
- 4 cups spinach
- 1 cup shredded red cabbage

Pour boiling water over edamame in a bowl, cover, and let steam for 5 minutes. Drain and cool. Pulse edamame, garlic, lime juice, mayo, herbs, mustard, salt, and pepper in a food processor until blended but still chunky. Chill. To serve, top beds of spinach and cabbage with the mash.

Pecans with Berries and Coconut

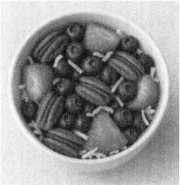

Serves: 1

- ¼ cup pecans
- ¼ cup blueberries
- ¼ cup strawberries
- 2 tbsp unsweetened coconut flakes

Combine all ingredients in a small bowl and enjoy.

Pecans and Dark Chocolate

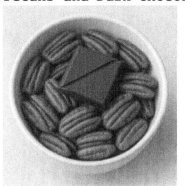

Serves: 1

- 1 oz piece of 70% or darker chocolate
- ¼ cup pecans

Eat the chocolate and pecans together or dip the nuts in melted chocolate.

Raspberries with Pecans

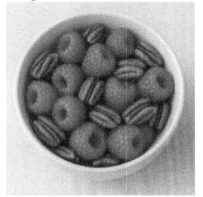

Serves: 1

- ½ cup fresh raspberries
- ¼ cup pecans

Mix raspberries and pecans in a bowl and enjoy.

Nutty Berry Bowl

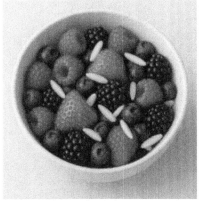

Serves: 1

- ¼ cup strawberries, halved
- ¼ cup raspberries
- ¼ cup blackberries
- ¼ cup blueberries
- 2 tbsp slivered almonds

Combine berries and almonds in a serving bowl.

Tropical Berries

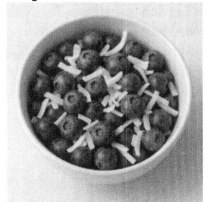

Serves: 1

- ½ cup blueberries
- 2 tbsp unsweetened coconut flakes

Toss blueberries with coconut in a bowl and serve.

Strawberries with Chia Cream

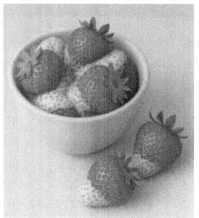

Serves: 1

- 1 cup halved strawberries
- 2 tbsp heavy cream
- 1 tbsp chia seeds
- 1 tbsp coconut flakes

Drizzle cream over strawberries, then sprinkle with chia seeds and coconut.

Pear Slices and Ricotta Cheese

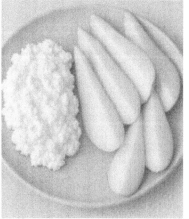

Serves: 1

- ½ ripe pear, sliced
- ¾ cup whole-milk ricotta (or dairy-free alternative)
- Dash of cinnamon (optional)

Arrange pear slices on a plate. Add a scoop of ricotta and sprinkle with cinnamon, if desired.

Chocolate Mocha Almonds with String Cheese

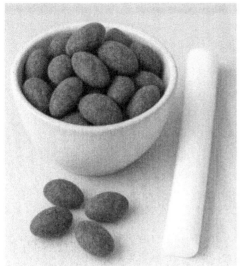

Serves: 6

- 1 cup raw almonds
- ½ tsp olive oil
- 1 tbsp unsweetened cocoa
- 1 tsp instant coffee granules
- 1 tsp Swerve powdered sweetener
- 6 string cheese sticks

Toast almonds in a skillet over low heat for 3 minutes. Add oil and toss to coat. In a processor, blend cocoa, coffee, and sweetener until smooth. Toss almonds in the mixture, shake off excess, and let cool on parchment. Serve with string cheese.

Blueberry Pie Smoothie

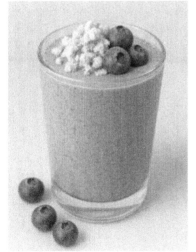

Serves: 1

- 2 scoops collagen powder
- 1 scoop MCT powder or 1 tbsp coconut oil
- 1 cup chopped spinach
- ½ cup blueberries
- 2 tbsp chia seeds
- 2 tbsp flax seeds
- 2 tbsp almond butter
- ½ tsp almond extract
- Dash of nutmeg (optional)

Blend all ingredients until smooth. Add almond extract and nutmeg at the end and pulse briefly.

Mixed Berry Smoothie

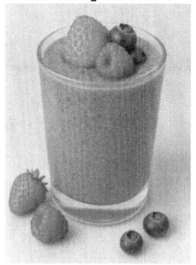

Serves: 1

- ¼ cup strawberries, halved
- ¼ cup blackberries
- ¼ cup raspberries
- ¼ cup full-fat plain Greek yogurt
- 1 cup spinach
- 1 tbsp chia seeds
- 1 tbsp flaxseed
- Ice cubes

Blend all ingredients with ice. Add water if needed to adjust thickness.

Raspberry Almond Smoothie

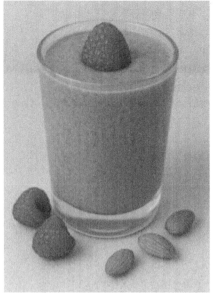

Serves: 1

- ½ cup full-fat Greek yogurt
- ½ cup chopped kale
- ¼ cup raspberries
- 1 tbsp almond butter
- 1 tbsp chia seeds

Blend until fully smooth and creamy.

Peanut Butter Cup Smoothie

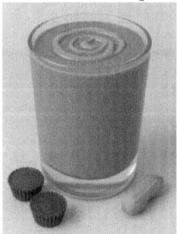

Serves: 1

- ¼ cup full-fat Greek yogurt
- 2 tbsp unsweetened cocoa powder
- 2 tbsp natural peanut butter
- 1 tbsp flaxseed
- ½ tsp vanilla extract
- Ice cubes (optional)

Combine all ingredients in a blender and process until smooth.

Peanut Butter-Mocha Smoothie

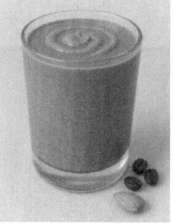

Serves: 1

- ½ cup unsweetened almond milk
- 2 tbsp chia seeds
- 2 tbsp flaxseed
- 1 tsp cocoa powder
- 2 tbsp natural peanut butter
- ¼ tsp vanilla extract
- ½ frozen banana
- 2 tbsp fresh espresso
- ⅓ cup crushed ice
- Pinch of salt

Blend all ingredients until smooth. Taste and adjust salt if needed.

Green Almond Butter Smoothie

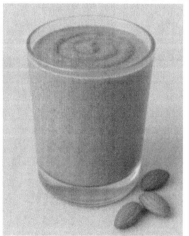

Serves: 1

- 1 scoop plant-based protein powder
- 1 cup almond milk
- ½ cup fresh blueberries
- 2 tbsp almond butter
- 2 tbsp ground flaxseed

Add all ingredients to a blender and blend until smooth.

Vegan Cinnamon Roll Smoothie

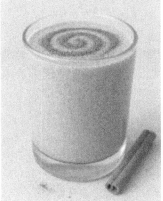

Serves: 1

- 2 scoops Carrington Farms Coconut Protein Blend (substituting may change macros)
- 1 tsp cinnamon
- ½ tsp vanilla extract
- 2 tbsp ground flaxseed
- ¾ cup Kite Hill unsweetened almond milk yogurt
- 1 cup unsweetened almond milk
- 1 cup ice

Combine all ingredients in a blender and process until smooth and creamy.

Chia Pudding

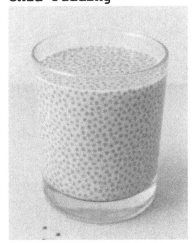

Serves: 1

- 1 tbsp flax seeds
- 2 tbsp chopped pecans
- Ground cinnamon, to taste
- ½ cup unsweetened coconut milk
- ¼ cup chia seeds

In a bowl, mix flax, pecans, and cinnamon. Slowly stir in the coconut milk until incorporated. Sprinkle in chia seeds and stir gently. Cover and refrigerate for 4-5 hours or overnight until set.

Coconut-Chia Pudding with Raspberries

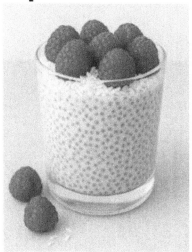

Serves: 2

- 1 (15 oz) can unsweetened coconut milk
- ½ tsp vanilla extract
- Pinch of stevia or monk fruit sweetener
- ¼ tsp pumpkin pie spice
- ½ cup chia seeds
- ½ cup fresh raspberries

In a bowl, whisk together the coconut milk, vanilla, sweetener, and spice until smooth. Stir in chia seeds and mix well. Cover and chill for 4+ hours. Serve topped with raspberries.

Coconut and Walnut Chia Pudding

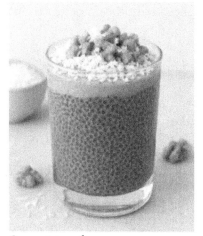

Serves: 4

- 4 cups unsweetened almond milk
- 4 tbsp chia seeds
- ½ tsp stevia

- ½ tsp cinnamon
- ½ cup chopped walnuts
- ½ cup chopped pecans
- ¼ cup sunflower seeds
- ¼ cup unsweetened coconut flakes

Mix almond milk, chia seeds, stevia, and cinnamon in a bowl. Cover and refrigerate for at least 2 hours or overnight. When ready to serve, top portions with nuts, seeds, and coconut.

Peanut Butter and Chocolate Chia Pudding

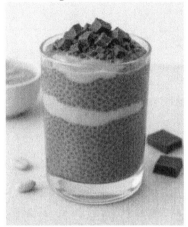

Serves: 2
Pudding Base:

- ¼ cup cacao or unsweetened cocoa powder
- 1 tbsp Swerve sweetener
- ½ tsp cinnamon (optional)
- Pinch of salt
- ½ tsp vanilla extract
- 1½ cups unsweetened almond milk
- ½ cup chia seeds

Toppings:

- 2 tbsp no-sugar-added peanut butter
- ¼ cup fresh raspberries

Whisk dry ingredients in a bowl. Gradually add almond milk, whisking to form a paste, then mix until smooth. Stir in chia seeds. Cover and refrigerate 3-5 hours or overnight, stirring once midway. Before serving, warm the peanut butter and drizzle over the pudding. Garnish with raspberries.

Chocolate Peanut Butter Yogurt

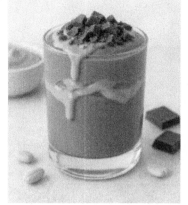

Serves: 1

- ½ cup full-fat plain Greek yogurt
- 1 tbsp no-sugar-added peanut butter
- 1 tbsp cocoa powder
- 2 tbsp chia seeds

Stir all ingredients together in a bowl until fully combined.

Vegan Yogurt Parfait

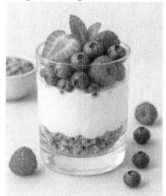

Serves: 1

- ½ cup plain unsweetened almond milk yogurt
- 1 scoop vanilla KOS Organic Plant Protein (macros may vary with other brands)
- 1 tbsp ground flaxseed
- ⅓ cup fresh blueberries
- ¼ cup chopped pecans

Mix yogurt, protein, and flax in a bowl. Top with blueberries and pecans.

Raspberry-Flax Muffin

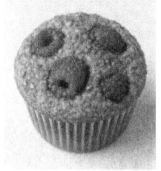

Serves: 1

- 1 large egg
- 1 tbsp melted coconut oil
- 1 tsp vanilla extract
- 4 tbsp ground flaxseed
- ½ tsp baking powder
- ¼ tsp cinnamon
- 3 tsp monk fruit sweetener
- 2 tbsp fresh raspberries
- 1 tbsp sugar-free dark chocolate chips
- 1 tbsp whipped cream

In a small microwave-safe bowl, mix egg, oil, and vanilla. Stir in flax, baking powder, cinnamon, and sweetener. Fold in raspberries and chocolate chips. Microwave for 90 seconds. Let cool slightly and top with whipped cream.

Chocolate-Cinnamon Apple Bites

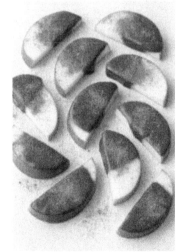

Makes ~6 mini muffins

- Nonstick baking spray
- ½ cup almond butter
- ¼ cup cocoa powder
- ¼ cup melted coconut oil
- 2 tbsp unsweetened apple butter

- Dash of salt
- ½ tsp almond extract
- Pinch of cinnamon

Preheat oven to 325°F and coat mini muffin tin with spray. Mix all ingredients in a bowl until smooth. Divide into muffin cups and fill unused wells with water. Bake for 10 minutes or until a toothpick comes out clean. Cool and serve 1 per person.

Chocolate Peanut Butter Mug Cake

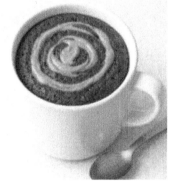

Serves: 1

- 1 tbsp butter
- 1 large egg
- 1 tbsp coconut flour
- 1 tbsp stevia or monk fruit sweetener
- 1 tbsp no-sugar-added peanut butter
- 1 tbsp cocoa powder
- ½ tsp baking powder
- 2 tbsp sugar-free dark chocolate chips

Melt butter in a large mug (15-30 sec). Stir in egg, flour, sweetener, peanut butter, cocoa, and baking powder. Mix in chocolate chips. Microwave for 1 minute. Let cool before serving.

Vegan Snack Bars

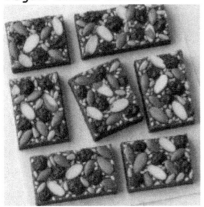

Yields: 16 bars

- Cooking spray
- ½ cup almonds
- ½ cup walnut halves
- ½ cup macadamia nuts
- ½ cup pumpkin seeds
- 1 cup unsweetened shredded coconut
- 1 tsp cinnamon
- ½ cup no-sugar-added peanut butter
- ¼ cup coconut oil
- 2 tsp vanilla bean paste

Line a 6x10-inch pan with parchment after spraying. Chop nuts and seeds in a food processor, then combine with coconut and cinnamon in a large bowl. In a saucepan, melt peanut butter, coconut oil, and vanilla over low heat. Stir into dry ingredients and press firmly into pan. Chill 2-3 hours. Slice into 16 bars.

Chocolate Banana "Nice" Cream

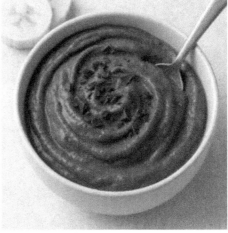

Serves: 2

- 2 ripe bananas
- 2 tbsp almond butter
- ¼ cup almond milk
- 1 tbsp cocoa powder
- 3 tbsp cacao nibs
- 1 tbsp chia seeds
- 2 tbsp ground flaxseed

Blend all ingredients until smooth. Pour into a freezer-safe container and freeze for several hours or overnight before serving.

Meze, Antipasti, Tapas, and Other Small Plates

Classic Hummus

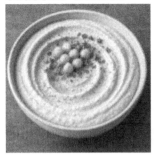

Makes about 2 cups | Vegetarian
Ingredients:
- ¼ cup water
- 3 tablespoons lemon juice
- 6 tablespoons tahini
- 2 tablespoons extra-virgin olive oil (plus more for drizzling)
- 1 (15-ounce) can chickpeas, rinsed
- 1 small garlic clove, minced
- ½ teaspoon salt
- ¼ teaspoon ground cumin
- Pinch of cayenne pepper

Directions:
1. In a small bowl, mix the water and lemon juice. In another bowl, whisk together the tahini and olive oil until smooth.
2. Add the chickpeas, garlic, salt, cumin, and cayenne to a food processor. Blend for about 15 seconds until it's mostly ground up. Scrape down the sides of the bowl.
3. With the machine running, slowly pour in the lemon-water mixture. Scrape down the sides again and process for another minute.
4. While it's still running, drizzle in the tahini-oil mixture. Blend for about 15 seconds more, or until the hummus is smooth and creamy. Scrape the sides as needed.

Serve it up with a drizzle of olive oil and whatever garnishes you like.

Quick Toasted Almonds

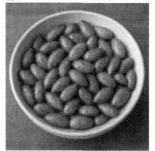

Makes 2 cups | Fast | Vegetarian
Ingredients:
- 1 tablespoon extra-virgin olive oil
- 2 cups raw whole almonds (with skin)
- 1 teaspoon salt
- ¼ teaspoon black pepper

Directions:
Heat the olive oil in a 12-inch nonstick skillet over medium-high heat until it starts to shimmer. Add the almonds, salt, and pepper, then lower the heat to medium-low. Cook, stirring often, for about 8 minutes—until the almonds smell toasty and turn a bit darker.
Transfer them to a paper towel-lined plate and let them cool completely before serving.
(You can store them in an airtight container at room temp for up to 5 days.)

Garlic and Rosemary White Bean Dip

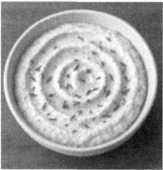

Makes about 1¼ cups | Fast | Vegetarian
Ingredients:
- 1 (15-ounce) can cannellini beans, rinsed
- ¼ cup extra-virgin olive oil, divided
- 2 tablespoons water

- 2 teaspoons lemon juice
- 1 teaspoon minced fresh rosemary
- 1 small garlic clove, minced
- Salt and pepper
- Pinch of cayenne pepper

Directions:
1. Add the beans, 3 tablespoons of the oil, water, lemon juice, rosemary, garlic, ¼ teaspoon salt, ¼ teaspoon pepper, and cayenne to a food processor. Blend until smooth, about 45 seconds, scraping down the sides as needed.
2. Scoop the dip into a bowl, cover, and let it sit at room temperature for about 30 minutes to let the flavors come together. (You can make it ahead and chill it for up to a day. If it's too thick after chilling, stir in a tablespoon of warm water.)
3. Taste and adjust the seasoning, then drizzle the last tablespoon of olive oil over the top before serving.

Tzatziki

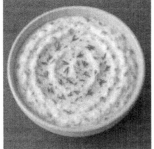

Makes about 2 cups | Vegetarian
Ingredients:
- 1 (12-ounce) cucumber, peeled, halved lengthwise, seeded, and shredded
- Salt and pepper
- 1 cup whole-milk Greek yogurt
- 2 tablespoons extra-virgin olive oil
- 2 tablespoons chopped fresh mint and/or dill
- 1 small garlic clove, minced

Directions:

1. Toss the shredded cucumber with ½ teaspoon salt in a colander and let it drain for 15 minutes.
2. In a bowl, whisk together the yogurt, olive oil, herbs, and garlic. Stir in the drained cucumber. Cover and refrigerate for at least 1 hour to chill (or up to 2 days).
3. Taste and season with salt and pepper before serving.

Caponata

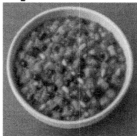

Makes about 3 cups | Vegetarian
Ingredients:
- 1 large eggplant (about 1½ pounds), cut into ½-inch cubes
- ½ teaspoon salt
- ¾ cup V8 juice (or tomato juice)
- ¼ cup red wine vinegar, plus more to taste
- 2 tablespoons brown sugar
- ¼ cup chopped fresh parsley
- 1½ teaspoons minced anchovy fillets (about 2-3 fillets)
- 1 large tomato, cored, seeded, and chopped
- ¼ cup raisins
- 2 tablespoons minced black olives
- 2 tablespoons extra-virgin olive oil, divided
- 1 celery rib, finely chopped
- 1 red bell pepper, seeded and finely chopped
- 1 small onion, finely chopped (about ½ cup)
- ¼ cup pine nuts, toasted

Directions:
1. Toss the eggplant with salt in a bowl. Line a large microwave-safe plate with a double layer of coffee filters (or undyed paper towels) and spray lightly with oil. Spread the eggplant

out evenly and microwave until it shrinks to about a third of its size—about 8 to 15 minutes. It should be dry but not browned. Transfer to a paper towel-lined plate right away.
2. While that's going, mix the V8 juice, vinegar, brown sugar, parsley, and anchovies in a medium bowl. Stir in the tomato, raisins, and olives.
3. Heat 1 tablespoon of oil in a large nonstick skillet over medium-high heat until hot. Add the eggplant and cook, stirring now and then, until the edges brown—about 4 to 8 minutes. If the pan gets dry, add a teaspoon more oil. Move the eggplant to a bowl when done.
4. Add the remaining 2 teaspoons oil to the same skillet. Toss in the celery, red pepper, and onion. Cook until they soften and start to brown at the edges, about 6 to 8 minutes.
5. serving

Creamy Turkish Nut Dip (Tarator)

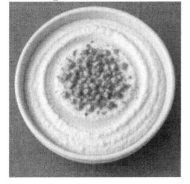

Makes about 1 cup | Fast | Vegetarian
Ingredients:
- 1 slice hearty white sandwich bread, crusts removed, torn into 1-inch pieces
- ¾ cup water (plus more if needed)
- 1 cup toasted blanched almonds, hazelnuts, pine nuts, or walnuts
- ¼ cup extra-virgin olive oil
- 2 tablespoons lemon juice (plus more to taste)
- 1 small garlic clove, minced

- Salt and pepper
- Pinch of cayenne pepper

Directions:
1. In a bowl, mash the bread and water together with a fork until it forms a paste.
2. Add the bread paste, nuts, olive oil, lemon juice, garlic, ½ teaspoon salt, ⅛ teaspoon pepper, and cayenne to a blender. Blend until smooth, about 2 minutes. If it's too thick, add a little extra water until it's just thicker than heavy cream.
3. Taste and adjust with more salt, pepper, or lemon juice if needed. Serve at room temperature.

(You can store it in the fridge for up to 2 days. Just let it come to room temp before serving.)

Baba Ghanoush

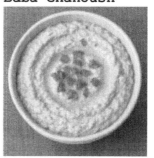

Makes about 2 cups | Vegetarian
Ingredients:
- 2 eggplants (about 1 pound each), pricked all over with a fork
- 2 tablespoons tahini
- 2 tablespoons extra-virgin olive oil (plus more for serving)
- 4 teaspoons lemon juice
- 1 small garlic clove, minced
- Salt and pepper
- 2 teaspoons chopped fresh parsley

Directions:
1. Move your oven rack to the middle and preheat to 500°F. Place eggplants on a foil-lined baking sheet and roast, turning them every 15 minutes, until they feel soft when pressed with

tongs—about 40 to 60 minutes. Let them cool for 5 minutes.

2. Set a colander over a bowl. Trim the tops and bottoms off the eggplants and slice them open lengthwise. Scoop out the hot pulp and place it in the colander. Discard the skins. Let the pulp drain for about 3 minutes.

3. Transfer the drained pulp to a food processor. Add tahini, olive oil, lemon juice, garlic, ¾ teaspoon salt, and ¼ teaspoon pepper. Pulse about 8 times until it's a coarse purée. Taste and adjust seasoning.

4. Spoon into a bowl, cover, and chill for about an hour. (You can refrigerate it for up to a day. Let it come to room temp before serving.)

Right before serving, adjust the seasoning, drizzle with a little olive oil, and sprinkle with parsley.

Olive Oil–Sea Salt Pita Chips

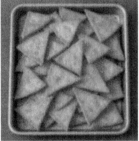

Serves 8 | Fast | Vegetarian
Ingredients:
- 4 (8-inch) pita breads
- ½ cup extra-virgin olive oil
- 1 teaspoon sea salt or kosher salt

Directions:
1. Set your oven racks to the upper-middle and lower-middle positions, then preheat to 350°F. Cut around the edge of each pita with kitchen shears and separate them into two thin rounds.

2. Working one at a time, brush the rough side of each round generously with olive oil and sprinkle with salt. Stack the rounds rough side up as you go. Once they're all coated, cut the

stack into 8 wedges using a chef's knife.

3. Lay the wedges in a single layer, rough side up, on two rimmed baking sheets. Bake for about 15 minutes, switching and rotating the sheets halfway through, until the chips are golden and crisp.

Let them cool completely before serving.

(They'll keep in an airtight container at room temp for up to 3 days.)

Muhammara

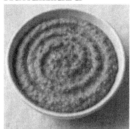

Makes about 2 cups | Fast | Vegetarian

Ingredients:
- 1½ cups jarred roasted red peppers, rinsed and patted dry
- 1 cup toasted walnuts
- ¼ cup plain wheat crackers, crumbled
- 3 tablespoons pomegranate molasses
- 2 tablespoons extra-virgin olive oil
- ¾ teaspoon salt
- ½ teaspoon ground cumin
- ⅛ teaspoon cayenne pepper
- Lemon juice, as needed
- 1 tablespoon chopped fresh parsley (optional)

Directions:
1. Add everything except the parsley to a food processor. Pulse about 10 times until smooth.

2. Scoop into a bowl, cover, and chill for 15 minutes to let the flavors come together. (You can refrigerate it for up to a day. Let it come to room temp before serving.)

3. Before serving, season with lemon juice, salt, or more

cayenne to taste. Top with parsley, if using.

Provençal-Style Anchovy Dip (Anchoïade)

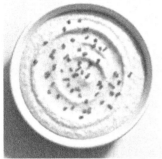

Makes about 1½ cups

Ingredients:
- ¾ cup whole blanched almonds
- 20 anchovy fillets (about 1½ ounces), rinsed, patted dry, and minced
- ¼ cup water
- 2 tablespoons raisins
- 2 tablespoons lemon juice (plus more to taste)
- 1 garlic clove, minced
- 1 teaspoon Dijon mustard
- Salt and pepper
- ¼ cup extra-virgin olive oil (plus more for serving)
- 1 tablespoon minced fresh chives

Directions:
1. Bring 4 cups of water to a boil in a medium saucepan. Add the almonds and cook until soft, about 20 minutes. Drain and rinse well.
2. In a food processor, blend the almonds, anchovies, water, raisins, lemon juice, garlic, mustard, ¼ teaspoon pepper, and ⅛ teaspoon salt until mostly smooth—about 2 minutes. Scrape down the sides as needed.
3. With the processor running, slowly pour in the olive oil. Continue blending for another 2 minutes until the dip is smooth.
4. Transfer to a bowl, stir in 2 teaspoons of chives, and season with more lemon juice, salt, or pepper to taste.

Top with the remaining chives and a drizzle of olive oil before serving. (Dip keeps in the fridge for up to 2 days—just let it come to room temp before serving.)

Skordalia

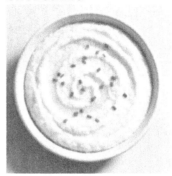

Makes about 2 cups | Vegetarian

Ingredients:
- 1 (10- to 12-ounce) russet potato, peeled and cut into 1-inch chunks
- 3 garlic cloves, minced into a paste
- 3 tablespoons lemon juice
- 2 slices hearty white sandwich bread, crusts removed and torn into 1-inch pieces
- 6 tablespoons warm water (plus more if needed)
- Salt and pepper
- ¼ cup extra-virgin olive oil
- ¼ cup plain Greek yogurt

Directions:
1. Place the potato in a small saucepan and cover with water by about an inch. Bring to a boil, then reduce to a simmer. Cook until the potato is tender and a knife slides in easily—about 15 to 20 minutes. Drain well, tossing to shake off any extra water.
2. While the potato cooks, mix the garlic and lemon juice in a bowl and let it sit for 10 minutes. In a separate bowl, mash the bread with ¼ cup warm water and ½ teaspoon salt using a fork to make a paste.
3. Run the potato through a ricer or food mill into the bowl with the bread. Stir in the lemon-

garlic mix, olive oil, yogurt, and remaining 2 tablespoons warm water until everything is smooth and well combined.

Season with salt and pepper to taste, and thin with a little more warm water if needed before serving.
(You can make it ahead—just refrigerate for up to 3 days and let it come to room temp before serving.)

Lavash Crackers

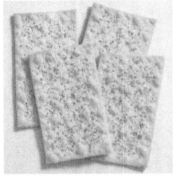

Serves 10 to 12 | Vegetarian

Ingredients:
- 1½ cups (8⅝ oz) semolina flour
- ¾ cup (4⅛ oz) whole-wheat flour
- ¾ cup (3¾ oz) all-purpose flour
- ¾ teaspoon salt
- 1 cup warm water
- ⅓ cup extra-virgin olive oil (plus more for brushing)
- 1 large egg, lightly beaten
- 2 tablespoons sesame seeds
- 2 teaspoons sea salt or kosher salt
- 1 teaspoon coarsely ground pepper

Directions:
1. In a stand mixer fitted with a dough hook, combine all three flours and the salt on low speed. Slowly add the warm water and olive oil. Knead for 7 to 9 minutes until the dough is smooth and elastic.
2. Turn the dough out onto a lightly floured surface, knead it briefly into a ball, then divide it into 4 equal pieces. Brush each with a little oil and cover with plastic wrap. Let rest at room temp for 1 hour.
3. Preheat oven to 425°F with racks in the upper-middle and lower-middle positions. Spray two large rimless (or inverted) baking sheets with oil.
4. Working with 2 dough pieces at a time (keep the rest covered), press each into a rough rectangle and place on the baking sheets. Roll and stretch the dough out to the edges of the sheets. Prick the dough all over with a fork every 2 inches.
5. Brush each sheet with beaten egg. Sprinkle each with 1½ teaspoons sesame seeds, ½ teaspoon salt, and ¼ teaspoon pepper. Press gently to help the toppings stick.
6. Bake for 15 to 18 minutes, switching and rotating the sheets halfway through, until the lavash is deeply golden brown.
7. Let the crackers cool on a wire rack. Cool the sheets completely before repeating with the rest of the dough.

Once cooled, break the lavash into large pieces.
(Store in an airtight container at room temp for up to 2 weeks.)

Marinated Green and Black Olives

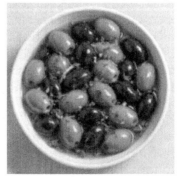

Serves 8 | Vegetarian

Ingredients:
- 1 cup brine-cured green olives with pits
- 1 cup brine-cured black olives with pits
- ¾ cup extra-virgin olive oil
- 1 shallot, minced
- 1 garlic clove, minced
- 2 teaspoons lemon zest

- 2 teaspoons minced fresh thyme
- 2 teaspoons minced fresh oregano
- ½ teaspoon red pepper flakes
- ½ teaspoon salt

Directions:
1. Rinse the olives well, then drain and pat them dry with paper towels.
2. In a bowl, toss the olives with all the remaining ingredients. Cover and refrigerate for at least 4 hours or up to 4 days.
3. Let them sit at room temperature for at least 30 minutes before serving.

Marinated Cauliflower and Chickpeas with Saffron

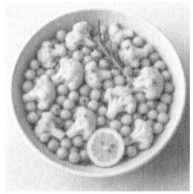

Serves 6 to 8 | Vegetarian

Ingredients:
- ½ head cauliflower (about 1 lb), cored and cut into 1-inch florets
- Salt and pepper
- ⅛ teaspoon saffron threads, crumbled
- ⅓ cup extra-virgin olive oil
- 5 garlic cloves, peeled and smashed
- 1½ teaspoons sugar
- 1½ teaspoons smoked paprika
- 1 small sprig fresh rosemary
- 2 tablespoons sherry vinegar
- 1 cup canned chickpeas, rinsed
- ½ lemon, thinly sliced
- 1 tablespoon chopped fresh parsley

Directions:
1. Bring 2 quarts of water to a boil. Add the cauliflower and 1 tablespoon of salt. Cook until just tender, about 3 minutes. Drain and spread on a paper towel-lined sheet to cool.
2. In a small bowl, mix the saffron with ¼ cup hot water and set aside.
3. In a small saucepan, heat the olive oil and garlic over medium-low heat until the garlic just begins to sizzle but doesn't brown, about 4-6 minutes. Stir in the sugar, paprika, and rosemary. Cook for about 30 seconds until fragrant, then remove from heat.
4. Stir in the saffron water, sherry vinegar, 1½ teaspoons salt, and ¼ teaspoon pepper.
5. In a large bowl, combine the cauliflower, chickpeas, lemon slices, and the saffron marinade. Cover and refrigerate for at least 4 hours or up to 3 days, stirring occasionally.

To serve, remove the rosemary sprig and transfer to a serving bowl using a slotted spoon. Sprinkle with parsley and enjoy.

Marinated Artichokes

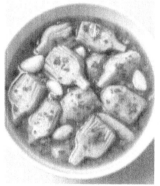

Serves 6 to 8 | Vegetarian

Ingredients:
- 2 lemons
- 2½ cups extra-virgin olive oil
- 3 pounds baby artichokes (2 to 4 oz each)
- 8 garlic cloves (6 smashed, 2 minced)
- ¼ teaspoon red pepper flakes
- 2 sprigs fresh thyme
- Salt and pepper
- 2 tablespoons minced fresh mint

Directions:
1. Use a vegetable peeler to remove three 2-inch strips of zest from one lemon. Grate ½ teaspoon zest from the second lemon and set aside. Juice both lemons to get ¼ cup of juice and save the used lemon halves.
2. Pour the oil into a large saucepan and add the lemon zest strips. Prepare each artichoke by cutting off the top quarter, snapping off the tough outer leaves, trimming the dark parts, and peeling the stem. Cut each one in half (or quarters if they're large), rub with a used lemon half to prevent browning, and drop into the saucepan.
3. Add the smashed garlic, red pepper flakes, thyme, 1 teaspoon salt, and ¼ teaspoon pepper. Bring to a rapid simmer over high heat. Lower the heat to medium-low and simmer gently, stirring occasionally, for about 5 minutes—just until the artichokes are starting to soften.
4. Remove from heat, cover, and let the mixture sit for about 20 minutes until the artichokes are fully tender.
5. Stir in the reserved grated lemon zest, lemon juice, and minced garlic. Transfer everything—including the oil—to a serving bowl and let it cool to room temperature.

Before serving, season with extra salt if needed and top with fresh mint. (They'll keep in the fridge for up to 4 days. Let them come to room temp before serving.)

Giardiniera

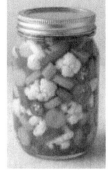

Makes Four 1-Pint Jars | Vegetarian

Ingredients:
- ½ head cauliflower (about 1 lb), cored and cut into ½-inch florets
- 3 carrots, peeled and sliced ¼ inch thick on the bias
- 3 celery ribs, cut into ½-inch pieces
- 1 red bell pepper, stemmed, seeded, and cut into ½-inch strips
- 2 serrano chiles, stemmed and thinly sliced
- 4 garlic cloves, thinly sliced
- 1 cup chopped fresh dill
- 2¾ cups white wine vinegar
- 2¼ cups water
- ¼ cup sugar
- 2 tablespoons salt

Directions:
1. In a large bowl, mix together the cauliflower, carrots, celery, bell pepper, serranos, and garlic. Pack the mixture evenly into four 1-pint jars with tight-fitting lids.
2. Wrap the chopped dill in cheesecloth and tie it into a bundle with kitchen twine. In a saucepan over medium-high heat, combine the vinegar, water, sugar, salt, and dill bundle. Bring to a boil, then remove from heat and let it steep for 10 minutes. Discard the dill.
3. Bring the brine back to a brief boil. Carefully pour it over the vegetables in the jars, dividing it evenly.

4. Let the jars cool to room temperature, then seal and refrigerate.

Let the giardiniera sit for at least 7 days before eating. It'll keep in the fridge for up to a month.

Yogurt Cheese (Labneh)

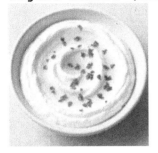

Makes about 1 cup | Vegetarian

Ingredients:
- 2 cups plain yogurt (not nonfat; no added starches or gums)

Directions:
1. Line a fine-mesh strainer with 3 basket-style coffee filters or a double layer of cheesecloth. Set the strainer over a bowl or large measuring cup, making sure there's room for at least 1 cup of liquid to drain.
2. Spoon the yogurt into the strainer, cover with plastic wrap, and refrigerate for at least 10 hours, or up to 2 days, until it has a thick, cream cheese-like texture.
3. Transfer the yogurt cheese to a clean container and discard the liquid.

(You can refrigerate it for up to 2 days.)

Spicy Whipped Feta with Roasted Red Peppers (Htipiti)

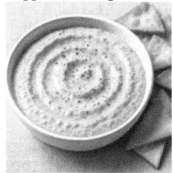

Makes about 2 cups | Fast | Vegetarian

Ingredients:
- 8 ounces feta cheese, crumbled (about 2 cups)
- 1 cup jarred roasted red peppers, rinsed, patted dry, and chopped
- ⅓ cup extra-virgin olive oil (plus more for drizzling)
- 1 tablespoon lemon juice
- ½ teaspoon cayenne pepper (use ¼ tsp for less heat)
- ¼ teaspoon black pepper

Directions:
1. Add the feta, roasted red peppers, olive oil, lemon juice, cayenne, and black pepper to a food processor.
2. Blend until smooth, about 30 seconds, scraping down the sides as needed.
3. Scoop into a serving bowl, drizzle with a bit more olive oil, and serve.

(Store in the fridge for up to 2 days—just let it come to room temp before serving.)

Broiled Feta with Olive Oil and Parsley

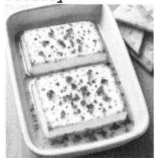

Serves 8 to 12 | Fast | Vegetarian

Ingredients:
- 2 (8-ounce) blocks of feta, sliced into ½-inch-thick slabs
- ¼ teaspoon red pepper flakes
- ¼ teaspoon black pepper
- 2 tablespoons extra-virgin olive oil
- 2 teaspoons minced fresh parsley

Directions:
1. Set your oven rack about 4 inches from the broiler and turn the broiler on.
2. Pat the feta slices dry with paper towels and lay them in a broiler-safe gratin dish.
3. Sprinkle the cheese with red pepper flakes and black pepper.
4. Broil until the edges start to turn golden—about 3 to 8 minutes, depending on your broiler's heat. Keep an eye on it!
5. Remove from the oven, drizzle with olive oil, sprinkle with parsley, and serve immediately.

Perfect with pita chips or warm slices of pita bread.

Pan-Fried Halloumi

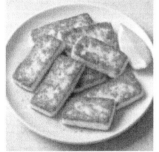

Serves 6 to 8 | Fast | Vegetarian

Ingredients:
- 2 tablespoons stone-ground cornmeal
- 1 tablespoon all-purpose flour
- 1 (8-ounce) block halloumi, sliced into ½-inch-thick slabs
- 2 tablespoons extra-virgin olive oil
- Lemon wedges, for serving

Directions:

1. In a shallow dish, mix the cornmeal and flour. Dredge each halloumi slice in the mixture, coating both sides well and pressing to help it stick. Set aside.
2. Heat the olive oil in a 12-inch nonstick skillet over medium heat until shimmering.
3. Add the halloumi slices in a single layer and cook until golden brown, about 2 to 4 minutes per side.
4. Transfer to a platter and serve hot with lemon wedges.

Toasted Bread for Bruschetta

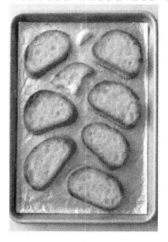

Serves 8 to 10 | Fast | Vegetarian

Ingredients:
- 1 (10x5-inch) loaf of country bread with a thick crust, ends discarded
- 1 garlic clove, peeled
- Extra-virgin olive oil
- Salt

Directions:
1. Move your oven rack about 4 inches from the broiler and preheat the broiler. Line a baking sheet with foil.
2. Slice the bread crosswise into ¾-inch-thick pieces and place on the prepared sheet.
3. Broil until the bread is deeply golden and crisp, about 1 to 2 minutes per side—keep a close eye on it.
4. Once toasted, rub one side of each slice lightly with the

garlic clove (you won't need all of it).

5. Brush with olive oil and sprinkle with salt to taste.

Serve immediately for best texture.

Bruschetta with Arugula Pesto and Goat Cheese

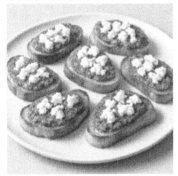

Serves 8 to 10 | Fast | Vegetarian

Ingredients:
- 5 ounces (about 5 cups) baby arugula
- ¼ cup extra-virgin olive oil (plus more for drizzling)
- ¼ cup toasted pine nuts
- 1 tablespoon minced shallot
- 1 teaspoon grated lemon zest
- 1 teaspoon lemon juice
- Salt and pepper
- 1 recipe Toasted Bread for Bruschetta
- 2 ounces goat cheese, crumbled

Directions:
1. In a food processor, combine the arugula, olive oil, pine nuts, shallot, lemon zest and juice, ½ teaspoon salt, and ¼ teaspoon pepper. Pulse until mostly smooth, about 8 pulses, scraping down the bowl as needed.
2. Spread the arugula pesto evenly over each piece of toasted bread.
3. Top with crumbled goat cheese and drizzle with a bit more olive oil to finish.

Serve right away for the best flavor and texture.

Bruschetta with Ricotta, Tomatoes, and Basil

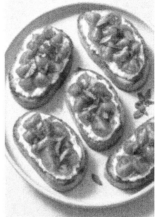

Serves 8 to 10 | Fast | Vegetarian

Ingredients:
- 1 pound cherry tomatoes, quartered
- Salt and pepper
- 1 tablespoon extra-virgin olive oil (plus more for drizzling)
- 5 tablespoons shredded fresh basil
- 10 ounces whole-milk ricotta cheese
- 1 recipe Toasted Bread for Bruschetta

Directions:
1. Toss the tomatoes with 1 teaspoon of salt in a colander and let them drain for 15 minutes.
2. Transfer the drained tomatoes to a bowl. Add the olive oil and ¼ cup (4 tablespoons) of the basil. Season with salt and pepper to taste.
3. In a separate bowl, mix the ricotta with the remaining 1 tablespoon basil. Season with salt and pepper.
4. Spread the ricotta mixture evenly on the toasted bread. Top with the tomato mixture and drizzle with a little more olive oil.

Serve right away for the best texture and flavor.

Bruschetta with Black Olive Pesto, Ricotta, and Basil

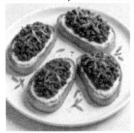

Serves 8 to 10 | Fast | Vegetarian

Ingredients:
- ¾ cup pitted kalamata olives
- 1 small shallot, minced
- 2 tablespoons extra-virgin olive oil (plus more for drizzling)
- 1½ teaspoons lemon juice
- 1 garlic clove, minced
- 10 ounces whole-milk ricotta cheese
- Salt and pepper
- 1 recipe Toasted Bread for Bruschetta
- 2 tablespoons shredded fresh basil

Directions:
1. In a food processor, pulse the olives, shallot, olive oil, lemon juice, and garlic until coarsely chopped—about 10 pulses. Scrape down the sides as needed.
2. In a separate bowl, season the ricotta with salt and pepper to taste.
3. Spread the ricotta onto each piece of toasted bread. Top with the olive pesto, then drizzle with a little more olive oil.
4. Sprinkle with fresh basil just before serving.

Best enjoyed right after assembling.

Bruschetta with Artichoke Hearts and Parmesan

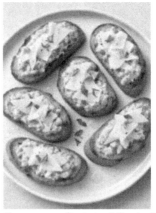

Serves 8 to 10 | Fast | Vegetarian

Ingredients:
- 1 cup jarred whole baby artichoke hearts (packed in water), rinsed and patted dry (or 6 oz frozen artichoke hearts, thawed and dried)
- 2 tablespoons extra-virgin olive oil (plus more for drizzling)
- 2 tablespoons chopped fresh basil
- 2 teaspoons lemon juice
- 1 garlic clove, minced
- Salt and pepper
- 2 ounces Parmesan cheese (1 oz grated, 1 oz shaved)
- 1 recipe Toasted Bread for Bruschetta

Directions:
1. In a food processor, pulse the artichoke hearts, olive oil, basil, lemon juice, garlic, ¼ teaspoon salt, and ¼ teaspoon pepper until coarsely puréed—about 6 pulses. Scrape down the bowl as needed.
2. Add the grated Parmesan and pulse just a couple more times to combine.
3. Spread the artichoke mixture over each piece of toasted bread. Top with shaved Parmesan.
4. Season with a bit more pepper and drizzle with olive oil to finish.

Serve immediately for best flavor and texture.

Prosciutto-Wrapped Stuffed Dates

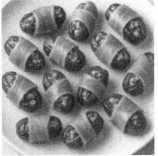

Serves 6 to 8 | Fast

Ingredients:
- ⅔ cup walnuts, toasted and finely chopped
- ½ cup minced fresh parsley
- 2 tablespoons extra-virgin olive oil
- ½ teaspoon grated orange zest
- Salt and pepper
- 12 large pitted Medjool dates, halved lengthwise
- 12 thin slices prosciutto, halved lengthwise

Directions:
1. In a bowl, mix the walnuts, parsley, olive oil, and orange zest. Season with salt and pepper to taste.
2. Fill each date half with a heaping teaspoon of the walnut mixture.
3. Wrap each stuffed date with a half slice of prosciutto, securing it snugly.

Serve at room temperature.
(You can make them up to 8 hours ahead—just refrigerate and bring to room temp before serving.)

Stuffed Grape Leaves (Dolmathes)

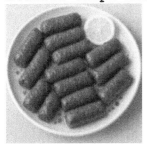

Makes about 24 | Vegetarian

Ingredients:
- 1 (16-ounce) jar grape leaves
- 2 tablespoons extra-virgin olive oil (plus more for serving)
- 1 large onion, finely chopped
- Salt and pepper
- ¾ cup short-grain white rice
- ⅓ cup chopped fresh dill
- ¼ cup chopped fresh mint
- 1½ tablespoons grated lemon zest
- 2 tablespoons lemon juice

Directions:
1. Prep the Leaves:
   Reserve 24 large grape leaves (around 6 inches wide); set the rest aside. Bring 6 cups of water to a boil in a medium saucepan. Blanch reserved leaves for 1 minute, then transfer to cold water to cool. Drain again and place on a plate, covered with plastic wrap.
2. Make the Filling:
   In the same saucepan, heat the oil over medium heat. Add the onion and ½ teaspoon salt and cook until softened and lightly browned, 5-7 minutes. Stir in the rice and cook until the edges of the grains turn translucent, about 2 minutes. Add ¾ cup water and bring to a boil. Cover, reduce heat, and simmer until the rice is tender but still firm and water is absorbed, about 10-12 minutes. Let cool for 10 minutes, then stir in dill, mint, and lemon zest.
3. Stuff the Leaves:
   Place a grape leaf smooth side down with the stem facing you. Trim the stem into a small triangle, then overlap the cut ends slightly. Pat dry. Add a heaping tablespoon of filling just above the stem cut, fold the bottom over the filling, tuck in the sides, and roll tightly. Repeat with remaining leaves and filling.
4. Cook the Dolmathes:
   Line a 12-inch skillet with the leftover grape leaves.

Place stuffed leaves seam side down in tight rows. Combine 1¼ cups water with the lemon juice and pour into the skillet. Bring to a simmer over medium heat, then cover and reduce to medium-low. Cook for 45 minutes to 1 hour, until the leaves and rice are tender and most of the liquid is absorbed.

5. Serve:
   Transfer dolmathes to a platter and let cool to room temperature, about 30 minutes. Drizzle with extra olive oil before serving.

Sizzling Garlic Shrimp (Gambas al Ajillo)

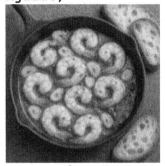

Serves 8

Ingredients:
- 1 pound medium-large shrimp (31-40 per pound), peeled, deveined, tails removed
- 14 garlic cloves, peeled (2 minced, 12 whole)
- ½ cup extra-virgin olive oil
- ¼ teaspoon salt
- 1 bay leaf
- 1 (2-inch) piece mild dried chile, roughly broken (seeds included)
- 1½ teaspoons sherry vinegar
- 1 tablespoon minced fresh parsley

Directions:
1. Marinate the Shrimp
   In a bowl, toss shrimp with the minced garlic, 2 tablespoons of the olive oil, and salt. Let it marinate at room temperature for 30 minutes to 1 hour.

2. Infuse the Oil
   Smash 4 of the garlic cloves. In a 12-inch skillet, combine them with the remaining 6 tablespoons olive oil and heat over medium-low. Stir occasionally until garlic turns light golden, 4 to 7 minutes. Let the oil cool slightly, then remove and discard the garlic.

3. Add Flavor Base
   Thinly slice the remaining 8 garlic cloves. Return the skillet to low heat and add the sliced garlic, bay leaf, and dried chile. Cook, stirring now and then, until garlic is soft but not browned—4 to 7 minutes. (If there's no sizzle after 3 minutes, bump the heat slightly.)

4. Cook the Shrimp
   Turn heat to medium-low and add the shrimp with its marinade. Let cook undisturbed until the oil begins to bubble gently, about 2 minutes. Flip the shrimp and cook another 2 minutes, until nearly done.

5. Finish with a Sizzle
   Increase heat to high. Add sherry vinegar and parsley and stir constantly until the shrimp are just cooked through and the oil is bubbling loudly—15 to 20 seconds. Remove the bay leaf.

Serve immediately—ideally in a hot cast-iron skillet—for that classic sizzling effect. Don't forget the bread!

Mussels Escabèche

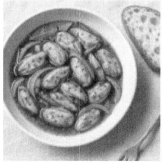

Serves 6 to 8

Ingredients:
- ⅔ cup white wine

- ⅔ cup water
- 2 pounds mussels, scrubbed and debearded
- ⅓ cup extra-virgin olive oil
- ½ small red onion, sliced ¼ inch thick
- 4 garlic cloves, thinly sliced
- 2 bay leaves
- 2 sprigs fresh thyme
- 2 tablespoons minced fresh parsley (divided)
- ¾ teaspoon smoked paprika
- ¼ cup sherry vinegar
- Salt and pepper

Directions:
1. In a Dutch oven, bring the wine and water to a boil over high heat. Add the mussels, cover, and steam, stirring occasionally, until they open—about 3 to 6 minutes. Discard any unopened mussels and the cooking liquid. Let the mussels cool slightly, then remove them from their shells and transfer to a large bowl.
2. In the same Dutch oven, heat the olive oil over medium heat until shimmering. Add the onion, garlic, bay leaves, thyme, 1 tablespoon of the parsley, and paprika. Cook, stirring often, for about 1 minute, just until the garlic is fragrant and the onion softens slightly.
3. Remove from heat and stir in the sherry vinegar, ¼ teaspoon salt, and ⅛ teaspoon pepper. Pour this mixture over the mussels and let them marinate for 15 minutes.
4. Before serving, season with more salt and pepper if needed and sprinkle with the remaining parsley.

(Mussels can be stored in the fridge for up to 2 days—just let them come to room temperature before serving to avoid congealed oil.)

Chili-Marinated Calamari with Oranges

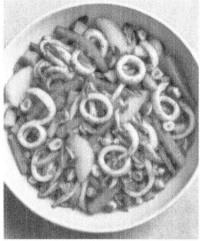

Serves 6 to 8

Ingredients:
- 2 tablespoons baking soda
- Salt and pepper
- 2 pounds small squid (bodies 3 to 4 inches long), bodies sliced into ¼-inch rings, tentacles halved
- ¼ cup extra-virgin olive oil
- 3 tablespoons red wine vinegar
- 2½ tablespoons harissa (store-bought or homemade)
- 2 garlic cloves, minced
- 1 teaspoon Dijon mustard
- 2 oranges
- 1 red bell pepper, sliced into 2-inch matchsticks
- 2 celery ribs, thinly sliced on the bias
- 1 shallot, thinly sliced
- ⅓ cup hazelnuts, toasted, skinned, and chopped
- 3 tablespoons chopped fresh mint

Directions:
1. Brine the Squid
   In a large container, dissolve baking soda and 1 tablespoon salt in 3 cups cold water. Submerge squid and refrigerate for 15 minutes. Drain and separate the bodies from the tentacles.
2. Cook the Squid
   Bring a large pot of salted water to a boil. Add the tentacles and cook for 30

seconds, then add the bodies
and cook everything for 30 to
45 seconds more until just
opaque. Drain and immediately
transfer to an ice bath to
cool. Drain again and pat dry.
3. Make the Marinade
   In a large bowl, whisk
   together olive oil, vinegar,
   harissa, garlic, and mustard.
   Season with salt and pepper to
   taste.
4. Prep the Salad
   Cut away the peel and pith
   from the oranges, then segment
   the fruit and cut segments into
   bite-size pieces. Add the
   oranges, bell pepper, celery,
   shallot, and squid to the bowl
   with the marinade. Toss to
   coat.
5. Marinate
   Cover and refrigerate for at
   least 1 hour, preferably 24
   hours, stirring occasionally.
Finish and Serve
 Right before serving, stir in the
hazelnuts and mint. Taste and adjust
seasoning as needed. Serve chilled
or at room temperature.

Stuffed Sardines (Sarde a Beccafico)

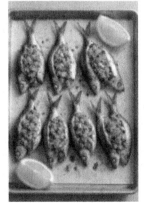

Serves 8

Ingredients:
- ⅓ cup capers, rinsed and
  minced
- ¼ cup golden raisins, finely
  chopped
- ¼ cup pine nuts, toasted and
  finely chopped
- 3 tablespoons extra-virgin
  olive oil, divided
- 2 tablespoons minced fresh
  parsley
- 2 teaspoons grated orange zest
  (plus orange wedges for
  serving)
- 2 garlic cloves, minced
- Salt and pepper
- ⅓ cup panko breadcrumbs
- 8 fresh sardines (2 to 3 oz
  each), scaled, gutted, with
  head and tail on

Directions:
1. Prep the Oven and Stuffing
   Heat oven to 450°F and
   position rack in the lower-
   middle. Line a rimmed baking
   sheet with foil. In a bowl, mix
   capers, raisins, pine nuts, 1
   tablespoon oil, parsley, orange
   zest, garlic, ¼ teaspoon salt,
   and ¼ teaspoon pepper. Add
   panko and stir gently to
   combine.
2. Prepare the Sardines
   With a paring knife, slit open
   each sardine's belly from gill
   to tail, keeping the spine
   intact. Rinse under cold water
   and pat dry. Rub the skins with
   the remaining 2 tablespoons oil
   and season with salt and
   pepper.
3. Stuff and Bake
   Arrange sardines skin-side
   down on the baking sheet,
   spaced about 1 inch apart. Fill
   each with about 2 tablespoons
   of the breadcrumb mixture,
   pressing gently to help it
   stick, then press the fish
   closed.
4. Bake and Serve
   Bake until the fish flakes
   easily and the stuffing is
   golden, about 15 minutes. Serve
   warm with orange wedges on the
   side.

Soups

Classic Gazpacho

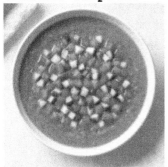

Serves: 8 to 10
Vegetarian

Ingredients:
- 1½ pounds tomatoes, cored and chopped into ¼-inch pieces
- 2 red bell peppers, stemmed, seeded, and chopped into ¼-inch pieces
- 2 small cucumbers (peel one), halved lengthwise, seeded, and chopped into ¼-inch pieces
- ½ small sweet onion or 2 large shallots, finely chopped
- ⅓ cup sherry vinegar
- 2 garlic cloves, minced
- Salt and pepper
- 5 cups tomato juice
- 8 ice cubes
- 1 teaspoon hot sauce (optional)
- Extra-virgin olive oil, for drizzling

Instructions:
1. In a large bowl (at least 4 quarts), mix the tomatoes, bell peppers, cucumbers, onion, vinegar, garlic, and 2 teaspoons of salt. Add pepper to taste. Let it sit for about 5 minutes until the veggies start to release some juice.
2. Stir in the tomato juice, ice cubes, and hot sauce if you're using it. Cover and chill in the fridge for at least 4 hours, or up to 2 days.
3. Before serving, toss out any ice cubes that haven't melted. Taste and adjust with more salt and pepper if needed. Ladle into chilled bowls and drizzle with olive oil.

Classic Croutons

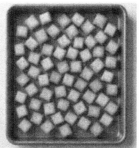

Makes: About 3 cups
Quick • Vegetarian
Ingredients:
- 6 slices hearty white sandwich bread, crusts removed and cut into ½-inch cubes (about 3 cups)
- 3 tablespoons extra-virgin olive oil
- Salt and pepper

Instructions:
1. Preheat your oven to 350°F and move the rack to the middle position.
2. Toss the bread cubes with the olive oil, then season with salt and pepper.
3. Spread them out on a rimmed baking sheet in an even layer.
4. Bake for 20 to 25 minutes, stirring about halfway through, until golden and crispy.
5. Let them cool before serving.

Store at room temp in an airtight container for up to 3 days.

White Gazpacho (Ajo Blanco)

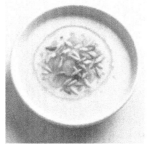

Ingredients:
- 6 slices hearty white sandwich bread, crusts removed

- 4 cups water
- 2½ cups (about 8¾ oz) + ⅓ cup sliced blanched almonds
- 1 garlic clove, peeled and smashed
- 3 tablespoons sherry vinegar
- Salt and pepper
- Pinch of cayenne pepper
- ½ cup plus 2 teaspoons extra-virgin olive oil, plus extra for drizzling
- ⅛ teaspoon almond extract
- 6 oz seedless green grapes, thinly sliced (about 1 cup)

Instructions:
1. Soak the bread in the water for 5 minutes. Meanwhile, blend 2½ cups almonds in a blender until finely ground (about 30 seconds), scraping the sides as needed.
2. Lightly squeeze the soaked bread, then add it to the blender. Measure out 3 cups of the soaking water and set it aside; pour the rest into the blender. Add garlic, vinegar, ½ teaspoon salt, and a pinch of cayenne. Blend until the mixture is smooth and thick like cake batter (30 to 45 seconds).
3. With the blender running, slowly drizzle in ½ cup olive oil over about 30 seconds. Add the reserved 3 cups of water and blend for another minute.
4. Taste and adjust with salt and pepper. Strain the soup through a fine-mesh sieve into a bowl, pressing on the solids to get every last bit of liquid. Discard the solids.
5. In a small bowl, mix 1 tablespoon of the soup with the almond extract. Stir 1 teaspoon of that mix back into the main soup, then discard the rest. Cover and chill for at least 4 hours, or up to a day.
6. Toast the remaining ⅓ cup almonds: heat 2 teaspoons olive oil in a skillet over medium-high heat until shimmering. Add the almonds and stir constantly until golden (3 to 4 minutes).

Transfer to a bowl, sprinkle with ¼ teaspoon salt, and let cool.
7. To serve, ladle the soup into shallow bowls. Pile some sliced grapes in the center, sprinkle with toasted almonds, and finish with a drizzle of olive oil. Serve right away.

Chilled Cucumber and Yogurt Soup

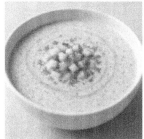

Serves: 6
Vegetarian

Ingredients:
- 5 pounds English cucumbers, peeled and seeded
  - Cut 1 cucumber into ½-inch pieces (for garnish)
  - Cut the rest into 2-inch chunks
- 4 scallions, green parts only, coarsely chopped
- 2 cups water
- 2 cups plain Greek yogurt
- 1 tablespoon lemon juice
- 1½ teaspoons salt, plus more to taste
- ¼ teaspoon sugar
- Freshly ground black pepper
- 1½ tablespoons minced fresh dill
- 1½ tablespoons minced fresh mint
- Extra-virgin olive oil, for drizzling

Instructions:
1. Combine the 2-inch cucumber chunks and scallions. In two batches, blend with the water until completely smooth (about 2 minutes per batch). Pour into a large bowl.
2. Whisk in the yogurt, lemon juice, 1½ teaspoons salt, sugar, and a pinch of pepper.

Cover and chill for at least 1 hour, or up to 12.

3. Before serving, stir in the dill and mint. Taste and adjust seasoning with more salt and pepper.
4. Ladle into bowls, top with the reserved ½-inch cucumber pieces, and drizzle with olive oil. Serve chilled.

Classic Chicken Broth

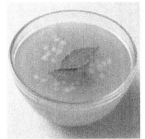

Makes: About 8 cups

Ingredients:
- 4 pounds chicken backs and wings
- 14 cups water
- 1 onion, chopped
- 2 bay leaves
- 2 teaspoons salt

Instructions:
1. In a large stockpot or Dutch oven, combine the chicken and water. Bring to a boil over medium-high heat, skimming off any foam that rises to the top.
2. Lower the heat and simmer gently for 3 hours.
3. Add the chopped onion, bay leaves, and salt. Keep simmering for another 2 hours.
4. Strain the broth through a fine-mesh strainer into a clean pot or container, pressing on the solids to get every last drop of liquid. Let it sit for about 5 minutes, then skim off the fat from the surface.You can refrigerate the cooled broth for up to 4 days or freeze it for up to a month.

Vegetable Broth Base

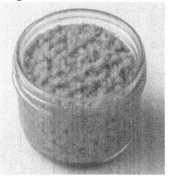

Makes: About 1¾ cups base (enough for around 1¾ gallons broth)
Quick • Vegetarian

Ingredients:
- 1 pound leeks (white and light green parts only), chopped and well-washed (about 2½ cups)
- 2 carrots, peeled and cut into ½-inch chunks (about ⅔ cup)
- ½ small celery root, peeled and chopped into ½-inch chunks (about ¾ cup)
- ½ cup (about ½ oz) fresh parsley leaves and tender stems
- 3 tablespoons dried minced onion
- 3 tablespoons kosher salt
- 1½ tablespoons tomato paste

Instructions:
1. In a food processor, combine the leeks, carrots, celery root, parsley, dried onion, and salt. Blend for 3 to 4 minutes, scraping down the sides often, until the mixture forms a fine paste.
2. Add the tomato paste and continue processing for another 2 minutes, scraping down every 30 seconds.
3. Scoop the paste into an airtight container, tap it on the counter to release air pockets, and press a piece of parchment paper directly onto the surface. Seal tightly and freeze for up to 6 months.

To Make 1 Cup of Broth:
Mix 1 tablespoon of the base (frozen or fresh) into 1 cup of boiling water. For a clearer broth,

let it sit for 5 minutes, then strain through a fine-mesh sieve.

Provençal Vegetable Soup (Soupe au Pistou)

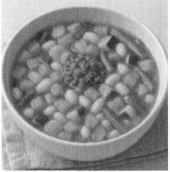

Serves 6 | Vegetarian

Pistou
- ½ cup fresh basil leaves
- 1 oz Parmesan cheese, grated (about ½ cup)
- ⅓ cup extra-virgin olive oil
- 1 garlic clove, minced

Soup
- 1 tbsp extra-virgin olive oil
- 1 leek (white and light green parts only), halved lengthwise, sliced ½ inch thick, and well washed
- 1 celery rib, cut into ½-inch pieces
- 1 carrot, peeled and sliced ¼ inch thick
- Salt and pepper
- 2 garlic cloves, minced
- 3 cups vegetable broth
- 3 cups water
- ½ cup orecchiette
- 8 oz haricots verts, trimmed and cut into ½-inch pieces
- 1 (15-oz) can cannellini or navy beans, rinsed
- 1 small zucchini, halved lengthwise, seeded, and cut into ¼-inch pieces
- 1 large tomato, cored, seeded, and chopped

How to Make It
1. Make the Pistou
   Toss everything into a food processor and blend until smooth, scraping down the sides if needed. You can stash it in the fridge for up to 4 hours.

2. Start the Soup
   In a large pot or Dutch oven, heat the olive oil over medium. Add the leek, celery, carrot, and ½ tsp of salt. Cook, stirring now and then, until the veggies are soft—about 8 to 10 minutes. Stir in the garlic and cook for another 30 seconds or so until fragrant.
3. Add Liquids and Pasta
   Pour in the broth and water, bring it to a simmer. Add the pasta and cook for about 5 minutes, just until it starts to soften.
4. Add Veggies and Beans
   Stir in the green beans and cook until they're bright green but still have some bite, about 3 minutes. Add the beans, zucchini, and tomato. Let everything simmer until the pasta and veggies are tender—about 3 more minutes. Taste and season with salt and pepper as needed.

Ladle the soup into bowls and top each with a spoonful of pistou.

Roasted Eggplant and Tomato Soup

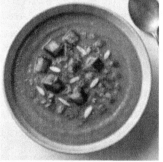

Serves 4 to 6 | Vegetarian

Ingredients
- 2 lbs eggplant, cut into ½-inch cubes
- 6 tbsp extra-virgin olive oil, plus more for serving
- 1 onion, chopped
- Salt and pepper
- 2 garlic cloves, minced
- 1½ tsp ras el hanout
- ½ tsp ground cumin
- 4 cups chicken or vegetable broth (plus extra if needed)

- 1 (14.5-oz) can diced tomatoes, drained
- ¼ cup raisins
- 1 bay leaf
- 2 tsp lemon juice
- 2 tbsp slivered almonds, toasted
- 2 tbsp fresh cilantro, minced

How to Make It
1. Roast the Eggplant
   Place an oven rack about 4 inches from the broiler and turn on the broiler. Toss the eggplant with 5 tbsp of olive oil and spread it out on a foil-lined baking sheet. Broil for 10 minutes, then give it a stir and broil for another 5 to 7 minutes until it's deep brown. Set aside 2 cups of the roasted eggplant for later.
2. Make the Soup Base
   In a large pot, heat the remaining 1 tbsp of oil over medium heat. Add the onion, ¾ tsp salt, and ¼ tsp pepper. Cook, stirring now and then, until the onion is soft and lightly browned—about 5 to 7 minutes. Add the garlic, ras el hanout, and cumin. Cook for about 30 seconds, just until it smells amazing. Stir in the broth, tomatoes, raisins, bay leaf, and the rest of the eggplant. Bring it to a simmer, then lower the heat, cover, and let it cook gently for about 20 minutes.
3. Blend and Finish
   Toss the bay leaf. Working in batches, blend the soup until it's smooth (about 2 minutes per batch). Pour it back into a clean pot, stir in the reserved eggplant, and reheat gently—don't let it boil. If it's too thick, thin it out with a bit of hot broth. Stir in the lemon juice, then taste and adjust the seasoning.

Ladle it into bowls and top each with some toasted almonds, chopped cilantro, and a drizzle of olive oil.

Roasted Red Pepper Soup with Smoked Paprika and Cilantro Yogurt

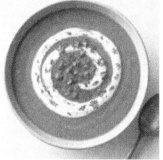

Serves 6 | Vegetarian

Ingredients
- ½ cup whole-milk yogurt
- 3 tbsp minced fresh cilantro
- 1 tsp lime juice
- Salt and pepper
- 8 red bell peppers, cored and flattened
- 1 tbsp extra-virgin olive oil
- 2 garlic cloves, minced
- 1 red onion, chopped
- ½ tsp ground cumin
- ½ tsp smoked paprika (or sweet paprika as a milder option)
- 2 tbsp tomato paste
- 1 tbsp all-purpose flour
- 4 cups chicken or vegetable broth (plus more if needed)
- 1 bay leaf
- ½ cup half-and-half
- 2 tbsp dry sherry

How to Make It
1. Make the Yogurt Topping
   In a bowl, mix the yogurt, 1 tablespoon of cilantro, and the lime juice. Add salt and pepper to taste. Cover and pop it in the fridge until you're ready to serve.
2. Roast the Peppers
   Move your oven rack about 3 inches from the broiler and turn the broiler on. Arrange half the peppers skin side up on a foil-lined baking sheet. Broil until the skins are blistered and blackened but the flesh is still firm—8 to 10 minutes, rotating the sheet halfway through. Transfer them

to a bowl, cover with foil or plastic wrap, and let them steam for about 10 to 15 minutes so the skins come off easily. Repeat with the other half of the peppers. Peel and roughly chop all the roasted peppers.

3. Start the Soup Base
   In a Dutch oven, heat the olive oil and garlic over low heat, stirring constantly, until the garlic is golden and sticky—about 6 to 8 minutes. Add the chopped onion and ¼ tsp salt, crank the heat up to medium, and cook until the onion is soft—about 5 minutes.

4. Build Flavor
   Stir in the cumin and smoked paprika and let them bloom for 30 seconds. Add the tomato paste and flour, cooking for another minute. Slowly whisk in the broth, scraping up any bits from the bottom and making sure there are no lumps. Add the bay leaf and chopped peppers. Bring to a simmer and cook until the peppers are super tender—about 5 to 7 minutes.

5. Blend and Finish
   Remove the bay leaf. Working in batches, blend the soup until smooth (about 2 minutes per batch). Pour it back into a clean pot and stir in the half-and-half and sherry. Warm it gently over low heat—don't let it boil. If it's too thick, thin it out with a little hot broth. Stir in the remaining cilantro and season to taste.

Ladle into bowls and top each with a generous spoonful of the cilantro-lime yogurt.

Turkish Tomato, Bulgur, and Red Pepper Soup

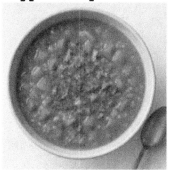

Serves 6 to 8 | Vegetarian

Ingredients
- 2 tbsp extra-virgin olive oil
- 1 onion, chopped
- 2 red bell peppers, stemmed, seeded, and chopped
- Salt and pepper
- 3 garlic cloves, minced
- 1 tsp dried mint, crumbled
- ½ tsp smoked paprika
- ⅛ tsp red pepper flakes
- 1 tbsp tomato paste
- ½ cup dry white wine
- 1 (28-oz) can diced fire-roasted tomatoes
- 4 cups chicken or vegetable broth
- 2 cups water
- ¾ cup medium-grind bulgur, rinsed
- ⅓ cup chopped fresh mint

How to Make It
1. Start the Base
   In a Dutch oven or large pot, heat the olive oil over medium. Add the onion, bell peppers, ¾ tsp salt, and ¼ tsp pepper. Cook, stirring occasionally, until the veggies are soft and starting to brown—about 6 to 8 minutes. Stir in the garlic, dried mint, smoked paprika, and red pepper flakes. Cook for about 30 seconds, just until everything smells amazing. Add the tomato paste and cook for another minute.

2. Add Wine and Tomatoes
   Pour in the white wine, scraping up any browned bits from the bottom. Let it simmer until it reduces by half—about

1 minute. Stir in the fire-roasted tomatoes and their juices. Let it cook for around 10 minutes, stirring now and then, until the tomatoes break down a bit.
   3. Simmer the Soup
      Add the broth, water, and rinsed bulgur. Bring everything to a simmer, then lower the heat, cover the pot, and let it gently cook until the bulgur is tender—about 20 minutes. Give it a taste and add more salt and pepper if needed.
Ladle into bowls and top each serving with a sprinkle of fresh mint.

Artichoke Soup à la Barigoule

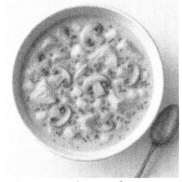

Serves 4 to 6
Ingredients
- 3 tbsp extra-virgin olive oil
- 3 cups jarred whole baby artichokes (in water), quartered, rinsed, and patted dry
- 12 oz white mushrooms, trimmed and thinly sliced
- 1 leek (white and light green parts only), halved, sliced ¼-inch thick, and washed
- 4 garlic cloves, minced
- 2 anchovy fillets, rinsed, dried, and minced
- 1 tsp fresh thyme (or ¼ tsp dried)
- 3 tbsp all-purpose flour
- ¼ cup dry white wine
- 3 cups chicken broth
- 3 cups vegetable broth
- 6 oz parsnips, peeled and cut into ½-inch pieces
- 2 bay leaves
- ¼ cup heavy cream
- 2 tbsp minced fresh tarragon
- 1 tsp white wine vinegar (plus more to taste)
- Salt and pepper

How to Make It
   1. Brown the Artichokes
      Heat 1 tbsp of oil in a Dutch oven over medium heat. Add the artichokes and cook until they're golden and browned—about 8 to 10 minutes. Transfer them to a cutting board, let them cool a bit, then give them a rough chop.
   2. Cook the Mushrooms
      Add another tablespoon of oil to the pot. Toss in the mushrooms, cover, and cook for about 5 minutes until they release their moisture. Uncover and keep cooking another 5 minutes until they're dry and starting to brown.
   3. Build the Base
      Stir in the leek and the last tablespoon of oil. Cook everything together until the leeks soften and the mushrooms are nicely browned—about 8 to 10 minutes. Add garlic, anchovies, and thyme; stir for about 30 seconds until fragrant. Sprinkle in the flour, stir, and cook for a minute. Pour in the wine and scrape up any browned bits; let it simmer down for about a minute.
   4. Simmer the Soup
      Add the broths, parsnips, bay leaves, and chopped artichokes. Bring it to a simmer, cover, and cook until the parsnips are tender—about 15 to 20 minutes. Remove bay leaves.
   5. Finish and Serve
      Stir in the cream, tarragon, and vinegar. Season with salt and pepper to taste, and adjust the vinegar if needed for a little more brightness.
Ladle it up and serve warm.

Risi e Bisi (Rice and Peas)

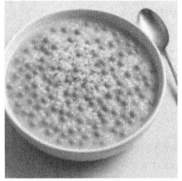

Serves 6
Quick Pea Broth
- 6 cups water
- 1¾ cups chicken broth
- 8 oz snow peas, chopped
- 1 small onion, chopped
- 1 carrot, chopped
- 1 garlic clove, lightly crushed
- 1 tsp salt
- 2 bay leaves

Soup
- 2 tbsp extra-virgin olive oil
- 1 onion, finely chopped
- 2 oz pancetta, finely chopped
- 1 garlic clove, minced
- 1 cup Arborio rice
- ½ cup dry white wine
- 20 oz frozen peas
- 1½ oz Parmesan cheese, grated (about ¾ cup)
- 4 tsp fresh parsley, minced
- 2 tsp lemon juice
- Salt and pepper

How to Make It
1. Make the Broth
   In a Dutch oven, combine all the broth ingredients. Bring to a boil over medium-high heat, then reduce to a gentle simmer. Partially cover and cook for 30 minutes. Strain the broth through a fine-mesh strainer into a medium saucepan, pressing on the solids to get out all the flavor. Keep the broth warm on low heat.
2. Start the Soup
   In the now-empty Dutch oven, heat the olive oil over medium. Add the onion and pancetta. Cook, stirring every so often, until the onion softens and starts to brown—about 5 to 7 minutes. Stir in the garlic and cook for 30 seconds until fragrant.
3. Cook the Rice
   Add the rice and stir often until the edges of the grains turn translucent—about 3 minutes. Pour in the wine and cook, stirring constantly, until it's fully absorbed, about 1 minute.
4. Simmer and Finish
   Stir in the warm broth. Bring it to a boil, then reduce to a simmer. Cover and cook, stirring now and then, until the rice is just tender—about 15 minutes. Stir in the frozen peas and cook until heated through, about 2 minutes more.
Take the pot off the heat and stir in the Parmesan, parsley, and lemon juice. Taste and season with salt and pepper. Serve right away while it's still creamy and warm.

French Lentil Soup

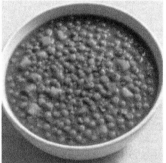

Serves 4 to 6
Ingredients
- 3 slices bacon, cut into ¼-inch pieces
- 1 large onion, finely chopped
- 2 carrots, peeled and chopped
- 3 garlic cloves, minced
- 1 tsp fresh thyme (or ¼ tsp dried)
- 1 (14.5-oz) can diced tomatoes, drained
- 1 bay leaf
- 1 cup lentilles du Puy (French green lentils), rinsed and picked over
- Salt and pepper
- ½ cup dry white wine

- 4½ cups chicken broth (plus more as needed)
- 1½ cups water
- 1½ tsp balsamic vinegar
- 3 tbsp fresh parsley, minced

How to Make It
1. Start with the Base
   In a Dutch oven, cook the bacon over medium-high heat until crisp—about 5 minutes. Stir in the onion and carrots and cook for 2 minutes, just until they start to soften. Add the garlic and thyme; cook for about 30 seconds until fragrant. Stir in the drained tomatoes and bay leaf and cook for another 30 seconds. Add the lentils and ¼ tsp salt. Cover the pot, reduce heat to medium-low, and cook for 8 to 10 minutes until the veggies are soft and the lentils have darkened slightly.
2. Add Liquid and Simmer
   Turn the heat up to high. Add the white wine and bring to a simmer. Pour in the broth and water and bring everything to a boil. Partially cover the pot, reduce heat to low, and simmer gently for 30 to 35 minutes, until the lentils are tender but still hold their shape.
3. Blend and Finish
   Toss out the bay leaf. Scoop out 3 cups of the soup and blend until smooth—about 30 seconds—then stir it back into the pot. Warm the soup gently over low heat (don't let it boil). Add extra hot broth if it's thicker than you like. Stir in the balsamic vinegar and parsley, and season to taste with salt and pepper.

Serve warm, with crusty bread on the side if you like.

Spanish-Style Lentil and Chorizo Soup

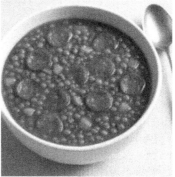

Serves 6 to 8
Ingredients
- 1 lb (about 2¼ cups) lentils, picked over and rinsed
- Salt and pepper
- 1 large onion
- 5 tbsp extra-virgin olive oil
- 1½ lbs Spanish-style chorizo, pricked with a fork
- 3 carrots, peeled and cut into ¼-inch pieces
- 3 tbsp fresh parsley, minced
- 3 tbsp sherry vinegar (plus more to taste)
- 2 bay leaves
- ⅛ tsp ground cloves
- 2 tbsp sweet smoked paprika
- 3 garlic cloves, minced
- 1 tbsp all-purpose flour

How to Make It
1. Soak the Lentils
   In a heatproof bowl, combine lentils with 2 tsp salt and 4 cups boiling water. Let them soak for 30 minutes, then drain well.
2. Prep the Onion and Cook the Sausage
   Chop three-quarters of the onion (you'll want about 1 cup), then grate the rest (around 3 tbsp). Heat 2 tbsp oil in a Dutch oven over medium heat. Add the chorizo and cook until nicely browned all over—about 6 to 8 minutes. Transfer it to a plate. Lower the heat and add the chopped onion, carrots, 1 tbsp parsley, and 1 tsp salt. Cover and cook, stirring now and then, until everything's super soft but not

browned—25 to 30 minutes. If it starts to brown, splash in 1 tbsp water.

3. Start the Soup
  Stir in the soaked lentils and vinegar. Raise the heat to medium-high and cook, stirring often, until the vinegar is mostly evaporated—about 3 to 4 minutes. Add 7 cups water, the chorizo, bay leaves, and cloves. Bring to a simmer, then lower the heat, cover, and cook until lentils are tender—about 30 minutes.

4. Make the Flavor Boost
  In a small saucepan, heat the remaining 3 tbsp oil over medium. Add the paprika, grated onion, garlic, and ½ tsp pepper. Cook, stirring constantly, until fragrant—about 2 minutes. Stir in the flour and cook for another minute, still stirring.

5. Finish the Soup
  Take the chorizo and bay leaves out of the soup. Stir the paprika mixture into the pot and let it all simmer gently for 10 to 15 minutes to meld the flavors and thicken up a bit. Slice the cooled chorizo in half lengthwise, then into ¼-inch pieces. Stir the sausage and remaining 2 tbsp parsley into the soup and heat through—about a minute. Taste and add more salt, pepper, or up to 2 tsp more vinegar if you'd like a little more tang.

This soup keeps great—make it up to 3 days ahead if you want, and reheat when you're ready to dig in.

Red Lentil Soup with North African Spices

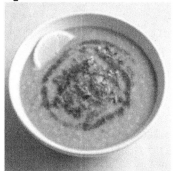

Serves 4 to 6 | Vegetarian
Ingredients
- ¼ cup extra-virgin olive oil
- 1 large onion, finely chopped
- Salt and pepper
- ¾ tsp ground coriander
- ½ tsp ground cumin
- ¼ tsp ground ginger
- ⅛ tsp ground cinnamon
- Pinch of cayenne pepper
- 1 tbsp tomato paste
- 1 garlic clove, minced
- 4 cups chicken or vegetable broth (plus more if needed)
- 2 cups water
- 10½ oz (about 1½ cups) red lentils, picked over and rinsed
- 2 tbsp lemon juice (plus more to taste)
- 1½ tsp dried mint, crumbled
- 1 tsp paprika
- ¼ cup chopped fresh cilantro

How to Make It
1. Build the Flavor Base
  In a large saucepan, heat 2 tbsp of the oil over medium heat until shimmering. Add the onion and 1 tsp salt. Cook, stirring now and then, until soft—about 5 minutes. Add the coriander, cumin, ginger, cinnamon, ¼ tsp pepper, and cayenne. Stir for about 2 minutes until the spices are fragrant. Mix in the tomato paste and garlic and cook for another minute.
2. Add Lentils and Simmer
  Pour in the broth, water, and lentils. Bring to a lively simmer and cook for about 15 minutes, stirring every so

often, until the lentils are tender and starting to fall apart.
3. Whisk and Finish
   Use a whisk to stir the soup vigorously for about 30 seconds until it's a coarse purée. Add more hot broth if you want it thinner. Stir in the lemon juice and taste—add more salt or lemon juice if needed. Keep warm, covered.
4. Make the Spiced Oil
   In a small skillet, heat the remaining 2 tbsp oil over medium. Remove from heat, then stir in the dried mint and paprika.

To serve, ladle soup into bowls, drizzle with about 1 tsp of the mint-paprika oil, and sprinkle with fresh cilantro.

Moroccan-Style Chickpea Soup

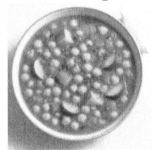

Serves 4 to 6 | Vegetarian
Ingredients
- 3 tbsp extra-virgin olive oil
- 1 onion, finely chopped
- 1 tsp sugar
- Salt and pepper
- 4 garlic cloves, minced
- ½ tsp hot paprika (or regular paprika + pinch of cayenne)
- ¼ tsp saffron threads, crumbled
- ¼ tsp ground ginger
- ¼ tsp ground cumin
- 2 (15-oz) cans chickpeas, rinsed
- 1 lb red potatoes, unpeeled, cut into ½-inch pieces
- 1 (14.5-oz) can diced tomatoes
- 1 zucchini, cut into ½-inch pieces
- 3½ cups chicken or vegetable broth

- ¼ cup fresh parsley or mint, minced
- Lemon wedges, for serving

How to Make It
1. Start the Soup
   In a Dutch oven, heat the olive oil over medium-high. Add the onion, sugar, and ½ tsp salt. Cook, stirring occasionally, until the onion softens—about 5 minutes.
2. Add Spices and Base Ingredients
   Stir in the garlic, paprika, saffron, ginger, and cumin. Cook for about 30 seconds until the spices smell amazing. Add the chickpeas, potatoes, tomatoes (with juice), zucchini, and broth. Bring everything to a simmer.
3. Simmer and Mash
   Cook, stirring now and then, until the potatoes are tender— about 20 to 30 minutes. Use the back of a spoon to mash some of the potatoes against the side of the pot to thicken the soup a bit.
4. Finish and Serve
   Off the heat, stir in the parsley or mint. Taste and season with salt and pepper as needed. Serve hot with lemon wedges on the side.

This one's comforting, colorful, and super satisfying.

Sicilian Chickpea and Escarole Soup

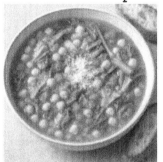

Serves 6 to 8 | Vegetarian
Ingredients
- Salt and pepper
- 1 lb (about 2¾ cups) dried chickpeas, picked over and rinsed

- 2 tbsp extra-virgin olive oil, plus more for serving
- 2 fennel bulbs (stalks discarded), halved, cored, and finely chopped
- 1 small onion, chopped
- 5 garlic cloves, minced
- 2 tsp fresh oregano (or ½ tsp dried)
- ¼ tsp red pepper flakes
- 5 cups chicken or vegetable broth
- 1 Parmesan rind (or 2-inch chunk of Parmesan)
- 2 bay leaves
- 1 (3-inch) strip orange zest
- 1 head escarole (about 1 lb), trimmed and cut into 1-inch pieces
- 1 large tomato, cored and chopped
- Grated Parmesan, for serving

How to Make It
1. Soak the Chickpeas
   In a large container, dissolve 3 tbsp salt in 4 quarts cold water. Add chickpeas and soak at room temp for 8 to 24 hours. Drain and rinse well.
2. Start the Soup Base
   Heat the oil in a Dutch oven over medium. Add the fennel, onion, and 1 tsp salt. Cook, stirring occasionally, until softened—about 7 to 10 minutes. Stir in the garlic, oregano, and pepper flakes; cook for about 30 seconds until fragrant.
3. Simmer the Chickpeas
   Add 7 cups water, the broth, soaked chickpeas, Parmesan rind, bay leaves, and orange zest. Bring to a boil, then lower the heat and let it simmer gently until the chickpeas are tender—about 1¼ to 1¾ hours.
4. Add Greens and Finish
   Stir in the escarole and tomato. Let it cook for another 5 to 10 minutes until the escarole wilts and softens. Remove from heat, fish out the

bay leaves and Parmesan rind (scrape and stir in any melted cheese clinging to it). Taste and adjust seasoning with more salt and pepper if needed.
Ladle into bowls, drizzle with a bit of olive oil, and finish with freshly grated Parmesan. This soup's humble ingredients turn into something pretty special.

Garlic Toasts

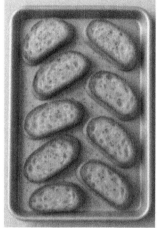

Makes 8 slices | Fast | Vegetarian
Ingredients
- 8 slices rustic bread, about 1-inch thick
- 1 large garlic clove, peeled
- 3 tbsp extra-virgin olive oil
- Salt and pepper

How to Make It
1. Adjust your oven rack so it's about 6 inches from the broiler and turn the broiler on.

2. Arrange the bread slices on a rimmed baking sheet. Broil until golden and crisp on both sides, flipping as needed—this should take about 4 minutes total.
3. Rub one side of each toast lightly with the garlic clove.
4. Drizzle with olive oil and sprinkle with salt and pepper to taste.

Serve warm, or at room temp if you're prepping ahead—they're great either way.

Greek White Bean Soup (Fasolatha)

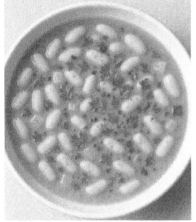

Serves 6 | Vegetarian
Ingredients

- Salt and pepper
- 1 lb (about 2½ cups) dried cannellini beans, picked over and rinsed
- 2 tbsp extra-virgin olive oil, plus more for serving
- 1 onion, chopped
- 2½ tsp fresh oregano (or ¾ tsp dried)
- 6 cups chicken or vegetable broth (plus more as needed)
- 4 celery ribs, cut into ½-inch pieces
- 3 tbsp lemon juice
- 1 tsp ground Aleppo pepper (or ¼ tsp paprika + ¼ tsp red pepper flakes)
- 2 tbsp fresh parsley, chopped

How to Make It
1. Soak the Beans
   In a large container, dissolve 3 tbsp salt in 4 quarts cold water. Add the beans and let them soak at room temperature for at least 8 hours or overnight. Drain and rinse well before cooking.
2. Cook the Soup
   In a Dutch oven, heat the olive oil over medium heat. Add the onion, ½ tsp salt, and ½ tsp pepper. Cook until the onion is soft and lightly browned—about 5 to 7 minutes. Stir in the oregano and cook for about 30 seconds until fragrant. Add the broth, celery, and soaked beans. Bring everything to a boil, then reduce heat to low, cover, and simmer until the beans are tender—about 45 to 60 minutes.
3. Blend and Finish
   Scoop out 2 cups of the soup and blend until smooth—about 30 seconds—then return it to the pot. Warm the soup gently over low heat (don't let it boil). Add more hot broth if you want it thinner. Stir in the lemon juice, Aleppo pepper, and parsley. Taste and adjust seasoning with more salt and pepper if needed.

Ladle into bowls, and finish each with a drizzle of olive oil. Serve with crusty bread for a cozy, satisfying meal.

Pasta e Fagioli with Orange and Fennel

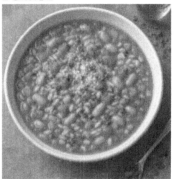

Serves 8 to 10
Ingredients

- 1 tbsp extra-virgin olive oil, plus more for serving
- 3 oz pancetta, finely chopped
- 1 onion, finely chopped
- 1 fennel bulb (stalks discarded), halved, cored, and chopped
- 1 celery rib, minced
- 4 garlic cloves, minced
- 3 anchovy fillets, rinsed and minced
- 1 tbsp fresh oregano (or 1 tsp dried)
- 2 tsp grated orange zest
- ½ tsp fennel seeds
- ¼ tsp red pepper flakes
- 1 (28-oz) can diced tomatoes, with juice

- 1 Parmesan rind (or a 2-inch chunk of cheese), plus grated Parmesan for serving
- 2 (15-oz) cans cannellini beans, rinsed
- 3½ cups chicken broth
- 2½ cups water
- Salt and pepper
- 1 cup orzo (or ditalini or tubettini)
- ¼ cup fresh parsley, minced

How to Make It
1. Sauté the Base
   Heat the olive oil in a Dutch oven over medium-high. Add pancetta and cook, stirring now and then, until it starts to brown—about 3 to 5 minutes. Add the onion, fennel, and celery. Cook until everything softens—around 5 to 7 minutes.
2. Add the Flavor Builders
   Stir in garlic, anchovies, oregano, orange zest, fennel seeds, and red pepper flakes. Cook for about 1 minute until everything smells amazing.
3. Simmer the Soup
   Stir in the diced tomatoes with their juice, scraping up any browned bits from the bottom. Add the Parmesan rind and the beans. Let it all simmer together for about 10 minutes so the flavors meld.
4. Add Broth and Pasta
   Pour in the chicken broth and water, plus 1 tsp salt. Crank up the heat and bring it to a boil. Stir in the orzo and cook until just al dente—about 10 minutes. Remove from heat and discard the Parmesan rind.
5. Finish and Serve
   Stir in the parsley, then season to taste with more salt and pepper. To serve, ladle into bowls and top with a drizzle of olive oil and a sprinkle of grated Parmesan.

This soup is bright, comforting, and packed with flavor—everything pasta e fagioli should be.

Spiced Fava Bean Soup (B'ssara)

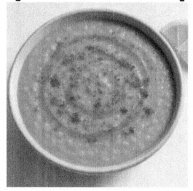

Serves 4 to 6 | Vegetarian
Ingredients
- 3 tbsp extra-virgin olive oil, plus more for serving
- 1 onion, chopped
- Salt and pepper
- 5 garlic cloves, minced
- 2 tsp paprika, plus more for serving
- 2 tsp ground cumin, plus more for serving
- 1 lb (about 3 cups) dried split fava beans, picked over and rinsed
- 6 cups chicken or vegetable broth (plus extra if needed)
- 2 cups water
- ¼ cup lemon juice (from about 2 lemons)

How to Make It
1. Sauté the Aromatics
   In a Dutch oven, heat the olive oil over medium. Add the onion, ¾ tsp salt, and ¼ tsp pepper. Cook, stirring occasionally, until soft and lightly browned—about 5 to 7 minutes. Stir in the garlic, paprika, and cumin. Cook for about 30 seconds, just until fragrant.
2. Simmer the Beans
   Stir in the rinsed fava beans, broth, and water. Bring everything to a boil, then cover, reduce heat to low, and simmer gently. Stir occasionally, and cook until the beans are soft and breaking down—about 1½ to 2 hours.

3. Blend and Finish
   Take the pot off the heat and whisk the soup vigorously for about 30 seconds to break down the beans into a coarse purée. If it's thicker than you'd like, stir in some hot broth to loosen it up. Add the lemon juice and adjust seasoning with more salt and pepper to taste.

To serve, ladle into bowls and finish each with a drizzle of olive oil and a pinch of extra paprika and cumin for a bold, aromatic touch.

Avgolemono (Greek Lemon-Egg Soup)

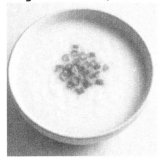

Serves 6 to 8
Ingredients
- 8 cups chicken broth
- ½ cup long-grain white rice
- 12 strips (about 4-inch long) lemon zest
- 4 green cardamom pods, crushed (or 2 whole cloves)
- 1 bay leaf
- 1½ tsp salt
- 2 large eggs + 2 large yolks, at room temperature
- ¼ cup lemon juice (from 2 lemons)
- 1 scallion, thinly sliced or 3 tbsp chopped fresh mint (for garnish)

How to Make It
1. Cook the Rice
   In a medium saucepan, bring the broth to a boil over high heat. Stir in the rice, lemon zest strips, cardamom pods, bay leaf, and salt. Lower the heat and let it simmer until the rice is tender and the broth is fragrant—about 16 to 20 minutes.

2. Temper the Eggs
   In a medium bowl, whisk together the whole eggs, yolks, and lemon juice. Remove the bay leaf, zest, and cardamom pods from the broth. Reduce heat to low. Slowly ladle about 2 cups of the hot broth into the egg mixture, whisking constantly to avoid curdling.

3. Finish the Soup
   Pour the tempered egg mixture back into the pot with the rest of the broth. Stir constantly over low heat until the soup thickens slightly and you see wisps of steam—about 5 minutes. Don't let it simmer or boil.

Serve immediately, garnished with scallions or fresh mint. This soup is best enjoyed fresh—it thickens as it sits and doesn't reheat quite the same.

Spicy Moroccan-Style Chicken and Lentil Soup (Harira)

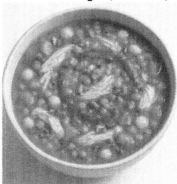

Serves 8
Ingredients
- 1½ lbs bone-in split chicken breasts, trimmed
- Salt and pepper
- 1 tbsp extra-virgin olive oil
- 1 onion, finely chopped
- 1 tsp grated fresh ginger
- 1 tsp ground cumin
- ½ tsp paprika
- ¼ tsp ground cinnamon
- ¼ tsp cayenne pepper
- Pinch of saffron threads, crumbled
- 1 tbsp all-purpose flour
- 10 cups chicken broth

- ¾ cup green or brown lentils (not French lentils), picked over and rinsed
- 1 (15-oz) can chickpeas, rinsed
- 4 plum tomatoes, cored and cut into ¾-inch chunks
- ⅓ cup fresh cilantro, minced
- ¼ cup harissa (plus more for serving)

How to Make It
1. Brown the Chicken
   Pat the chicken dry with paper towels and season with salt and pepper. In a large Dutch oven, heat the olive oil over medium-high until just smoking. Brown the chicken for about 3 minutes per side, then transfer to a plate.
2. Build the Flavor Base
   Add the onion to the fat left in the pot. Cook over medium heat until softened—about 5 minutes. Stir in the ginger, cumin, paprika, cinnamon, cayenne, saffron, and ¼ tsp black pepper. Cook for 30 seconds until fragrant. Stir in the flour and cook for 1 minute more.
3. Simmer the Soup
   Slowly whisk in the chicken broth, scraping up any browned bits and smoothing out the flour. Bring it to a boil.
4. Add Lentils and Chicken
   Return the browned chicken to the pot along with the lentils. Lower the heat and simmer gently until the chicken is cooked through and the lentils are tender—about 20 to 25 minutes.
5. Finish the Soup
   Remove the chicken, shred it, and discard the bones. Stir the shredded chicken back into the pot along with the chickpeas and tomatoes. Simmer another 10 minutes. Off heat, stir in the cilantro and harissa. Taste and season with more salt, pepper, or harissa if desired.

Ladle into bowls and serve with extra harissa on the side for anyone who wants more heat.

Spicy Moroccan-Style Lamb and Lentil Soup

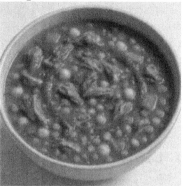

Serves 6 to 8
Ingredients
- 1 lb lamb shoulder chops (blade or round bone), 1–1½ inches thick, trimmed and halved
- Salt and pepper
- 1 tbsp extra-virgin olive oil
- 1 onion, finely chopped
- 1 tsp grated fresh ginger
- 1 tsp ground cumin
- ½ tsp paprika
- ¼ tsp ground cinnamon
- ¼ tsp cayenne pepper
- Pinch of saffron threads, crumbled
- 1 tbsp all-purpose flour
- 10 cups chicken broth
- ¾ cup green or brown lentils (not French lentils), picked over and rinsed
- 1 (15-oz) can chickpeas, rinsed
- 4 plum tomatoes, cored and cut into ¾-inch pieces
- ⅓ cup fresh cilantro, minced
- ¼ cup harissa (plus more for serving)

How to Make It
1. Prep and Brown the Lamb
   Adjust your oven rack to the lower-middle position and preheat the oven to 325°F. Pat lamb dry with paper towels and season with salt and pepper. Heat olive oil in a Dutch oven over medium-high heat. Once hot, brown the lamb for about 4 minutes per side, then transfer

to a plate. Pour off all but 2 tbsp of the fat from the pot.

2. Build the Flavor Base

   Add the onion to the pot and cook over medium heat until softened—about 5 minutes. Stir in ginger, cumin, paprika, cinnamon, cayenne, ¼ tsp black pepper, and saffron. Cook for about 30 seconds until fragrant. Stir in the flour and cook 1 minute more.

3. Simmer the Soup

   Slowly whisk in the broth, scraping up any browned bits and smoothing out the flour. Bring to a boil. Return the lamb (with juices) to the pot, reduce heat to simmer, and cook for 10 minutes. Stir in the lentils and chickpeas, cover the pot, and transfer to the oven. Bake until the lamb is tender and the lentils are cooked—about 50 minutes to 1 hour.

4. Finish and Serve

   Remove the lamb from the pot and let it cool slightly. Shred the meat into bite-size pieces, discarding fat and bones. Return the shredded lamb to the pot and let it sit for a couple minutes to warm through. Stir in the tomatoes, cilantro, and harissa. Taste and adjust seasoning with salt and pepper.

Ladle into bowls and serve with extra harissa on the side for an added kick.

Spicy Moroccan Lamb and Lentil Soup

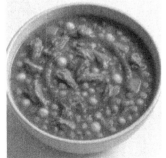

Serves 6 to 8

What You'll Need

- 1 lb lamb shoulder chops (blade or round bone), 1 to 1½ inches thick, trimmed and halved
- Salt and pepper
- 1 tbsp extra-virgin olive oil
- 1 onion, finely chopped
- 1 tsp fresh ginger, grated
- 1 tsp ground cumin
- ½ tsp paprika
- ¼ tsp ground cinnamon
- ¼ tsp cayenne pepper
- A pinch of saffron threads, crumbled
- 1 tbsp all-purpose flour
- 10 cups chicken broth
- ¾ cup green or brown lentils (avoid French lentils)
- 1 (15 oz) can chickpeas, rinsed
- 4 plum tomatoes, cored and chopped into ¾-inch pieces
- ⅓ cup chopped fresh cilantro
- ¼ cup harissa (plus more for serving)

How to Make It

1. Brown the Lamb

   Preheat your oven to 325°F and move the rack to the lower-middle position. Pat the lamb dry and season it with salt and pepper. Heat the oil in a Dutch oven over medium-high. Brown the lamb for about 4 minutes per side, then transfer it to a plate. Pour off all but 2 tablespoons of the fat.

2. Sauté the Aromatics

   Add the onion to the pot and cook until soft, about 5 minutes. Stir in the ginger, cumin, paprika, cinnamon, cayenne, saffron, and a little black pepper. Let the spices bloom for 30 seconds, then stir in the flour and cook another minute.

3. Simmer the Soup

   Slowly whisk in the broth, scraping up any brown bits from the bottom. Once it comes to a boil, return the lamb and any juices to the pot. Simmer for 10 minutes. Add the lentils and chickpeas, cover the pot, and transfer to the oven. Cook until the lamb is tender and lentils are soft—about 50 minutes to an hour.

4. Finish It Off

   Take the lamb out of the pot and let it cool a bit. Shred it into bite-sized pieces, discarding any fat and bones, and return the meat to the soup. Stir in the chopped tomatoes, cilantro, and harissa. Let everything warm through for a couple minutes. Taste and adjust seasoning as needed.

Serve hot, with extra harissa on the side for anyone who wants a little more heat.

Spanish-Style Meatball Soup with Saffron

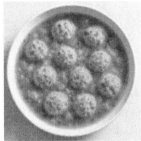

Serves 6 to 8
Ingredients
Meatballs

- 2 slices white sandwich bread, torn
- ⅓ cup whole milk
- 8 oz ground pork
- 1 oz Manchego cheese, grated (½ cup)
- 3 tbsp fresh parsley, minced
- 1 shallot, minced
- 2 tbsp extra-virgin olive oil
- ½ tsp salt
- ½ tsp black pepper
- 8 oz ground beef (80% lean)

Soup

- 1 tbsp extra-virgin olive oil
- 1 onion, finely chopped
- 1 red bell pepper, cut into ¾-inch pieces
- 2 garlic cloves, minced
- 1 tsp paprika
- ¼ tsp saffron threads, crumbled
- ⅛ tsp red pepper flakes
- 1 cup dry white wine
- 8 cups chicken broth
- 1 recipe Picada (see below)
- 2 tbsp fresh parsley, minced

- Salt and pepper

How to Make It
1. Make the Meatballs

   In a large bowl, mash the bread and milk with a fork to form a paste. Mix in the pork, Manchego, parsley, shallot, olive oil, salt, and pepper. Add the beef and mix gently with your hands until just combined. Roll into 2-teaspoon-size balls (you should get 30-35). Place on a baking sheet, cover, and refrigerate for at least 30 minutes to firm up.

2. Build the Broth

   Heat the olive oil in a Dutch oven over medium-high. Add onion and bell pepper and cook until softened and lightly browned, about 8 to 10 minutes. Stir in garlic, paprika, saffron, and red pepper flakes. Cook for 30 seconds until fragrant. Add wine and scrape up any browned bits. Let it cook down until nearly evaporated—about 1 minute.

3. Simmer the Soup

   Pour in the broth and bring to a simmer. Gently drop in the chilled meatballs and cook until they're done—about 10 to 12 minutes. Off the heat, stir in the picada and parsley. Season with salt and pepper to taste.

Serve hot, with extra parsley or a drizzle of olive oil if you like.

Provençal Fish Soup

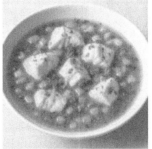

Serves 6 to 8
Ingredients

- 1 tbsp extra-virgin olive oil, plus more for drizzling
- 6 oz pancetta, finely chopped
- 1 fennel bulb, stalks discarded, bulb halved, cored, and chopped into ½-inch pieces, plus 2 tbsp fronds minced for garnish

- 1 onion, chopped
- 2 celery ribs, halved lengthwise and chopped into ½-inch pieces
- Salt and pepper
- 4 garlic cloves, minced
- 1 tsp paprika
- ⅛ tsp red pepper flakes
- Pinch saffron threads, crumbled
- 1 cup dry white wine or dry vermouth
- 4 cups water
- 2 (8-oz) bottles clam juice
- 2 bay leaves
- 2 lbs skinless hake fillets (1 to 1½ inches thick), cut into 6 pieces
- 2 tbsp fresh parsley, minced
- 1 tbsp orange zest

How to Make It
1. Sauté the Base
   Heat the olive oil in a Dutch oven over medium. Add pancetta and cook until starting to brown, about 3 to 5 minutes. Add the fennel, onion, celery, and 1½ tsp salt. Cook, stirring occasionally, until the veggies are soft and lightly browned—around 12 to 14 minutes.
2. Layer the Flavor
   Stir in garlic, paprika, red pepper flakes, and saffron. Cook for about 30 seconds, just until fragrant. Pour in the wine, scraping up any bits from the bottom of the pot. Add the water, clam juice, and bay leaves. Bring to a simmer and cook for 15 to 20 minutes to let the flavors come together.
3. Poach the Fish
   Turn off the heat and discard the bay leaves. Nestle the fish pieces into the hot broth, cover the pot, and let it sit for 8 to 10 minutes, or until the fish flakes easily and registers about 140°F.
4. Finish and Serve
   Gently stir in the parsley, fennel fronds, and orange zest. Break up the fish into large chunks without shredding it.

Taste and season with salt and pepper as needed.
Ladle into bowls and drizzle with a little more olive oil before serving. Serve with crusty bread for a complete, soul-warming meal.

Shellfish Soup with Leeks and Turmeric

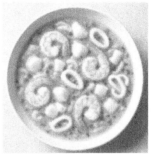

Serves 6 to 8
Ingredients
- 2 tbsp extra-virgin olive oil, plus more for serving
- 12 oz large shrimp (26–30 per lb), peeled and deveined, shells reserved
- 1 cup dry white wine or dry vermouth
- 4 cups water
- 1½ lbs leeks (white/light green parts only), halved lengthwise, thinly sliced and thoroughly washed
- 4 oz pancetta, finely chopped
- 3 tbsp tomato paste
- 2 garlic cloves, minced
- 1 tsp grated fresh ginger
- 1 tsp ground coriander
- ½ tsp ground turmeric
- ⅛ tsp red pepper flakes
- Salt and pepper
- 2 (8-oz) bottles clam juice
- 12 oz large sea scallops, tendons removed
- 12 oz squid, sliced into ½-inch rings and tentacles halved (or sub 1½ lbs total shrimp)
- ⅓ cup minced fresh parsley

How to Make It
1. Make the Shrimp Broth
   Heat 1 tbsp oil in a Dutch oven over medium heat. Add shrimp shells and cook, stirring often, until spotty brown and the pot begins to

173

brown—about 2 to 4 minutes. Add
the wine and simmer for 2
minutes, scraping up bits from
the bottom. Stir in the water,
bring to a simmer, and cook for
another 4 minutes. Strain the
mixture through a fine-mesh
strainer into a bowl, pressing
on the solids to extract all
the liquid. Discard the shells.

2. Build the Soup Base
   Wipe out the pot and heat the
remaining 1 tbsp oil over
medium. Add leeks and pancetta
and cook until the leeks soften
and begin to brown—about 8
minutes. Stir in tomato paste,
garlic, salt, ginger,
coriander, turmeric, and red
pepper flakes. Cook until
fragrant—about 1 minute. Pour
in the shrimp broth and clam
juice, scraping up any browned
bits. Simmer for 15 to 20
minutes to let the flavors
meld.

3. Add the Seafood
   Turn the heat down to a gentle
simmer. Add scallops and cook
for 2 minutes. Stir in shrimp
and cook until just opaque—
about 2 minutes more. Turn off
the heat, add squid, cover, and
let sit for 1 to 2 minutes
until opaque and just tender.

4. Finish and Serve
   Stir in the parsley. Taste and
season with more salt and
pepper as needed. Ladle into
bowls and finish with a drizzle
of olive oil.

This soup is perfect with warm,
crusty bread—or just as is, spooned
straight from the bowl.

Salads

GREEN SALADS

Basic Green Salad

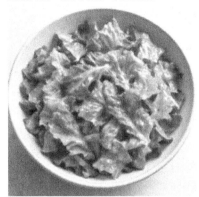

Serves 4 | Fast | Vegetarian
Ingredients
- ½ garlic clove, peeled
- 8 oz (about 8 cups) lettuce, torn into bite-size pieces if needed
- Extra-virgin olive oil
- Vinegar (any kind you like—red wine, balsamic, or sherry)
- Salt and pepper

How to Make It
1. Rub the inside of your salad bowl with the garlic clove to lightly scent it, then discard the garlic.
2. Add the lettuce to the bowl.
3. Slowly drizzle a small amount of olive oil over the greens— use your thumb to control the pour. Toss the greens gently.
4. Keep adding oil and tossing just until the leaves are lightly coated and glistening, not greasy.
5. Sprinkle with a little vinegar, salt, and pepper to taste. Toss gently again to coat.

Serve right away while the greens are fresh and crisp.

Tricolor Salad with Balsamic Vinaigrette

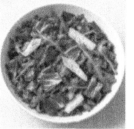

Serves 4 to 6 | Fast | Vegetarian
Ingredients
- 1 small head radicchio (about 6 oz), cored and chopped into 1-inch pieces
- 1 head Belgian endive (about 4 oz), chopped into 2-inch pieces
- 3 oz (about 3 cups) baby arugula
- 1 tbsp balsamic vinegar
- 1 tsp red wine vinegar
- Salt and pepper
- 3 tbsp extra-virgin olive oil

How to Make It
1. In a large bowl, combine the radicchio, endive, and arugula.
2. In a small bowl, whisk together the balsamic vinegar, red wine vinegar, ⅛ tsp salt, and a pinch of pepper.
3. While whisking, slowly drizzle in the olive oil to form a smooth vinaigrette.
4. Drizzle the dressing over the salad and gently toss to coat.
5. Taste and adjust seasoning with more salt and pepper if needed.

Serve right away for the freshest flavor and texture.

Green Salad with Marcona Almonds and Manchego Cheese

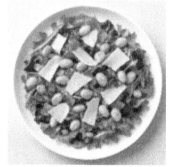

Serves 4 to 6 | Fast | Vegetarian
Ingredients

- 6 oz (about 6 cups) mesclun greens
- 5 tsp sherry vinegar
- 1 shallot, minced
- 1 tsp Dijon mustard
- Salt and pepper
- ¼ cup extra-virgin olive oil
- ⅓ cup Marcona almonds, coarsely chopped
- 2 oz Manchego cheese, shaved

How to Make It

1. Place the mesclun greens in a large bowl.
2. In a small bowl, whisk together the sherry vinegar, minced shallot, Dijon mustard, ¼ tsp salt, and ¼ tsp pepper.
3. While whisking, slowly drizzle in the olive oil until the dressing is well blended.
4. Pour the vinaigrette over the greens and toss gently until evenly coated.
5. Taste and adjust with more salt and pepper if needed.
6. Plate the salad and top each portion with Marcona almonds and shaved Manchego cheese.

Serve right away for the best texture and flavor.

Arugula Salad with Fennel and Shaved Parmesan

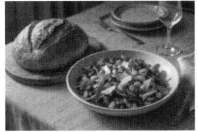

Serves 4 to 6 | Fast | Vegetarian

Ingredients
- 6 oz (about 6 cups) baby arugula
- 1 large fennel bulb, stalks removed, halved, cored, and thinly sliced
- 1½ tbsp lemon juice
- 1 small shallot, minced
- 1 tsp Dijon mustard
- 1 tsp fresh thyme, minced
- 1 small garlic clove, minced
- Salt and pepper

- ¼ cup extra-virgin olive oil
- 1 oz Parmesan cheese, shaved

Instructions

1. Add arugula and fennel to a large bowl.
2. In a small bowl, whisk together lemon juice, shallot, mustard, thyme, garlic, a pinch of salt, and pepper.
3. Slowly drizzle in the olive oil while whisking until the dressing is smooth.
4. Pour the vinaigrette over the greens and toss gently to coat.
5. Taste and adjust with more salt and pepper if needed.
6. Top each plate with shaved Parmesan and serve right away.

Light, zesty, and super simple—this one's a keeper.

SALAD DRESSINGS

Lemon Vinaigrette

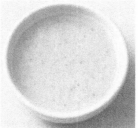

Makes ¼ cup | Fast | Vegetarian

This light and tangy dressing is perfect for delicate greens. A touch of mayo and mustard help it emulsify smoothly, while lemon zest and juice bring bright, fresh flavor.

Ingredients
- ¼ tsp grated lemon zest
- 1 tbsp fresh lemon juice
- ½ tsp mayonnaise
- ½ tsp Dijon mustard
- ⅛ tsp salt
- Pinch of pepper
- Pinch of sugar
- 3 tbsp extra-virgin olive oil

How to Make It

1. In a small bowl, whisk together the lemon zest and juice, mayo, mustard, salt, pepper, and sugar until smooth.

2. While whisking, slowly drizzle
   in the olive oil until the
   vinaigrette is fully blended
   and emulsified.

Use right away, or store in the
fridge for up to 2 weeks—just give
it a good stir before using again.

Balsamic-Mustard Vinaigrette

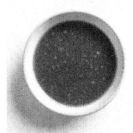

Makes ¼ cup | Fast | Vegetarian
Ingredients

- 1 tbsp balsamic vinegar
- 2 tsp Dijon mustard
- 1½ tsp minced shallot
- ½ tsp mayonnaise
- ½ tsp fresh thyme, minced
- ⅛ tsp salt
- Pinch of pepper
- 3 tbsp extra-virgin olive oil

How to Make It
1. In a small bowl, whisk together
   the vinegar, mustard, shallot,
   mayonnaise, thyme, salt, and
   pepper until well combined.
2. While whisking, slowly drizzle
   in the olive oil until the
   dressing is smooth and
   emulsified.

Keep in the fridge for up to 2
weeks. Give it a quick whisk before
using again.

Walnut Vinaigrette

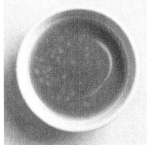

Makes ¼ cup | Fast | Vegetarian
Ingredients

- 1 tbsp wine vinegar (red or
  white)

- 1½ tsp minced shallot
- ½ tsp mayonnaise
- ½ tsp Dijon mustard
- ⅛ tsp salt
- Pinch of pepper
- 1½ tbsp roasted walnut oil
- 1½ tbsp extra-virgin olive oil

How to Make It
1. In a small bowl, whisk together
   the vinegar, shallot,
   mayonnaise, mustard, salt, and
   pepper until smooth.
2. Slowly drizzle in the walnut
   oil and olive oil while
   whisking constantly, until
   fully emulsified.

Store in the fridge for up to 2
weeks. Stir or shake before using.

Herb Vinaigrette

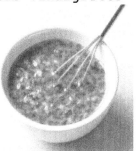

Makes ¼ cup | Fast | Vegetarian
Ingredients

- 1 tbsp wine vinegar (red or
  white)
- 1 tbsp minced fresh parsley or
  chives
- 1½ tsp minced shallot
- ½ tsp minced fresh thyme,
  tarragon, marjoram, or oregano
- ½ tsp mayonnaise
- ½ tsp Dijon mustard
- ⅛ tsp salt
- Pinch of pepper
- 3 tbsp extra-virgin olive oil

How to Make It
1. In a small bowl, whisk together
   the vinegar, herbs, shallot,
   mayo, mustard, salt, and pepper
   until smooth.
2. While whisking, slowly drizzle
   in the olive oil until the
   vinaigrette is well blended and
   emulsified.

Use immediately for the freshest flavor.

Tahini-Lemon Dressing

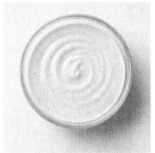

Makes about ½ cup | Fast | Vegetarian

Ingredients
- 2½ tbsp lemon juice
- 2 tbsp tahini
- 1 tbsp water
- 1 garlic clove, minced
- ½ tsp salt
- ⅛ tsp pepper
- ¼ cup extra-virgin olive oil

How to Make It
1. In a small bowl, whisk together the lemon juice, tahini, water, garlic, salt, and pepper until smooth.
2. While whisking, slowly drizzle in the olive oil until the dressing is creamy and fully emulsified

Refrigerate for up to 1 week. Stir before using if it separates.

VEGETABLE SALADS

Arugula Salad with Figs, Prosciutto, Walnuts, and Parmesan

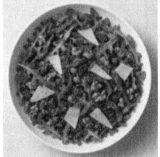

Serves 6 | Fast

Ingredients
- ¼ cup extra-virgin olive oil
- 2 oz thinly sliced prosciutto, cut into ¼-inch-wide ribbons
- 3 tbsp balsamic vinegar
- 1 tbsp raspberry jam (or honey)
- 1 small shallot, minced
- Salt and pepper
- ½ cup dried figs, stemmed and chopped
- 8 oz (about 8 cups) baby arugula
- ½ cup walnuts, toasted and chopped
- 2 oz Parmesan cheese, shaved

How to Make It
1. Crisp the Prosciutto
   Heat 1 tbsp oil in a nonstick skillet over medium heat. Add prosciutto and cook, stirring often, until crisp—about 7 minutes. Transfer to a paper towel-lined plate and set aside.
2. Make the Vinaigrette
   In a large bowl, whisk together balsamic vinegar, raspberry jam, shallot, ¼ tsp salt, and ⅛ tsp pepper. Stir in chopped figs, cover the bowl, and microwave until steaming—about 1 minute. Whisk in the remaining 3 tbsp olive oil slowly until the dressing emulsifies. Let sit for 15 minutes to allow the figs to soften and the flavors to meld.
3. Toss and Serve
   Re-whisk the vinaigrette just before serving. Add arugula and toss gently to coat. Season to taste with salt and pepper. Plate and top each serving with the crisped prosciutto, chopped walnuts, and shaved Parmesan.

This salad is bold, elegant, and comes together quickly—perfect for a dinner party or a special lunch.

Arugula Salad with Pear, Almonds, Goat Cheese, and Apricots

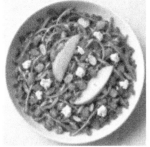

Serves 6 | Fast | Vegetarian

Ingredients

- 3 tbsp white wine vinegar
- 1 tbsp apricot jam (or honey)
- 1 small shallot, minced
- Salt and pepper
- ½ cup dried apricots, chopped
- 3 tbsp extra-virgin olive oil
- ¼ small red onion, thinly sliced
- 8 oz (about 8 cups) baby arugula
- 1 ripe but firm pear, halved, cored, and sliced ¼ inch thick
- ⅓ cup sliced almonds, toasted
- 3 oz goat cheese, crumbled (about ¾ cup)

How to Make It

1. Make the Dressing
   In a large bowl, whisk together vinegar, apricot jam, shallot, ¼ tsp salt, and ⅛ tsp pepper. Stir in the chopped apricots, cover the bowl, and microwave until steaming—about 1 minute. Slowly whisk in the olive oil until emulsified. Stir in the red onion and let sit for about 15 minutes, until the apricots soften and the dressing cools.
2. Toss and Serve
   Re-whisk the vinaigrette just before using. Add the arugula and sliced pear to the bowl and gently toss to coat. Season to taste with more salt and pepper if needed. Plate the salad and top each serving with toasted almonds and crumbled goat cheese.

Light, flavorful, and full of texture—this salad is perfect on its own or served alongside roasted meats or grilled chicken.

Asparagus and Arugula Salad with Cannellini Beans

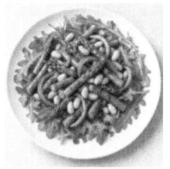

Serves 4 to 6 | Fast | Vegetarian

Ingredients

- 5 tbsp extra-virgin olive oil
- ½ red onion, thinly sliced
- 1 lb asparagus, trimmed and sliced on the bias into 1-inch pieces (use spears no thicker than ½ inch)
- Salt and pepper
- 1 (15-oz) can cannellini beans, rinsed
- 2 tbsp + 2 tsp balsamic vinegar
- 6 oz (about 6 cups) baby arugula

How to Make It

1. Cook the Veggies
   Heat 2 tbsp oil in a 12-inch nonstick skillet over high heat until just smoking. Add the onion and cook until lightly browned, about 1 minute. Stir in asparagus, ¼ tsp salt, and ¼ tsp pepper. Cook, stirring occasionally, until browned and crisp-tender—about 4 minutes. Transfer to a bowl, stir in the beans, and let cool slightly.
2. Make the Dressing
   In a small bowl, whisk together the balsamic vinegar, ¼ tsp salt, and ⅛ tsp pepper. While whisking, slowly drizzle in the remaining 3 tbsp oil until emulsified.
3. Assemble the Salad
   Toss arugula with 2 tbsp of the dressing and season with salt and pepper to taste. Divide among plates. Toss the asparagus mixture with the remaining dressing and spoon

over the arugula. Serve right
away.

Asparagus, Red Pepper, and Spinach Salad with Goat Cheese

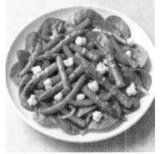

Serves 4 to 6 | Fast | Vegetarian
Ingredients
- 5 tbsp extra-virgin olive oil
- 1 red bell pepper, stemmed, seeded, and cut into 2-inch matchsticks
- 1 lb asparagus, trimmed and cut on the bias into 1-inch pieces
- Salt and pepper
- 1 shallot, halved and thinly sliced
- 1 tbsp + 1 tsp sherry vinegar
- 1 garlic clove, minced
- 6 oz (about 6 cups) baby spinach
- 2 oz goat cheese, crumbled (about ½ cup)

How to Make It
1. Sauté the Veggies
   Heat 1 tbsp oil in a 12-inch skillet over high heat. Add bell pepper and cook until lightly browned, about 2 minutes. Add asparagus, ¼ tsp salt, and ⅛ tsp pepper. Cook for 2 more minutes, stirring occasionally. Stir in the shallot and cook until softened and asparagus is just tender, about 1 more minute. Transfer to a bowl and let cool slightly.
2. Make the Dressing
   Whisk vinegar, garlic, ¼ tsp salt, and ⅛ tsp pepper together. Slowly whisk in the remaining ¼ cup olive oil.
3. Build the Salad
   Toss spinach with 2 tbsp of the dressing and season with

salt and pepper to taste. Divide onto plates. Toss the asparagus mixture with the remaining dressing and spoon over the spinach. Top with crumbled goat cheese and serve.

Citrus Salad with Radicchio, Dates, and Smoked Almonds

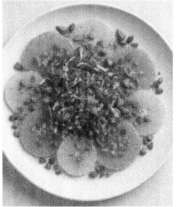

Serves 4 to 6 | Fast | Vegetarian
Ingredients
- 2 red grapefruits
- 3 oranges (navel, Cara Cara, or tangelos work best)
- 1 tsp sugar
- Salt and pepper
- 3 tbsp extra-virgin olive oil
- 1 small shallot, minced
- 1 tsp Dijon mustard
- 1 small head radicchio (about 6 oz), cored and thinly sliced
- ⅔ cup chopped pitted dates
- ½ cup smoked almonds, chopped coarse

How to Make It
1. Prep the Citrus
   Cut away the peel and white pith from the grapefruits and oranges. Halve each fruit from top to bottom, then slice crosswise into ¼-inch rounds. Transfer the slices to a bowl and toss with the sugar and ½ tsp salt. Let sit for 15 minutes to draw out excess juice.
2. Make the Vinaigrette
   Drain the fruit in a fine-mesh strainer set over a bowl, reserving 2 tbsp of the juice. Arrange the drained citrus slices on a serving platter and

drizzle with olive oil. In a separate bowl, whisk the reserved juice with the minced shallot and mustard.

3. Assemble the Salad
   Add radicchio, ⅓ cup of the dates, and ¼ cup of the almonds to the vinaigrette and toss gently to coat. Season with salt and pepper to taste. Spoon the radicchio mixture over the citrus slices, leaving a 1-inch border of fruit around the edge. Sprinkle the salad with the remaining dates and almonds.

Serve immediately for the freshest flavor and best texture.

Bitter Greens Salad with Olives and Feta

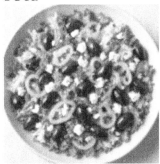

Serves 4 to 6 | Fast | Vegetarian
Ingredients

- 1 head escarole (about 1 lb), trimmed and chopped into 1-inch pieces
- 1 small head frisée (about 4 oz), trimmed and torn into 1-inch pieces
- ½ cup pitted kalamata olives, halved
- 2 oz feta cheese, crumbled (about ½ cup)
- ⅓ cup pepperoncini, seeded and sliced into ¼-inch strips (leave seeds in for extra heat)
- ⅓ cup chopped fresh dill
- 2 tbsp lemon juice
- 1 garlic clove, minced
- Salt and pepper
- 3 tbsp extra-virgin olive oil

How to Make It

1. In a large bowl, gently toss together the escarole, frisée, olives, feta, and pepperoncini.

2. In a small bowl, whisk together the dill, lemon juice, garlic, ¼ tsp salt, and ⅛ tsp pepper.
3. While whisking, slowly drizzle in the olive oil until the vinaigrette is fully blended.
4. Pour the dressing over the salad and toss gently to coat.

Serve immediately for maximum crunch and freshness.

Kale Salad with Sweet Potatoes and Pomegranate Vinaigrette

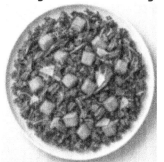

Serves 6 to 8 | Vegetarian
Ingredients
Salad

- 1½ lbs sweet potatoes, peeled and cut into ½-inch pieces
- 2 tsp extra-virgin olive oil
- Salt and pepper
- 12 oz Tuscan kale, stems removed, sliced into ½-inch strips (about 7 cups)
- ½ head radicchio (about 5 oz), cored and thinly sliced
- ⅓ cup toasted pecans, chopped
- Shaved Parmesan, to taste

Pomegranate Vinaigrette

- 2 tbsp water
- 1½ tbsp pomegranate molasses (or see note for substitute)
- 1 small shallot, minced
- 1 tbsp honey
- 1 tbsp cider vinegar
- ¼ tsp salt
- ¼ tsp pepper
- ¼ cup extra-virgin olive oil

How to Make It

1. Roast the Sweet Potatoes
   Preheat oven to 400°F and adjust rack to the middle position. Toss sweet potatoes with olive oil, salt, and pepper. Spread in a single layer on a baking sheet and

roast for 25–30 minutes, flipping halfway through, until golden and tender. Let cool for 20 minutes.
2. Massage the Kale
   Meanwhile, place kale in a large bowl and massage it with your hands—firmly squeeze and rub—for about 1 minute, until the leaves darken and feel softer.
3. Make the Vinaigrette
   In a large bowl, whisk together water, pomegranate molasses, shallot, honey, vinegar, salt, and pepper. While whisking, slowly drizzle in the olive oil until well blended.
4. Assemble the Salad
   Add the cooled sweet potatoes, massaged kale, and sliced radicchio to the bowl with the vinaigrette. Gently toss to coat. Taste and season with additional salt and pepper if needed. Transfer to a serving platter and top with chopped pecans and shaved Parmesan.

Tip: If you can't find pomegranate molasses, you can make a quick substitute by simmering pomegranate juice with a little sugar and lemon juice until thickened.

Mâche Salad with Cucumber and Mint

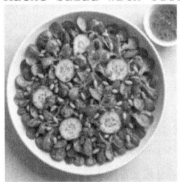

Serves 6 to 8 | Fast | Vegetarian
Ingredients
- 12 oz (about 12 cups) mâche
- 1 cucumber, thinly sliced
- ½ cup fresh mint, chopped
- ⅓ cup pine nuts, toasted
- 1 tbsp lemon juice
- 1 tbsp fresh parsley, minced

- 1 tbsp capers, rinsed and minced
- 1 tsp fresh thyme, minced
- 1 garlic clove, minced
- ¼ tsp salt
- ¼ tsp black pepper
- ¼ cup extra-virgin olive oil

How to Make It
1. Mix the Salad
   In a large bowl, gently toss together the mâche, cucumber, mint, and pine nuts.
2. Make the Dressing
   In a small bowl, whisk together the lemon juice, parsley, capers, thyme, garlic, salt, and pepper. While whisking, slowly drizzle in the olive oil until the dressing is smooth and emulsified.
3. Toss and Serve
   Drizzle the vinaigrette over the salad and gently toss to coat. Season with more salt and pepper to taste, and serve right away.

Salade Niçoise

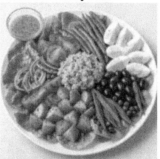

Serves 6
Ingredients
Dressing
- ¼ cup lemon juice (from about 2 lemons)
- 1 shallot, minced
- 2 tbsp fresh basil, minced
- 2 tsp each: fresh thyme and fresh oregano, minced
- 1 tsp Dijon mustard
- ½ tsp salt
- ¼ tsp pepper
- ½ cup extra-virgin olive oil
Salad
- 1¼ lbs small red potatoes, unpeeled and quartered

- Salt and pepper
- 2 tbsp dry vermouth
- 2 heads Boston or Bibb lettuce (about 1 lb), torn into bite-size pieces
- 2 (5-oz) cans solid white tuna in water, drained and flaked
- 3 small tomatoes, cored and cut into ½-inch wedges
- 1 small red onion, thinly sliced
- 8 oz green beans, trimmed and halved
- 3 hard-cooked eggs, peeled and quartered
- ¼ cup pitted niçoise olives
- 10-12 anchovy fillets, rinsed (optional)
- 2 tbsp capers, rinsed (optional)

How to Make It
1. Make the Dressing
   In a small bowl, whisk together the lemon juice, shallot, basil, thyme, oregano, mustard, salt, and pepper. Slowly drizzle in olive oil while whisking until the dressing is emulsified. Set aside.
2. Cook and Dress the Potatoes
   In a large saucepan, cover potatoes with water by 1 inch. Bring to a boil over high heat. Add 1 tbsp salt, reduce heat, and simmer until tender, 5-8 minutes. Transfer potatoes to a bowl using a slotted spoon (keep the water). Toss warm potatoes with ¼ cup vinaigrette and vermouth. Season with salt and pepper. Set aside.
3. Prepare the Lettuce and Tuna
   Toss lettuce with ¼ cup vinaigrette and arrange in a bed on a large platter. In the same bowl, toss tuna with ¼ cup vinaigrette and mound it in the center of the lettuce.
4. Tomatoes and Onion
   In the same bowl, toss tomatoes and onion with 2 tbsp vinaigrette. Season with salt and pepper and arrange in a mound on the platter.
5. Cook and Dress the Green Beans
   Bring the reserved water back to a boil. Add 1 tbsp salt and green beans. Cook until just tender, 3-5 minutes. Transfer to ice water to cool, then dry thoroughly. Toss beans with remaining 2 tbsp vinaigrette and arrange on platter.
6. Finish the Salad
   Add mounds of the dressed potatoes, eggs, olives, and anchovies (if using) around the platter. Sprinkle the whole salad with capers, if using.

Serve immediately, and let everyone admire before digging in.

Spinach Salad with Feta and Pistachios

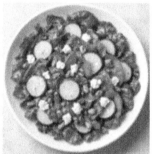

Serves 6 | Fast | Vegetarian
Ingredients
- 1½ oz feta cheese, crumbled (about ⅓ cup)
- 3 tbsp extra-virgin olive oil
- 1 (2-inch) strip lemon zest + 1½ tbsp lemon juice
- 1 shallot, minced
- 2 tsp sugar
- 10 oz curly-leaf spinach, stemmed and torn into bite-size pieces
- 6 radishes, thinly sliced
- 3 tbsp chopped toasted pistachios
- Salt and pepper

How to Make It
1. Chill the Feta
   Place the crumbled feta on a plate and freeze for about 15 minutes to firm it up.
2. Make the Warm Dressing
   In a Dutch oven, heat the olive oil, lemon zest, shallot,

and sugar over medium-low heat until the shallot softens—about 5 minutes. Remove from heat, discard the zest, and stir in the lemon juice.

3. Wilt the Spinach
   Add the spinach to the pot, cover, and let it sit off the heat for about 30 seconds until just beginning to wilt.

4. Assemble the Salad
   Transfer the spinach and any dressing from the pot to a large bowl. Add the radishes, pistachios, and chilled feta. Toss gently to combine. Season with salt and pepper to taste.

Serve right away while warm for the best texture and flavor.

Seared Tuna Salad with Olive Dressing

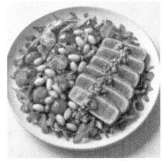

Serves 4 to 6 | Fast
Ingredients
- ½ cup pimento-stuffed green olives, chopped
- 3 tbsp lemon juice
- 1 tbsp fresh parsley, chopped
- 1 garlic clove, minced
- 6 tbsp extra-virgin olive oil
- Salt and pepper
- 2 (12-oz) tuna steaks, 1 to 1¼ inches thick
- 5 oz (about 5 cups) baby arugula
- 12 oz cherry tomatoes, halved
- 1 (15-oz) can cannellini beans, rinsed

How to Make It
1. Make the Dressing
   In a large bowl, whisk together olives, lemon juice, parsley, and garlic. While whisking, slowly drizzle in 5 tbsp olive oil until the dressing is emulsified. Season with salt and pepper to taste.

2. Sear the Tuna
   Pat the tuna dry and season with salt and pepper. Heat the remaining 1 tbsp oil in a 12-inch nonstick skillet over medium-high heat until just smoking. Sear the tuna about 2 minutes per side, until browned on the outside and still red in the center (110°F for rare). Transfer to a cutting board and slice into ½-inch-thick pieces.

3. Assemble the Salad
   Re-whisk the dressing if needed. Drizzle 1 tbsp of the dressing over the sliced tuna. Add arugula, cherry tomatoes, and cannellini beans to the remaining dressing in the bowl and toss gently to combine. Season to taste with salt and pepper.

4. Serve
   Divide the salad among plates and top with the sliced tuna. Serve immediately for the freshest flavor and best texture.

Asparagus Salad with Oranges, Feta, and Hazelnuts

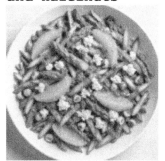

Serves 4 to 6 | Fast | Vegetarian
Ingredients
Pesto
- 2 cups fresh mint leaves
- ¼ cup fresh basil leaves
- ¼ cup grated Pecorino Romano
- 1 tsp lemon zest + 2 tsp lemon juice
- 1 garlic clove, minced
- ¾ tsp salt, plus more to taste
- ½ cup extra-virgin olive oil
- Pepper, to taste

Salad
- 2 lbs thick asparagus, trimmed
- 2 oranges, peeled and segmented
- 4 oz feta cheese, crumbled (about 1 cup)
- ¾ cup hazelnuts, toasted, skinned, and chopped
- Salt and pepper

How to Make It
1. Make the Pesto
   In a food processor, combine mint, basil, Pecorino, lemon zest and juice, garlic, and ¾ tsp salt. Pulse until finely chopped, about 20 seconds, scraping down sides as needed. Transfer to a large bowl. Stir in olive oil and season with salt and pepper to taste.
2. Prep the Salad
   Cut asparagus tips into ¾-inch pieces. Slice the stalks thinly on a diagonal (about ⅛ inch thick) into 2-inch pieces.
   Cut away the peel and pith from the oranges. Over a bowl to catch the juice, cut between the membranes to release segments.
3. Assemble
   Add sliced asparagus, orange segments, crumbled feta, and chopped hazelnuts to the bowl with pesto. Gently toss to coat everything evenly. Season with salt and pepper to taste.

Serve immediately for a crisp, colorful, and refreshing salad.

Roasted Beet Salad with Blood Oranges and Almonds

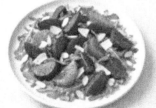

Serves 4 to 6 | Vegetarian
Ingredients
- 2 lbs beets (similar size, 2-3 inches), trimmed
- 4 tsp sherry vinegar
- Salt and pepper
- 2 tbsp extra-virgin olive oil
- 2 blood oranges (or substitute with 1 large navel orange or tangelo)
- 2 oz baby arugula (about 2 cups)
- 2 oz ricotta salata cheese, shaved
- 2 tbsp sliced almonds, toasted

How to Make It
1. Roast the Beets
   Preheat oven to 400°F and adjust rack to the middle position. Wrap each beet individually in foil and place on a rimmed baking sheet. Roast until a skewer slides into the center with little resistance—about 45 to 60 minutes. Larger beets may take longer.
2. Peel and Slice
   Unwrap and let beets cool just enough to handle. Use a paper towel to rub off the skins. Slice beets into ½-inch wedges. If they're large, cut the wedges in half.
3. Make the Dressing
   In a large bowl, whisk together vinegar, ¼ tsp salt, and ¼ tsp pepper. While whisking, slowly drizzle in olive oil to emulsify. Add warm beets and toss to coat. Let cool to room temperature, about 20 minutes.
4. Prep the Oranges
   Slice off peel and pith from oranges. Cut into quarters, then slice into ½-inch thick pieces.
5. Assemble the Salad
   Add oranges and arugula to the bowl with the beets and toss gently. Season with more salt and pepper to taste. Transfer to a serving platter and top with shaved ricotta salata and toasted almonds.

Serve at room temperature for the best flavor and texture.

Fava Bean and Radish Salad

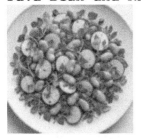

Serves 4 to 6 | Fast | Vegetarian
Ingredients
- 3 lbs fava beans in pods, shelled (about 3 cups beans)
- 3 tbsp lemon juice
- 2 garlic cloves, minced
- ½ tsp salt
- ¼ tsp pepper
- ¼ tsp ground coriander
- ¼ cup extra-virgin olive oil
- 10 radishes, halved and thinly sliced
- 1½ oz (about 1½ cups) pea shoots
- ¼ cup fresh basil, chopped

How to Make It
1. Blanch the Fava Beans
   Bring a large pot of water to a boil. Meanwhile, prepare a large bowl of ice water. Add shelled fava beans to the boiling water and cook for 1 minute. Drain and transfer immediately to the ice bath to cool—about 2 minutes. Pat dry on paper towels.
2. Peel the Beans
   Use a paring knife to make a small slit in the waxy coating of each bean, then gently squeeze to pop the bean out. Discard the outer sheaths.
3. Make the Dressing
   In a large bowl, whisk together the lemon juice, garlic, salt, pepper, and coriander. While whisking, slowly drizzle in the olive oil until combined.
4. Toss the Salad
   Add the peeled fava beans, sliced radishes, pea shoots, and basil to the bowl with the vinaigrette. Toss gently to coat everything evenly.

Serve right away for maximum freshness and crunch.

Green Bean Salad with Cilantro Sauce

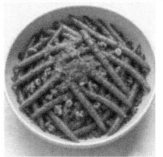

Serves 6 to 8 | Fast | Vegetarian
Ingredients
- ¼ cup walnuts
- 2 garlic cloves, unpeeled
- 2½ cups fresh cilantro leaves and tender stems (from about 2 bunches)
- ½ cup extra-virgin olive oil
- 4 tsp lemon juice
- 1 scallion, thinly sliced
- Salt and pepper
- 2 lbs green beans, trimmed

How to Make It
1. Toast the Nuts and Garlic
   In a small skillet over medium heat, toast the walnuts and garlic cloves, stirring often, until fragrant and golden—about 5 to 7 minutes. Transfer to a bowl. Let garlic cool slightly, then peel and roughly chop.
2. Make the Cilantro Sauce
   In a food processor, blend the toasted walnuts, garlic, cilantro, olive oil, lemon juice, scallion, ½ tsp salt, and ⅛ tsp pepper until smooth, about 1 minute. Scrape down the sides as needed. Transfer to a large bowl.
3. Blanch the Green Beans
   Bring a large pot of water to a boil. While it heats, fill a large bowl with ice water. Add 1 tbsp salt to the boiling water and cook the green beans until crisp-tender, 3 to 5 minutes. Drain and transfer to the ice water to chill, about 2 minutes. Drain again.

4. Toss and Serve
   Add the cooled green beans to the bowl with the cilantro sauce and toss gently to coat. Season with salt and pepper to taste.

Serve right away, or refrigerate for up to 4 hours for a cool, refreshing make-ahead side.

Brussels Sprout Salad with Pecorino and Pine Nuts

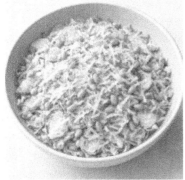

Serves 4 to 6 | Fast | Vegetarian

Ingredients
- 2 tbsp lemon juice
- 1 tbsp Dijon mustard
- 1 small shallot, minced
- 1 garlic clove, minced
- ½ tsp salt
- ¼ cup extra-virgin olive oil
- 1 lb Brussels sprouts, trimmed, halved, and very thinly sliced
- 2 oz Pecorino Romano, shredded (about ⅔ cup)
- ¼ cup pine nuts, toasted
- Black pepper, to taste

How to Make It
1. Make the Dressing
   In a large bowl, whisk together the lemon juice, mustard, shallot, garlic, and salt. While whisking, slowly drizzle in the olive oil until fully combined.
2. Toss and Marinate
   Add the sliced Brussels sprouts to the bowl and toss well to coat. Let the mixture sit for at least 30 minutes or up to 2 hours to soften and absorb flavor.

3. Finish the Salad
   Just before serving, stir in the shredded Pecorino and toasted pine nuts. Season with additional salt and black pepper to taste.
Serve chilled or at room temperature for a fresh, nutty, and tangy side salad.

Moroccan-Style Carrot Salad

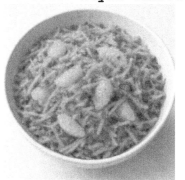

Serves 4 to 6 | Fast | Vegetarian
Ingredients
- 2 oranges
- 1 tbsp lemon juice
- 1 tsp honey
- ¾ tsp ground cumin
- ⅛ tsp cayenne pepper
- ⅛ tsp ground cinnamon
- Salt and pepper
- 1 lb carrots, peeled and shredded (use large holes of a box grater)
- 3 tbsp fresh cilantro, minced
- 3 tbsp extra-virgin olive oil

How to Make It
1. Prep the Oranges
   Cut off the peel and pith from both oranges. Working over a large bowl, slice between the membranes to release the segments. Cut segments in half crosswise and place in a fine-mesh strainer set over the bowl to collect the juice.
2. Make the Dressing
   To the reserved orange juice, whisk in the lemon juice, honey, cumin, cayenne, cinnamon, and ½ tsp salt.
3. Toss and Marinate
   Add the drained orange pieces and shredded carrots to the dressing. Toss gently to coat

and let sit for 3 to 5 minutes,
until some liquid collects in
the bottom of the bowl.
4. Drain and Finish
   Drain the salad again using
   the strainer, then return it to
   the bowl. Stir in cilantro and
   olive oil. Season with
   additional salt and pepper to
   taste.
Serve chilled or at room
temperature.

North African Cauliflower Salad with Chermoula

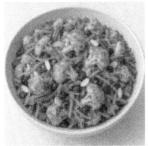

Serves 4 to 6 | Vegetarian

Ingredients
Salad
- 1 head cauliflower (about 2
  lbs), cored and cut into 2-inch
  florets
- 2 tbsp extra-virgin olive oil
- Salt and pepper
- ½ red onion, sliced ¼ inch
  thick
- 1 cup shredded carrot (use
  large holes of box grater)
- ½ cup raisins
- 2 tbsp chopped fresh cilantro
- 2 tbsp sliced almonds, toasted

Chermoula
- ¾ cup fresh cilantro leaves
- ¼ cup extra-virgin olive oil
- 2 tbsp lemon juice
- 4 garlic cloves, minced
- ½ tsp ground cumin
- ½ tsp paprika
- ¼ tsp salt
- ⅛ tsp cayenne pepper

How to Make It
1. Roast the Vegetables
   Preheat oven to 475°F and
   place rack in the lowest
   position. Toss cauliflower

florets with 2 tbsp olive oil,
salt, and pepper. Spread in a
single layer on a parchment-
lined baking sheet and cover
tightly with foil. Roast for 5
to 7 minutes.
   Remove foil, scatter sliced
onion over the cauliflower, and
roast uncovered for 10 to 15
minutes more, stirring halfway
through, until cauliflower is
golden and onions are slightly
charred.
2. Make the Chermoula
   While the vegetables roast,
blend all chermoula ingredients
in a food processor until
smooth, about 1 minute. Scrape
down sides as needed. Transfer
to a large bowl.
3. Assemble the Salad
   Let the roasted vegetables
cool slightly (about 5
minutes), then toss them with
the chermoula, shredded carrot,
raisins, and cilantro until
well coated. Transfer to a
serving platter and sprinkle
with toasted almonds.
Serve warm or at room temperature—
either way, it's packed with bold
flavor and texture.

Mediterranean Chopped Salad

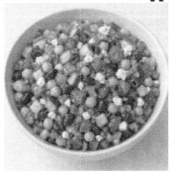

Serves 4 | Vegetarian
Ingredients
- 1 cucumber, peeled, halved
  lengthwise, seeded, and chopped
  into ½-inch pieces
- 10 oz grape tomatoes, quartered
  (or cherry tomatoes)
- Salt and pepper
- 3 tbsp red wine vinegar
- 1 garlic clove, minced
- 3 tbsp extra-virgin olive oil
- 1 (15-oz) can chickpeas, rinsed

- ½ cup pitted kalamata olives, chopped
- ½ small red onion, finely chopped
- ½ cup chopped fresh parsley
- 1 romaine heart (6 oz), chopped into ½-inch pieces
- 4 oz feta cheese, crumbled (about 1 cup)

How to Make It
1. Prep the Veggies
   Toss the cucumber and tomatoes with 1 tsp salt and let them drain in a colander for 15 minutes to release excess moisture.
2. Make the Dressing
   In a large bowl, whisk together the red wine vinegar and garlic. Slowly whisk in the olive oil until combined.
3. Marinate the Mix
   Add the drained cucumber and tomato, along with the chickpeas, olives, onion, and parsley, to the bowl. Toss to coat with the dressing. Let sit for 5 to 20 minutes for the flavors to meld.
4. Finish the Salad
   Add chopped romaine and crumbled feta. Toss gently to combine. Season with salt and pepper to taste.

Serve right away for the best crunch and freshness.

Sesame-Lemon Cucumber Salad

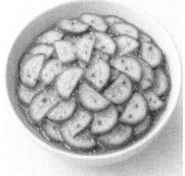

Serves 4 | Vegetarian
Ingredients
- 3 cucumbers, peeled, halved lengthwise, seeded, and sliced ¼ inch thick
- Salt and pepper

- ¼ cup rice vinegar
- 2 tbsp toasted sesame oil
- 1 tbsp lemon juice
- 1 tbsp sesame seeds, toasted
- 2 tsp sugar
- ⅛ tsp red pepper flakes, plus extra to taste

How to Make It
1. Drain the Cucumbers
   Toss the sliced cucumbers with 1 tbsp salt in a colander set over a large bowl. Place a gallon-sized zip-top bag filled with water on top to weigh them down. Let drain for 1 to 3 hours. Rinse and pat dry.
2. Make the Dressing
   In a large bowl, whisk together rice vinegar, sesame oil, lemon juice, sesame seeds, sugar, and red pepper flakes.
3. Toss and Serve
   Add the drained cucumbers to the dressing and toss to coat. Season with salt and pepper to taste. Serve at room temperature or chilled.

Algerian-Style Fennel, Orange, and Olive Salad

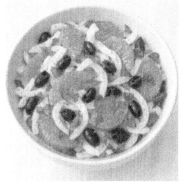

Serves 4 to 6 | Fast | Vegetarian
Ingredients
- 4 blood oranges (or 3 larger oranges like navels or Cara Caras)
- 2 fennel bulbs, stalks discarded, bulbs halved, cored, and thinly sliced
- ½ cup pitted oil-cured black olives, quartered
- ¼ cup fresh mint, coarsely chopped
- 2 tbsp lemon juice
- Salt and pepper

- ¼ cup extra-virgin olive oil

How to Make It
1. Prep the Oranges
   Cut away the peel and white pith from the oranges. Quarter the fruit, then slice crosswise into ¼-inch pieces.
2. Assemble the Salad
   In a large bowl, gently combine the orange slices, fennel, olives, and mint.
3. Make the Dressing
   In a small bowl, whisk together the lemon juice, ¼ tsp salt, and ⅛ tsp pepper. Slowly whisk in the olive oil until emulsified.
4. Toss and Serve
   Drizzle the dressing over the salad and toss gently to coat. Taste and adjust seasoning with more salt and pepper if needed.

Serve right away for the freshest flavor and texture.

Fennel and Apple Salad with Smoked Mackerel

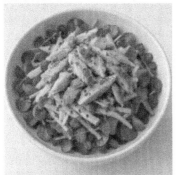

Serves 4 to 6
Ingredients
- 3 tbsp lemon juice
- 1 tbsp whole-grain mustard
- 1 small shallot, minced
- 2 tsp fresh tarragon, minced (divided)
- Salt and pepper
- ¼ cup extra-virgin olive oil
- 5 oz (about 5 cups) watercress
- 2 Granny Smith apples, peeled, cored, cut into 3-inch matchsticks
- 1 fennel bulb, stalks discarded, halved, cored, and sliced thin

- 6 oz smoked mackerel, skin and pin bones removed, flaked

How to Make It
1. Make the Dressing
   In a large bowl, whisk together lemon juice, mustard, shallot, 1 tsp tarragon, ½ tsp salt, and ¼ tsp pepper. Slowly whisk in olive oil until emulsified.
2. Toss the Salad
   Add watercress, apples, and fennel to the bowl. Toss gently to coat everything in the vinaigrette. Taste and season with more salt and pepper if needed.
3. Plate and Top with Mackerel
   Divide the salad among plates and top each with flaked mackerel. Drizzle any leftover dressing over the fish and sprinkle with the remaining 1 tsp of tarragon.

Serve immediately while everything is crisp and fresh.

Country-Style Greek Salad

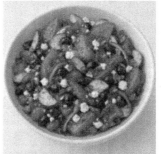

Serves 6 to 8 | Fast | Vegetarian
Ingredients
- 6 tbsp extra-virgin olive oil
- 1½ tbsp red wine vinegar
- 2 tsp fresh oregano, minced
- 1 tsp lemon juice
- 1 garlic clove, minced
- Salt and pepper
- 2 cucumbers, peeled, halved lengthwise, seeded, and thinly sliced
- ½ red onion, thinly sliced
- 6 large ripe tomatoes, cored, seeded, and cut into ½-inch wedges

- 1 cup jarred roasted red peppers, rinsed, patted dry, and cut into ½-inch strips
- ½ cup pitted kalamata olives, quartered
- ¼ cup fresh parsley, chopped
- ¼ cup fresh mint, chopped
- 5 oz feta cheese, crumbled (about 1¼ cups)

How to Make It
1. Make the Dressing & Marinate
   In a large bowl, whisk together olive oil, vinegar, oregano, lemon juice, garlic, ½ tsp salt, and ⅛ tsp pepper. Add the cucumbers and onion, toss to coat, and let sit for 20 minutes to marinate.
2. Assemble the Salad
   Add tomatoes, red peppers, olives, parsley, and mint to the bowl. Toss gently to combine everything.
3. Finish and Serve
   Taste and season with more salt and pepper if needed. Transfer to a serving platter or shallow bowl and sprinkle with feta.

Serve immediately for the freshest flavor and best texture.

Shaved Mushroom and Celery Salad

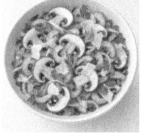

Serves 6 | Fast | Vegetarian
Ingredients
- ¼ cup extra-virgin olive oil
- 1½ tbsp lemon juice
- Salt and pepper
- 8 oz cremini mushrooms, trimmed and thinly sliced
- 1 shallot, halved and thinly sliced
- 4 celery ribs, thinly sliced
- ½ cup celery leaves (or substitute with parsley if needed)
- 2 oz Parmesan cheese, shaved

- ½ cup fresh parsley leaves
- 2 tbsp chopped fresh tarragon

How to Make It
1. Marinate the Mushrooms
   In a large bowl, whisk together olive oil, lemon juice, and ¼ tsp salt. Add mushrooms and shallot, toss to coat, and let sit for exactly 10 minutes—no longer, to avoid a watery salad.
2. Toss the Salad
   Add celery, celery leaves, Parmesan, parsley, and tarragon to the marinated mushroom mixture. Gently toss everything together.
3. Season and Serve
   Taste and adjust seasoning with salt and pepper. Serve immediately for the best texture.

This salad is all about freshness—serve it shortly after assembling to keep it crisp and flavorful.

Panzanella Salad with White Beans and Arugula

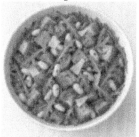

Serves 6 | Vegetarian
Ingredients
- 12 oz rustic Italian bread, cut into 1-inch pieces (about 4 cups)
- 5 tbsp extra-virgin olive oil
- Salt and pepper
- 3 tbsp red wine vinegar
- 1½ lbs ripe tomatoes, cored and chopped (reserve seeds and juice)
- 1 (15-oz) can cannellini beans, rinsed
- 1 small red onion, halved and thinly sliced
- 3 tbsp chopped fresh basil, divided

- 2 tbsp minced fresh oregano, divided
- 3 oz baby arugula (about 3 cups)
- 2 oz Parmesan cheese, shaved

How to Make It
1. Toast the Bread

   Preheat oven to 350°F. Toss bread cubes with 1 tbsp olive oil, season with salt and pepper, and spread on a rimmed baking sheet. Bake, stirring occasionally, until golden and crisp, 15-20 minutes. Let cool.

2. Make the Dressing & Marinate Veggies

   In a large bowl, whisk red wine vinegar with ¼ tsp salt. While whisking, slowly drizzle in the remaining ¼ cup oil. Stir in the chopped tomatoes with their seeds and juices, beans, onion, 1½ tbsp basil, and 1 tbsp oregano. Let marinate for 20 minutes.

3. Assemble the Salad

   Add the cooled bread, arugula, and remaining herbs to the bowl. Gently toss to combine and season with salt and pepper to taste.

4. Serve

   Transfer to a platter and top with shaved Parmesan. Serve right away for the best texture.

Fattoush

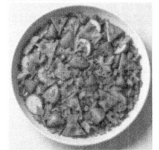

Serves 4 to 6 | Vegetarian
Ingredients
- 2 (8-inch) pita breads
- 7 tbsp extra-virgin olive oil
- Salt and pepper
- 3 tbsp lemon juice
- 4 tsp ground sumac, plus more for sprinkling

- ¼ tsp minced garlic
- 1 lb ripe tomatoes, cored and cut into ¾-inch pieces
- 1 English cucumber, peeled and thinly sliced
- 1 cup arugula, coarsely chopped
- ½ cup fresh cilantro, chopped
- ½ cup fresh mint, chopped
- 4 scallions, thinly sliced

How to Make It
1. Toast the Pita

   Preheat oven to 375°F. Cut around each pita to separate into 2 thin rounds, then cut each in half. Place smooth-side down on a wire rack over a baking sheet. Brush with 3 tbsp olive oil and season with salt and pepper. Bake until crisp and golden, about 10-14 minutes. Let cool.

2. Make the Dressing

   In a small bowl, whisk lemon juice, sumac, garlic, and ¼ tsp salt. Let sit 10 minutes. Slowly whisk in remaining ¼ cup olive oil until emulsified.

3. Assemble the Salad

   Break toasted pita into bite-size pieces and place in a large bowl. Add tomatoes, cucumber, arugula, cilantro, mint, and scallions. Drizzle with dressing and gently toss to coat. Season with salt and pepper to taste.

4. Serve

   Sprinkle individual servings with a little extra sumac for added zing. Enjoy immediately while the pita is still crisp.

French Potato Salad with Dijon and Fines Herbes

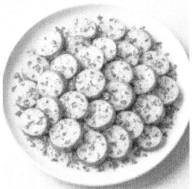

Serves 4 to 6 | Vegetarian

Ingredients
- 2 lbs small red potatoes, unpeeled, sliced ¼-inch thick
- 2 tbsp salt
- 1 garlic clove, peeled and skewered
- ¼ cup extra-virgin olive oil
- 1½ tbsp white wine vinegar or Champagne vinegar
- 2 tsp Dijon mustard
- ½ tsp pepper
- 1 small shallot, minced
- 1 tbsp minced fresh chervil*
- 1 tbsp minced fresh parsley
- 1 tbsp minced fresh chives
- 1 tsp minced fresh tarragon

*If no chervil: Add ½ tbsp more parsley + ½ tsp more tarragon.

How to Make It
1. Cook the Potatoes
   Place sliced potatoes in a large saucepan and add water to cover by 1 inch. Bring to a boil, then add salt and reduce to a simmer. Cook until just tender, about 6 minutes. Drain, reserving ¼ cup of the cooking water.
2. Blanch and Mince the Garlic
   While potatoes cook, blanch the garlic by lowering it (on a skewer) into the simmering water for 45 seconds. Rinse under cold water, remove from skewer, and mince.
3. Dress the Potatoes
   Spread warm, drained potatoes in a tight single layer on a rimmed baking sheet. In a bowl, whisk the oil, minced garlic, vinegar, mustard, pepper, and reserved cooking water. Drizzle this mixture evenly over the potatoes. Let sit for 10 minutes so the flavor soaks in.
4. Add Herbs and Finish
   Transfer potatoes to a large bowl. Combine shallot and fresh herbs in a small bowl, then gently fold into the potatoes. Season to taste with salt and pepper. Serve at room temperature.

Roasted Winter Squash Salad with Za'atar and Parsley

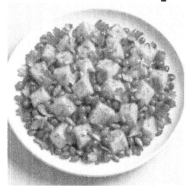

Serves 4 to 6 | Vegetarian
Ingredients
- 3 lbs butternut squash, peeled, seeded, and cut into ½-inch cubes (about 8 cups)
- ¼ cup extra-virgin olive oil, divided
- Salt and pepper
- 1 tsp za'atar (store-bought or homemade)
- 1 small shallot, minced
- 2 tbsp lemon juice
- 2 tbsp honey
- ¾ cup fresh parsley leaves
- ⅓ cup roasted, unsalted pepitas (pumpkin seeds)
- ½ cup pomegranate seeds

How to Make It
1. Roast the Squash
   Preheat oven to 450°F and position rack on the lowest level. Toss squash with 1 tbsp oil, season with salt and pepper, and spread in a single layer on a rimmed baking sheet.

Roast until browned and tender, stirring halfway through, about 30–35 minutes. Sprinkle roasted squash with za'atar and let cool for 15 minutes.

2. Make the Dressing
   In a large bowl, whisk together shallot, lemon juice, honey, and ¼ tsp salt. While whisking, slowly drizzle in the remaining 3 tbsp oil to form an emulsified vinaigrette.

3. Assemble the Salad
   Add the roasted squash, parsley, and pepitas to the bowl with the dressing and gently toss to coat. Transfer to a serving platter and sprinkle with pomegranate seeds.

Serve warm or at room temperature. Sub chopped grapes or blueberries if pomegranate seeds aren't available.

Tomato Salad with Feta and Cumin-Yogurt Dressing

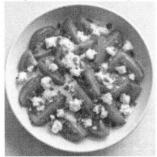

Serves 6 | Fast | Vegetarian
Ingredients
- 2½ lbs ripe tomatoes, cored and cut into ½-inch wedges
- Salt and pepper
- 1 tbsp extra-virgin olive oil
- 1 garlic clove, minced
- 1 tsp ground cumin
- ¼ cup plain Greek yogurt (not nonfat)
- 1 tbsp lemon juice
- 1 scallion, thinly sliced
- 1 tbsp fresh oregano, minced
- 3 oz feta cheese, crumbled (about ¾ cup)

How to Make It
1. Prep the Tomatoes
   Toss the tomato wedges with ½ tsp salt and let them sit in a colander over a bowl for 15–20 minutes. This draws out excess liquid and concentrates the tomato flavor.

2. Bloom the Spices
   In a small bowl, microwave the olive oil with the garlic and cumin until fragrant—about 30 seconds. Let it cool slightly.

3. Make the Dressing
   Measure 1 tbsp of the reserved tomato juice into a large bowl (discard the rest). Whisk in the yogurt, lemon juice, scallion, oregano, and the garlic-cumin oil until smooth.

4. Finish the Salad
   Add the drained tomatoes and crumbled feta to the bowl and gently toss everything to coat. Taste and season with more salt and pepper as needed.

Serve right away while the salad is fresh and the tomatoes are at their juiciest.

Tomato Salad with Tuna, Capers, and Black Olives

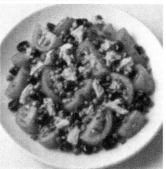

Serves 6 | Fast
Ingredients
- 2½ lbs ripe tomatoes, cored and cut into ½-inch-thick wedges
- Salt and pepper
- ¼ cup extra-virgin olive oil
- ⅓ cup kalamata olives, pitted and chopped
- ¼ cup capers, rinsed and minced
- ¼ cup finely chopped red onion
- 2 tbsp chopped fresh parsley
- 1 tbsp lemon juice
- 1 (5-oz) can solid white tuna in water, drained and flaked

How to Make It

1. Salt the Tomatoes
   Toss the tomato wedges with ½ tsp salt and let them sit in a colander set over a bowl for 15 to 20 minutes. This helps draw out excess moisture for a more concentrated flavor.
2. Make the Dressing
   Transfer 1 tbsp of the tomato juice to a large bowl and discard the rest. Whisk in the olive oil, olives, capers, red onion, parsley, and lemon juice.
3. Assemble the Salad
   Add the drained tomatoes and tuna to the bowl and gently toss to coat with the dressing. Season with more salt and pepper to taste.

Serve right away for the freshest flavor.

Cherry Tomato Salad with Feta and Olives

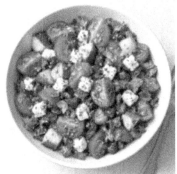

Serves 4 to 6 | Vegetarian
Ingredients
- 1½ lbs cherry tomatoes, quartered
- ½ tsp sugar
- Salt and pepper
- 1 small cucumber, peeled, halved, seeded, and cut into ½-inch pieces
- ½ cup pitted kalamata olives, chopped
- 4 oz feta cheese, crumbled (1 cup)
- 3 tbsp fresh parsley, chopped
- 1 shallot, minced
- 1 tbsp red wine vinegar
- 2 garlic cloves, minced
- 2 tsp fresh oregano, minced
- 2 tbsp extra-virgin olive oil

How to Make It
1. Prep the Tomatoes
   Toss tomatoes with sugar and ¼ tsp salt in a bowl and let sit for 30 minutes. Transfer to a salad spinner and spin until most seeds and juice are removed—about 45 to 60 seconds, shaking occasionally.
2. Build the Salad
   Add the drained tomatoes, cucumber, olives, feta, and parsley to a large bowl.
3. Make the Dressing
   Strain ½ cup of the tomato liquid into a measuring cup. In a small saucepan, bring that juice, shallot, vinegar, garlic, and oregano to a simmer. Cook until reduced to about 3 tbsp, 6 to 8 minutes. Let cool, then whisk in olive oil until smooth.
4. Finish and Serve
   Drizzle the dressing over the salad and toss gently to combine. Season with salt and pepper to taste. Serve fresh.

Tomato and Burrata Salad with Pangrattato and Basil

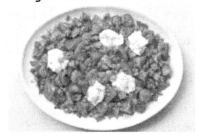

Serves: 4 to 6
 Vegetarian
Ingredients
- 1½ lbs ripe tomatoes, cored and cut into 1-inch chunks
- 8 oz cherry tomatoes, halved
- Salt and pepper
- 3 oz rustic Italian bread, cut into 1-inch pieces (about 1 cup)
- 6 tbsp extra-virgin olive oil
- 1 garlic clove, minced
- 1 shallot, halved and thinly sliced
- 1½ tbsp white balsamic vinegar
- ½ cup fresh basil, chopped

- 8 oz burrata cheese, at room temperature

Instructions

1. Prep tomatoes:
   Toss tomatoes with ¼ tsp salt. Let drain in a colander for 30 minutes.
2. Make pangrattato:
   Pulse bread into large crumbs (⅛–¼ inch). In a skillet, combine crumbs with 2 tbsp oil, salt, and pepper. Cook over medium heat, stirring until golden and crisp (about 10 minutes). Push crumbs aside, add garlic to center, mash and cook until fragrant (30 seconds). Stir garlic into crumbs. Let cool.
3. Make vinaigrette & assemble:
   In a large bowl, whisk shallot, vinegar, and ¼ tsp salt. Slowly whisk in remaining ¼ cup oil. Add tomatoes and basil, toss gently. Season to taste.
4. Finish & serve:
   Arrange salad on a platter. Cut burrata into 1-inch pieces and scatter over tomatoes, including the creamy interior. Top with pangrattato. Serve immediately.

Grilled Vegetable and Halloumi Salad

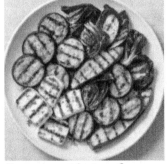

Serves: 4 to 6
Fast | Vegetarian
Ingredients
- 3 tbsp honey
- 1 tbsp fresh thyme, minced
- ½ tsp lemon zest + 3 tbsp lemon juice
- 1 garlic clove, minced
- Salt and pepper, to taste

- 1 lb eggplant, sliced into ½-inch rounds
- 1 head radicchio (about 10 oz), quartered
- 1 zucchini, halved lengthwise
- 8 oz halloumi cheese, sliced into ½-inch slabs
- ¼ cup extra-virgin olive oil

Instructions

1. Make vinaigrette:
   In a large bowl, whisk honey, thyme, lemon zest and juice, garlic, ⅛ tsp salt, and ⅛ tsp pepper. Set aside.
2. Prep grill and vegetables:
   Brush eggplant, radicchio, zucchini, and halloumi with 2 tbsp oil. Season with salt and pepper.
3. Grill setup:
   o Charcoal: Light coals, spread evenly, and preheat with lid on (about 5 minutes).
   o Gas: Preheat on high for 15 minutes, then reduce to medium.
4. Grill veggies and cheese:
   Clean and oil grate well (5–10 times until glossy). Grill radicchio for 3–5 minutes; grill eggplant, zucchini, and halloumi about 10 minutes, flipping as needed, until softened and charred. Transfer to a board, let cool, then chop into 1-inch pieces.
5. Assemble salad:
   Slowly whisk remaining 2 tbsp oil into the vinaigrette. Toss chopped vegetables and cheese gently to coat. Season to taste and serve.

Zucchini Ribbon Salad with Shaved Parmesan

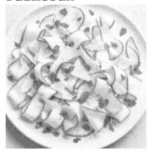

Serves: 6 to 8
Fast | Vegetarian
Ingredients

- 1½ lbs small zucchini, trimmed and sliced lengthwise into ribbons
- Salt and pepper, to taste
- ½ cup extra-virgin olive oil
- ¼ cup fresh lemon juice (about 2 lemons)
- 6 oz Parmesan cheese, shaved
- 2 tbsp fresh mint, minced

Instructions

1. Season zucchini:
   Toss ribbons with salt and pepper to taste.
2. Assemble salad:
   Arrange zucchini ribbons on a platter. Drizzle with olive oil and lemon juice. Top with Parmesan shavings and mint.
3. Serve immediately.

Rice and Grains

Basmati Rice Pilaf with Currants and Toasted Almonds

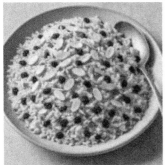

Serves: 4 to 6
Vegetarian
Ingredients

- 1 tbsp extra-virgin olive oil
- 1 small onion, finely chopped
- Salt and pepper, to taste
- 1½ cups basmati rice, rinsed
- 2 garlic cloves, minced
- ½ tsp ground turmeric
- ¼ tsp ground cinnamon
- 2¼ cups water
- ¼ cup currants
- ¼ cup sliced almonds, toasted

Instructions
1. Build flavor:
   In a saucepan over medium heat, heat oil until shimmering. Add onion and ¼ tsp salt; cook until soft, about 5 minutes. Stir in rice, garlic, turmeric, and cinnamon. Cook, stirring, until rice edges turn translucent, about 3 minutes.
2. Simmer rice:
   Add water, bring to a simmer. Reduce heat to low, cover, and cook until rice is tender and liquid is absorbed, 16-18 minutes.
3. Steam & finish:
   Remove from heat. Sprinkle currants over rice, cover with a clean dish towel under the lid, and let sit for 10 minutes. Add toasted almonds and fluff gently with a fork. Season to taste and serve.

Spiced Basmati Rice with Cauliflower and Pomegranate

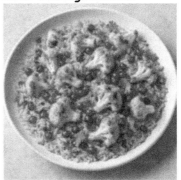

Serves: 8 to 10
Vegetarian
Ingredients

- 1 head cauliflower (2 lbs), cut into ¾-inch florets
- ¼ cup extra-virgin olive oil
- Salt and pepper, to taste
- ½ tsp ground cumin, divided
- 1 onion, coarsely chopped
- 1½ cups basmati rice, rinsed
- 4 garlic cloves, minced
- ½ tsp ground cinnamon
- ½ tsp ground turmeric
- 2¼ cups water
- ½ cup pomegranate seeds
- 2 tbsp chopped fresh cilantro
- 2 tbsp chopped fresh mint

Instructions
1. Roast cauliflower:
   Preheat oven to 475°F (rack in lowest position). Toss cauliflower with 2 tbsp oil, ½ tsp salt, ½ tsp pepper, and ¼ tsp cumin. Spread on a rimmed baking sheet in a single layer. Roast until tender and caramelized, 10-15 minutes. Set aside.
2. Build flavor base:
   In a large saucepan, heat remaining 2 tbsp oil over medium heat until shimmering. Add onion and ¼ tsp salt; cook until soft and lightly browned, 5-7 minutes. Add rice, garlic, cinnamon, turmeric, and remaining ¼ tsp cumin. Cook, stirring, until rice edges turn translucent, about 3 minutes.
3. Simmer rice:
   Stir in water. Bring to a simmer, then reduce heat to

low. Cover and cook until rice is tender and water is absorbed, 16–18 minutes.

4. Finish and serve:
   Remove from heat. Place a clean dish towel under the lid and let sit 10 minutes. Add roasted cauliflower and fluff gently with a fork. Season to taste. Transfer to a platter and top with pomegranate seeds, cilantro, and mint. Serve.

Herbed Basmati Rice and Pasta Pilaf

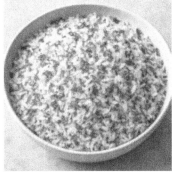

Serves: 4 to 6
Vegetarian
Ingredients
- 1½ cups basmati rice
- 3 tbsp extra-virgin olive oil
- 2 oz vermicelli pasta, broken into 1-inch pieces
- 1 onion, finely chopped
- 1 garlic clove, minced
- Salt and pepper, to taste
- 2½ cups chicken or vegetable broth
- 3 tbsp fresh parsley, minced

Instructions
1. Soak rice:
   Place rice in a bowl and cover with 2 inches of hot tap water. Let stand 15 minutes. Swish gently to release starch, then drain. Rinse with cold water 4–5 times until water runs nearly clear. Drain thoroughly in a fine-mesh strainer.
2. Toast pasta & build base:
   In a large saucepan over medium heat, heat oil until shimmering. Add pasta and cook, stirring, until golden brown (about 3 minutes). Add onion and garlic, and cook until

softened but not browned (about 4 minutes).

3. Cook rice:
   Stir in rice and cook until edges turn translucent (about 3 minutes). Add broth and 1¼ tsp salt. Bring to a boil, then reduce to low. Cover and simmer until rice and pasta are tender and liquid is absorbed (about 10 minutes).
4. Steam & finish:
   Remove from heat, lay a clean dish towel under the lid, and let sit for 10 minutes. Add parsley and fluff gently with a fork. Season to taste. Serve.

Spiced Baked Rice with Roasted Sweet Potatoes and Fennel

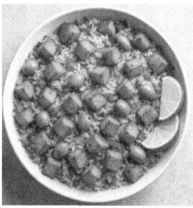

Serves: 6 to 8
Vegetarian
Ingredients
- 1½ lbs sweet potatoes, peeled and cut into 1-inch chunks
- ¼ cup extra-virgin olive oil, divided
- Salt and pepper, to taste
- 1 fennel bulb, cored and finely chopped
- 1 small onion, finely chopped
- 1½ cups long-grain white rice, rinsed
- 4 garlic cloves, minced
- 2 tsp ras el hanout (store-bought or homemade)
- 2¾ cups chicken or vegetable broth
- ¾ cup large brine-cured green olives, halved
- 2 tbsp fresh cilantro, minced
- Lime wedges, for serving

Instructions

1. Roast sweet potatoes:
   Preheat oven to 400°F. Toss sweet potatoes with 2 tbsp oil and ½ tsp salt. Spread on a baking sheet in a single layer. Roast for 25-30 minutes, stirring halfway through, until browned and tender. Remove and reduce oven to 350°F.
2. Build aromatic base:
   In a Dutch oven over medium heat, heat remaining 2 tbsp oil. Sauté fennel and onion until soft, 5-7 minutes. Stir in rice, garlic, and ras el hanout. Cook, stirring, until rice edges turn translucent, about 3 minutes.
3. Add broth and bake:
   Stir in broth and olives. Bring to a boil, cover, and transfer to the oven. Bake 12-15 minutes, until rice is tender and liquid is absorbed.
4. Finish & serve:
   Let rice sit, covered, for 10 minutes. Add roasted potatoes and gently fluff with a fork. Season to taste. Garnish with cilantro and serve with lime wedges.

Stovetop White Rice

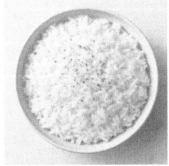

Serves: 4 to 6
Fast | Vegetarian

Ingredients

- 1 tbsp extra-virgin olive oil
- 2 cups long-grain white rice, rinsed
- 3 cups water
- Salt and pepper, to taste

Instructions

1. Cook rice:
   In a large saucepan, heat oil over medium heat until shimmering. Add rice and stir until the edges of the grains turn translucent (about 2 minutes).
2. Simmer:
   Add water and 1 tsp salt. Bring to a simmer. Cover, reduce heat to low, and cook for about 20 minutes, until rice is tender and water is absorbed.
3. Rest & fluff:
   Remove from heat. Place a clean dish towel under the lid and let the rice sit for 10 minutes. Fluff gently with a fork, season with salt and pepper, and serve.

Baked Brown Rice with Roasted Red Peppers and Onions

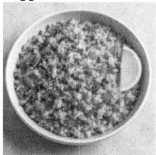

Serves: 4 to 6
Vegetarian

Ingredients

- 4 tsp extra-virgin olive oil
- 2 onions, finely chopped
- Salt and pepper, to taste
- 2¼ cups water
- 1 cup chicken or vegetable broth
- 1½ cups long-grain brown rice, rinsed
- ¾ cup jarred roasted red peppers, rinsed, patted dry, and chopped
- ½ cup fresh parsley, minced
- Grated Parmesan cheese, for serving
- Lemon wedges, for serving

Instructions

1. Prepare the Onions:

- In a Dutch oven, heat 2 teaspoons of olive oil over medium heat until shimmering.
- Add the chopped onions and 1 teaspoon of salt.
- Cook, stirring occasionally, until the onions are softened and well-browned, about 12 to 14 minutes.
2. Combine Ingredients:
- Stir in the water, broth, and rinsed rice.
- Bring the mixture to a boil.
- Cover the Dutch oven and transfer it to the oven.
- Bake at 375°F (190°C) until the rice is tender and the liquid is absorbed, about 65 to 70 minutes.
3. Finish the Dish:
- Remove the pot from the oven.
- Sprinkle the chopped roasted red peppers over the cooked rice.
- Cover and let the dish sit for 5 minutes.
- Stir in the minced parsley.
- Gently fluff the rice with a fork to combine.
- Season with additional salt and pepper to taste.
4. Serve:
- Serve the rice warm, topped with grated Parmesan cheese and accompanied by lemon wedges.

Brown Rice with Tomatoes and Chickpeas

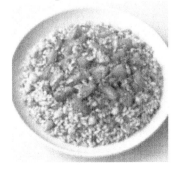

Serves: 6
Vegetarian
Why This Recipe Works
Ingredients
- 12 oz grape tomatoes, quartered
- 5 scallions, thinly sliced
- ¼ cup fresh cilantro, minced
- 4 tsp extra-virgin olive oil, divided
- 1 tbsp lime juice
- Salt and pepper, to taste
- 2 red bell peppers, seeded and finely chopped
- 1 onion, finely chopped
- 1 cup long-grain brown rice, rinsed
- 4 garlic cloves, minced
- Pinch of saffron threads, crumbled
- Pinch of cayenne pepper
- 3¼ cups chicken or vegetable broth
- 2 (15 oz) cans chickpeas, drained and rinsed

Instructions
1. Prepare the Tomato Mixture:
- In a bowl, combine the quartered tomatoes, sliced scallions, minced cilantro, 2 teaspoons of olive oil, and lime juice.
- Season with salt and pepper to taste.
- Set aside to allow flavors to meld.
2. Cook the Vegetables and Rice:
- In a large saucepan, heat the remaining 2 teaspoons of olive oil over medium-high heat until shimmering.
- Add the chopped bell peppers and onion.
- Cook, stirring occasionally, until softened and lightly browned, about 8 to 10 minutes.
- Stir in the rinsed rice, minced garlic, crumbled saffron, and cayenne pepper.

o Cook, stirring
  frequently, until
  fragrant, about 30
  seconds.
3. Simmer the Rice:
   o Pour in the broth and
     bring the mixture to a
     simmer.
   o Reduce heat to medium-
     low, cover, and simmer,
     stirring occasionally,
     for 25 minutes.
4. Add Chickpeas:
   o Stir in the drained
     chickpeas.
   o Cover and continue to
     simmer until the rice is
     tender and most of the
     liquid is absorbed, about
     25 to 30 minutes.
   o Season with salt and
     pepper to taste.
5. Serve:
   o Spoon the rice mixture
     onto serving plate,
   o Top each serving with the
     prepared tomato mixture.
   o Serve warm.

Rice Salad with Oranges, Olives, and Almonds

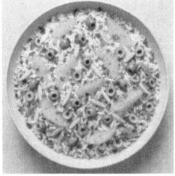

Serves: 4 to 6
Vegetarian
Ingredients
- 1½ cups basmati rice
- Salt and pepper, to taste
- 2 oranges, plus ¼ teaspoon grated orange zest and 1 tablespoon juice
- 2 tablespoons extra-virgin olive oil
- 2 teaspoons sherry vinegar
- 1 small garlic clove, minced
- ⅓ cup large pitted brine-cured green olives, chopped

- ⅓ cup slivered almonds, toasted
- 2 tablespoons fresh oregano, minced

Instructions
1. Cook the Rice:
   o Bring 4 quarts of water
     to a boil in a Dutch
     oven.
   o Meanwhile, toast the rice
     in a 12-inch skillet over
     medium heat until faintly
     fragrant and some grains
     turn opaque, about 5 to 8
     minutes.
   o Add the toasted rice and
     1½ teaspoons of salt to
     the boiling water.
   o Cook, stirring
     occasionally, until the
     rice is tender but not
     overly soft,
     approximately 15 minutes.
   o Drain the rice and spread
     it onto a rimmed baking
     sheet to cool completely,
     about 15 minutes.
2. Prepare the Orange Components:
   o Cut away the peel and
     white pith from the
     oranges.
   o Holding the fruit over a
     bowl, use a paring knife
     to slice between the
     membranes to release the
     segments, collecting any
     juice.
3. Make the Vinaigrette:
   o In a large bowl, whisk
     together the orange zest
     and juice, olive oil,
     sherry vinegar, minced
     garlic, 1 teaspoon of
     salt, and ½ teaspoon of
     pepper until well
     combined.
4. Assemble the Salad:
   o Add the cooled rice,
     orange segments, chopped
     olives, toasted almonds,
     and minced oregano to the
     bowl with the
     vinaigrette.

- o Gently toss to combine, ensuring all ingredients are well coated.
- o Let the salad sit for 20 minutes before serving to allow the flavors to meld.

Brown Rice Salad with Asparagus, Goat Cheese, and Lemon

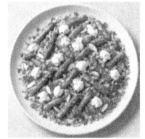

Serves: 4 to 6
 Vegetarian
Ingredients
- 1½ cups long-grain brown rice
- Salt and pepper, to taste
- 1 teaspoon grated lemon zest
- 3 tablespoons fresh lemon juice, divided
- 3½ tablespoons extra-virgin olive oil, divided
- 1 pound asparagus, trimmed and cut into 1-inch pieces
- 1 shallot, minced
- 2 ounces goat cheese, crumbled (about ½ cup)
- ¼ cup slivered almonds, toasted
- ¼ cup fresh parsley, minced

Instructions
1. Cook the Rice:
   - o Bring 4 quarts of water to a boil in a Dutch oven.
   - o Add the rice and 1½ teaspoons of salt; cook, stirring occasionally, until tender, about 25 to 30 minutes.
   - o Drain the rice, spread it onto a rimmed baking sheet, and drizzle with 1 tablespoon of lemon juice.
   - o Let the rice cool completely, approximately 15 minutes.
2. Sauté the Asparagus:

- o Heat 1 tablespoon of olive oil in a 12-inch skillet over high heat until shimmering.
- o Add the asparagus, season with ¼ teaspoon each of salt and pepper, and cook, stirring occasionally, until browned and crisp-tender, about 4 minutes.
- o Transfer the asparagus to a plate and let it cool slightly.
3. Prepare the Dressing:
   - o In a large bowl, whisk together the remaining 2½ tablespoons of olive oil, lemon zest, the remaining 2 tablespoons of lemon juice, minced shallot, ½ teaspoon of salt, and ½ teaspoon of pepper until well combined.
4. Assemble the Salad:
   - o Add the cooled rice and asparagus to the bowl with the dressing; gently toss to combine.
   - o Stir in 2 tablespoons of crumbled goat cheese, 3 tablespoons of toasted almonds, and 3 tablespoons of minced parsley.
   - o Let the salad sit for 10 minutes to allow flavors to meld.
   - o Season with additional salt and pepper to taste.
5. Serve:
   - o Transfer the salad to a serving platter.
   - o Sprinkle with the remaining 2 tablespoons of goat cheese, 1 tablespoon of toasted almonds, and 1 tablespoon of parsley.
   - o Serve immediately.

Seafood risotto

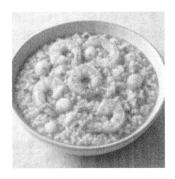

Ingredients:
- 1 tablespoon extra-virgin olive oil
- 1 onion, chopped fine
- 2 cups Arborio rice
- 5 garlic cloves, minced
- 1 teaspoon minced fresh thyme
- Pinch of saffron threads, crumbled
- 1 cup dry white wine
- 12 ounces large shrimp (26 to 30 per pound), peeled and deveined
- 12 ounces small bay scallops
- 2 tablespoons minced fresh parsley
- 1 tablespoon lemon juice
- Salt and pepper to taste

Seafood Broth:
- Shrimp shells from the peeled shrimp
- 2 cups chicken broth
- 2½ cups water
- 4 (8-ounce) bottles clam juice
- 1 (14.5-ounce) can diced tomatoes, drained
- 2 bay leaves

Instructions:
1. Prepare the Seafood Broth:
   - In a large saucepan, combine shrimp shells, chicken broth, water, clam juice, diced tomatoes, and bay leaves. Bring to a boil, then reduce to a simmer and cook for 20 minutes. Strain the broth through a fine-mesh strainer into a bowl, pressing on solids to extract as much liquid as possible. Return the broth to the saucepan, cover, and keep warm over low heat.

2. Cook the Aromatics:
   - In a Dutch oven or large saucepan, heat olive oil over medium heat until shimmering. Add chopped onion and cook until softened, about 5 minutes. Add Arborio rice, minced garlic, thyme, and saffron. Cook, stirring frequently, until the rice grains begin to turn translucent at the edges, about 3 minutes.

3. Deglaze and Simmer:
   - Pour in the white wine, stirring until fully absorbed, about 3 minutes. Add 3½ cups of the warm seafood broth, bring to a simmer, and cook, stirring occasionally, until the liquid is almost fully absorbed, 13 to 17 minutes.

4. Continue Cooking the Risotto:
   - Continue to cook the rice, adding the remaining warm broth, one cup at a time, and stirring frequently, until the rice is creamy and cooked through but still firm to the bite, about 13 to 17 minutes.

5. Cook the Seafood:
   - In a separate skillet, heat a bit of oil over medium heat. Add the shrimp and scallops, cooking until just opaque throughout, about 3 minutes.

6. Combine and Rest:
   - Stir the cooked shrimp and scallops into the risotto. Remove the pot from heat, cover, and let it sit for 5 minutes.

7. Finish the Dish:
   - Stir in the remaining 3 tablespoons of olive oil, minced parsley, and lemon juice. Season with salt

and pepper to taste.
Serve the risotto hot,
garnished with additional
parsley if desired.

Paniscia

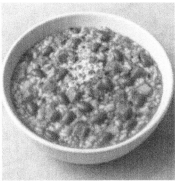

Ingredients:
For the bean and vegetable broth:
- 8 ounces (1¼ cups) dried
  cranberry beans, picked over
  and rinsed
- 1 tablespoon extra-virgin olive
  oil
- 2 ounces pancetta, chopped fine
- 1 leek, white and light green
  parts only, halved lengthwise,
  chopped fine, and washed
  thoroughly
- 1 carrot, peeled and chopped
  fine
- 1 celery rib, chopped fine
- 1 zucchini, cut into ½-inch
  pieces
- 1 small head green cabbage,
  chopped
- 1 small sprig fresh rosemary
- Salt and pepper to taste

For the risotto:
- 2 tablespoons extra-virgin
  olive oil
- 1 small onion, chopped fine
- 6 ounces Italian-style salami,
  cut into ½-inch pieces
- 1½ cups carnaroli rice
- 1 tablespoon tomato paste
- 1 cup dry red wine
- 2 teaspoons red wine vinegar
- Salt and pepper to taste
- 1 ounce Parmesan cheese, grated
  (½ cup), plus extra for serving
- 2 tablespoons unsalted butter
- 2 tablespoons chopped fresh
  parsley

Instructions:
- o Soak the cranberry beans in
  water with dissolved salt for
  at least 8 hours or overnight.
  Drain and rinse well.
- o In a large saucepan, heat olive
  oil over medium-high heat. Add
  pancetta and cook until
  beginning to brown, about 3-5
  minutes.
- o Stir in leek, carrot, celery,
  zucchini, cabbage, and
  rosemary. Cook until vegetables
  are softened, 5-7 minutes.
- o Add soaked beans and 8 cups of
  water. Bring to a boil, then
  reduce heat to medium-low.
  Simmer, stirring occasionally,
  until beans are tender, about
  45 minutes to 1 hour.
- o Strain the mixture, reserving
  the broth. Discard the rosemary
  and transfer the vegetables and
  beans to a separate bowl. Keep
  the broth warm over low heat.
2. Prepare the Risotto:
- o In a Dutch oven, heat
  olive oil over medium
  heat. Add onion and
  salami. Cook until onion
  is softened, about 5
  minutes.
- o Stir in rice and cook,
  stirring frequently,
  until grain edges begin
  to turn translucent,
  about 3 minutes.
- o Add tomato paste and cook
  until fragrant, about 1
  minute.
- o Pour in red wine and
  cook, stirring
  constantly, until fully
  absorbed, 2-3 minutes.
- o Stir in 2 cups of the
  warm broth. Bring to a
  simmer, cover, and cook
  for 10 minutes, stirring
  halfway through.
- o Add the reserved bean and
  vegetable mixture to the
  risotto. Continue
  cooking, covered, until
  almost all liquid has
  been absorbed and rice is

just al dente, 6-9 minutes.
- o Stir in beans and hot water, cooking gently until the risotto is creamy, about 3 minutes.
- o Remove from heat, cover, and let sit for 5 minutes.
- o Stir in Parmesan and butter. Adjust consistency with additional warm broth if needed.
- o Stir in red wine vinegar and season with salt and pepper to taste.
- o Garnish with chopped parsley and serve, passing extra Parmesan at the table.

Grilled Paella

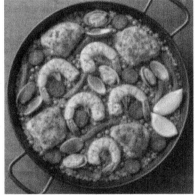

Ingredients:
For the proteins:
- 1½ pounds boneless, skinless chicken thighs, trimmed and halved crosswise
- 12 ounces jumbo shrimp (16 to 20 per pound), peeled and deveined
- 1 pound littleneck clams, scrubbed
- 8 ounces Spanish-style chorizo sausage, cut into ½-inch pieces

For the rice and aromatics:
- 5 tablespoons extra-virgin olive oil
- 1 onion, chopped fine
- ½ cup jarred roasted red peppers, rinsed, patted dry, and chopped fine
- 6 garlic cloves, minced, divided
- 1¾ teaspoons hot smoked paprika, divided
- 3 tablespoons tomato paste
- 3 cups Bomba rice (or Arborio rice as a substitute)
- 1 cup frozen peas, thawed
- Lemon wedges, for serving

For the liquids:
- 4½ cups chicken broth
- ⅔ cup dry sherry
- 1 (8-ounce) bottle clam juice
- Pinch saffron threads, crumbled (optional)

Instructions:
1. Prepare the proteins:
   - o Pat the chicken dry with paper towels and season both sides with salt and pepper.
   - o Toss the shrimp with 1½ teaspoons of olive oil, ½ teaspoon of minced garlic, ¼ teaspoon of paprika, and a pinch of salt. Set aside to marinate.
2. Prepare the broth:
   - o In a medium saucepan, heat 1½ teaspoons of olive oil over medium heat until shimmering.
   - o Add the remaining 5½ cloves of minced garlic and cook, stirring constantly, until the garlic begins to brown, about 1 minute.
   - o Stir in the tomato paste and the remaining 1½ teaspoons of paprika, cooking until the mixture darkens slightly, about 1 minute.
   - o Add the chicken broth, sherry, clam juice, and saffron (if using). Bring to a boil, then remove from heat and set aside.
3. Grill the chicken:
   - o Light a large grill and heat it to medium-high.
   - o Clean and oil the cooking grate.
   - o Place the chicken on the grill and cook until both sides are lightly

browned, about 5 to 7 minutes. Transfer the chicken to a plate and clean the cooking grate.

4. Cook the paella:
   o Place a large paella pan or heavy-duty roasting pan on the grill and add the remaining ¼ cup of olive oil. Heat until shimmering.
   o Add the chopped onion and roasted red peppers to the pan, season with salt and pepper, and cook, stirring frequently, until the onion begins to brown, about 4 to 7 minutes.
   o Stir in the rice, ensuring each grain is well coated with the oil and vegetable mixture.
   o Arrange the grilled chicken pieces around the perimeter of the pan.
   o Pour the prepared broth mixture over the rice, ensuring the liquid covers the rice evenly.
   o When the liquid reaches a gentle simmer, place the marinated shrimp in the center of the pan in a single layer.
   o Arrange the clams in the center, slightly pushing them into the rice so they stand upright.
   o Distribute the chorizo evenly over the surface of the rice.
   o Cover the grill and cook, rotating the pan occasionally to ensure even heating, until the rice is almost cooked through, about 12 to 18 minutes.

5. Add peas and finish cooking:
   o Sprinkle the thawed peas evenly over the paella.
   o Cover the grill and cook until the liquid is fully absorbed and the rice at the bottom of the pan

sizzles, about 5 to 8 minutes.
   o Continue cooking, uncovered, until a golden-brown crust forms on the bottom of the pan, known as "socarrat," about 8 to 15 minutes longer.

6. Rest and serve:
   o Remove the pan from the grill and cover with aluminum foil. Let the paella rest for 10 minutes.
   o Serve with lemon wedges on the side.

Enjoy your homemade Grilled Paella, a delightful blend of smoky flavors and tender textures, perfect for sharing with friends and family.

Vegetable paella

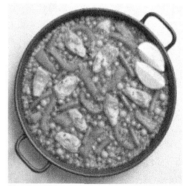

Key Components of Vegetable Paella:
- Rice: Short-grain varieties like Bomba or Arborio are traditional choices, as they absorb flavors well and contribute to the dish's characteristic texture.
- Vegetables: Common additions include artichokes, bell peppers, fennel, peas, green beans, and tomatoes. These provide a mix of textures and flavors, from tender to crunchy, and sweet to savory.
- Legumes: Chickpeas are frequently included, offering a hearty bite and a boost of protein.
- Aromatics and Spices: Sautéed onions and garlic form a

flavorful base, while spices like smoked paprika and saffron impart depth and the signature golden hue.

- Cooking Method: The ingredients are typically cooked together in a wide, shallow pan, allowing the rice to cook evenly and form a desirable crust known as "socarrat" on the bottom. This crust is cherished for its crispy texture and intensified flavor.

Recipe Overview:
1. Sauté Aromatics: Begin by cooking onions, garlic, and fennel in olive oil until softened and caramelized.
2. Add Vegetables and Spices: Incorporate chopped tomatoes, bell peppers, and other chosen vegetables. Stir in smoked paprika, saffron, and any additional spices, cooking until fragrant.
3. Toast the Rice: Add the rice to the pan, stirring to coat the grains with the flavorful mixture.
4. Add Liquids: Pour in vegetable broth, white wine, and any other liquids. Bring the mixture to a simmer.
5. Cook the Rice: Let the rice absorb the liquids over medium heat without stirring, allowing the socarrat to form.
6. Add Delicate Ingredients: Once the rice is nearly tender, scatter peas, artichoke hearts, and chickpeas over the surface. Continue cooking until the rice is fully cooked and the liquid is absorbed.
7. Rest and Serve: Remove the pan from heat, cover, and let it rest for a few minutes. Garnish with fresh parsley and serve with lemon wedges for added brightness.

Creamy Parmesan Polenta

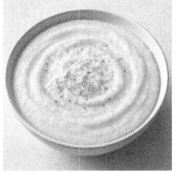

Ingredients:
- 7½ cups water
- 1½ teaspoons salt
- Pinch of baking soda
- 1½ cups coarse-ground cornmeal
- 2 ounces Parmesan cheese, grated (about 1 cup), plus extra for serving
- 2 tablespoons extra-virgin olive oil
- Freshly ground black pepper, to taste

Instructions:
1. Prepare the Polenta Base:
   o In a large saucepan, bring the water to a boil over medium-high heat.
   o Stir in the salt and baking soda.
   o Slowly pour the cornmeal into the boiling water in a steady stream, stirring constantly with a wooden spoon or rubber spatula.
   o Return the mixture to a boil, then reduce the heat to the lowest setting and cover the saucepan.
2. Cooking Process:
   o After 5 minutes, uncover and whisk the polenta to smooth out any lumps, scraping down the sides and bottom of the saucepan.
   o Re-cover and continue to cook on low heat without stirring for about 25 minutes, or until the grains are tender but slightly al dente.
   o The polenta should be loose and barely hold its

shape; it will thicken further as it cools.
3. Finish the Polenta:
   o Remove the saucepan from heat.
   o Stir in the grated Parmesan cheese and olive oil until fully incorporated.
   o Season with freshly ground black pepper to taste.
   o Cover and let the polenta sit for 5 minutes before serving.
   o Serve warm, passing additional Parmesan at the table if desired.

Enjoy your creamy Parmesan polenta!

Sautéed Cherry Tomato and Fresh Mozzarella Topping

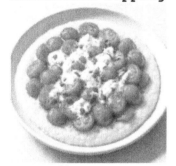

Ingredients:
- 3 tablespoons extra-virgin olive oil
- 2 garlic cloves, thinly sliced
- Pinch of red pepper flakes
- Pinch of sugar
- 1½ pounds cherry tomatoes, halved
- Salt and pepper to taste
- 3 ounces fresh mozzarella cheese, shredded (¾ cup)
- 2 tablespoons shredded fresh basil

Instructions:
1. In a 12-inch nonstick skillet over medium-high heat, warm the olive oil until shimmering.
2. Add the sliced garlic, red pepper flakes, and sugar; cook, stirring constantly, until the garlic becomes fragrant and slightly golden, about 1 minute.

3. Stir in the halved cherry tomatoes; cook until they begin to soften, approximately 1 minute. Season with salt and pepper to taste.
4. Spoon the tomato mixture over individual servings of polenta.
5. Top each serving with shredded mozzarella and a sprinkle of fresh basil. Serve immediately.

Broccoli Rabe, Sun-Dried Tomato, and Pine Nut Topping

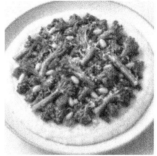

Ingredients:
- ½ cup oil-packed sun-dried tomatoes, chopped coarse
- 3 tablespoons extra-virgin olive oil
- 6 garlic cloves, minced
- ½ teaspoon red pepper flakes
- Salt and pepper to taste
- 1 pound broccoli rabe, trimmed and cut into 1½-inch pieces
- ¼ cup chicken or vegetable broth
- 2 tablespoons pine nuts, toasted
- ¼ cup grated Parmesan cheese

Instructions:
1. In a 12-inch nonstick skillet over medium-high heat, combine the sun-dried tomatoes, olive oil, minced garlic, red pepper flakes, and ½ teaspoon salt. Cook, stirring frequently, until the garlic becomes fragrant and slightly toasted, about 2 minutes.
2. Add the broccoli rabe and broth to the skillet. Cover and cook until the broccoli rabe turns bright green, approximately 2 minutes.
3. Uncover and continue cooking, stirring frequently, until most

of the broth has evaporated and the broccoli rabe is just tender, about 3 minutes. Season with salt and pepper to taste.
4. Spoon the broccoli rabe mixture over individual servings of polenta.
5. Garnish each serving with toasted pine nuts and a sprinkle of grated Parmesan cheese. Serve immediately.

Barley with Roasted Carrots, Snow Peas, and Lemon-Yogurt Sauce

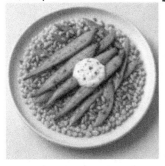

Ingredients:
For the Lemon-Yogurt Sauce:
- ½ cup plain yogurt
- 1½ teaspoons grated lemon zest
- 1½ tablespoons lemon juice
- 1½ tablespoons minced fresh mint
- Salt and pepper to taste

For the Barley and Vegetables:
- 1 cup pearl barley
- 5 carrots, peeled
- 3 tablespoons extra-virgin olive oil
- ¾ teaspoon ground coriander
- 8 ounces snow peas, strings removed, halved lengthwise
- ⅔ cup raw sunflower seeds
- ½ teaspoon ground cumin
- ⅛ teaspoon ground cardamom

Instructions:
1. Prepare the Lemon-Yogurt Sauce:
   o In a small bowl, whisk together the yogurt, lemon zest, lemon juice, minced mint, salt, and pepper.
   o Cover and refrigerate until ready to serve.
2. Cook the Barley:
   o Bring 4 quarts of water to a boil in a Dutch oven.
   o Add the barley and 1 tablespoon of salt.
   o Return to a boil and cook until tender, about 20 to 40 minutes.
   o Drain the barley and return it to the pot.
   o Cover to keep warm.
3. Roast the Carrots:
   o Halve the carrots crosswise, then halve or quarter lengthwise to create uniformly sized pieces.
   o Heat 1 tablespoon of olive oil in a 12-inch skillet over medium-high heat until shimmering.
   o Add the carrots and ½ teaspoon of ground coriander.
   o Cook, stirring occasionally, until lightly charred and just tender, about 5 to 7 minutes.
   o Transfer the carrots to a plate.
4. Sauté the Snow Peas:
   o In the same skillet, add the halved snow peas.
   o Cook, stirring occasionally, until spotty brown, about 3 to 5 minutes.
   o Transfer the snow peas to the plate with the carrots.
5. Toast the Sunflower Seeds:
   o In the now-empty skillet, heat 1½ teaspoons of olive oil over medium heat until shimmering.
   o Add the sunflower seeds, ground cumin, ground cardamom, the remaining ¼ teaspoon of ground coriander, and ¼ teaspoon of salt.
   o Cook, stirring constantly, until the seeds are toasted, about 2 minutes.

- o Transfer the toasted seeds to a small bowl.
6. Combine the Ingredients:
   - o In a large bowl, whisk together the remaining 1 teaspoon of lemon zest, 1 tablespoon of lemon juice, 1 tablespoon of minced mint, and the remaining 1½ tablespoons of olive oil.
   - o Add the cooked barley, roasted carrots, and sautéed snow peas.
   - o Gently toss to combine.
   - o Season with salt and pepper to taste.
7. Serve:
   - o Top individual portions with the toasted sunflower seeds.
   - o Drizzle with the prepared lemon-yogurt sauce.
   - o Serve and enjoy!

This dish combines a variety of textures and flavors, from the chewy barley to the tender carrots and crisp snow peas, all complemented by the refreshing lemon-yogurt sauce.

Barley with Lentils, Mushrooms, and Tahini-Yogurt Sauce

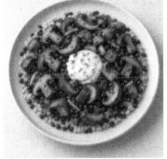

Ingredients:
For the dish:
- 1 cup pearl barley
- ½ cup black lentils, picked over and rinsed
- 2 tablespoons extra-virgin olive oil
- 1 onion, chopped finely
- 2 large portobello mushroom caps, cut into 1-inch pieces
- ½ ounce dried porcini mushrooms, rinsed
- 3 strips lemon zest, sliced thin lengthwise
- ¾ teaspoon ground coriander
- 2 tablespoons chopped fresh dill
- Salt and pepper to taste

For the tahini-yogurt sauce:
- ½ cup plain yogurt
- 1½ teaspoons grated lemon zest
- 1½ tablespoons minced fresh mint
- Salt and pepper to taste

Instructions:
1. Prepare the Porcini Mushrooms: Microwave 1½ cups water and the dried porcini mushrooms in a covered bowl until steaming, about 1 minute. Let them sit until softened, about 5 minutes. Drain, reserving the soaking liquid, and chop the mushrooms.
2. Cook the Barley and Lentils: Bring 4 quarts of water to a boil in a Dutch oven. Add the pearl barley, black lentils, and 1 tablespoon of salt. Return to a boil and cook until tender, 20 to 40 minutes. Drain and return to the pot, covering to keep warm.
3. Sauté the Vegetables: Heat the olive oil in a 12-inch nonstick skillet over medium heat until shimmering. Add the chopped onion and cook until softened, about 5 minutes. Stir in the portobello mushrooms, cover, and cook until they release their liquid and begin to brown, about 4 minutes.
4. Combine Ingredients: Uncover the skillet, add the lemon zest, ground coriander, ½ teaspoon of salt, and ¼ teaspoon of pepper. Cook until fragrant, about 30 seconds. Stir in the chopped porcini mushrooms and their soaking liquid. Bring to a boil and cook, stirring occasionally, until the liquid is slightly reduced, about 5 minutes.
5. Mix and Serve: Stir the mushroom mixture and chopped fresh dill into the cooked barley and lentils. Season with

salt and pepper to taste. Serve individual portions drizzled with the prepared tahini-yogurt sauce.

Tahini-Yogurt Sauce Preparation:
1. Whisk together the yogurt, grated lemon zest, minced fresh mint, ¼ teaspoon of salt, and ⅛ teaspoon of pepper in a small bowl. Cover and refrigerate until ready to serve.

This dish offers a delightful combination of flavors and textures, making it a perfect choice for a nutritious and satisfying meal.

Egyptian Barley Salad

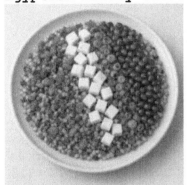

Ingredients:
- 1½ cups pearl barley
- Salt and pepper, to taste
- 3 tablespoons extra-virgin olive oil, plus extra for serving
- 2½ tablespoons pomegranate molasses
- 1 teaspoon fresh lemon juice
- 1 tablespoon sugar
- ½ teaspoon ground cinnamon
- ½ teaspoon ground cumin
- ½ cup coarsely chopped fresh cilantro
- ½ cup golden raisins
- ½ cup unsalted shelled pistachios, chopped coarse
- 4 ounces feta cheese, cut into ½-inch cubes
- 4 to 6 scallions, green parts only, sliced thin
- ½ cup pomegranate seeds

Instructions:
1. Cook the Barley: Bring 4 quarts of water to a boil in a large pot. Add the barley and 1 tablespoon of salt; return to a boil and cook until tender, about 45 minutes. Drain the barley, spread it on a rimmed baking sheet, and let it cool completely, about 15 minutes.
2. Prepare the Dressing: In a large bowl, whisk together the olive oil, pomegranate molasses, lemon juice, sugar, cinnamon, cumin, and ¼ teaspoon of salt.
3. Combine Ingredients: Add the cooled barley to the bowl with the dressing. Stir in the chopped cilantro, golden raisins, and chopped pistachios. Gently toss to combine. Season with salt and pepper to taste.
4. Assemble the Salad: Spread the barley mixture evenly on a serving platter. Arrange the feta cubes, sliced scallions, and pomegranate seeds in separate diagonal rows on top. Drizzle with extra olive oil before serving.

This salad can be made ahead and refrigerated for up to 3 days. Bring it to room temperature and toss gently before serving.

Barley risotto

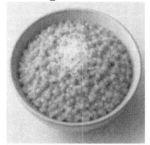

Ingredients:
- 4 cups chicken or vegetable broth
- 4 cups water
- 2 tablespoons extra-virgin olive oil
- 1 onion, finely chopped
- 1 carrot, peeled and finely chopped
- 1½ cups pearl barley
- 1 cup dry white wine

- 1 teaspoon minced fresh thyme
- 2 ounces Parmesan cheese, grated (about 1 cup)
- Salt and freshly ground black pepper, to taste

Instructions:

1. Prepare the Broth: In a medium saucepan, combine the chicken or vegetable broth and water. Bring to a simmer over medium heat, then reduce the heat to low to keep it warm.
2. Sauté Vegetables: In a large Dutch oven, heat the olive oil over medium heat until shimmering. Add the chopped onion and carrot. Cook, stirring occasionally, until the vegetables are softened, about 5 to 7 minutes.
3. Toast the Barley: Add the pearl barley to the pot with the sautéed vegetables. Cook, stirring frequently, until the barley is lightly toasted and aromatic, approximately 4 minutes.
4. Deglaze with Wine: Pour in the white wine, stirring constantly, and cook until the wine is fully absorbed, about 2 minutes.
5. Cook the Risotto: Stir in 3 cups of the warm broth along with the minced thyme. Bring the mixture to a simmer. Cook, stirring occasionally, until the liquid is absorbed and the bottom of the pot is dry, about 22 to 25 minutes.
6. Continue Adding Broth: Add the remaining 2 cups of warm broth to the barley mixture. Return to a simmer and cook, stirring occasionally, until the liquid is absorbed and the bottom of the pot is dry, about 15 to 18 minutes.
7. Final Cooking: Continue cooking, adding more broth as needed, until the barley is tender but still slightly firm in the center, approximately 15 to 20 minutes.
8. Finish the Dish: Remove the pot from heat. Stir in the grated Parmesan cheese and the remaining tablespoon of olive oil. Season with salt and freshly ground black pepper to taste. If the risotto is too thick, adjust the consistency with additional warm broth.
9. Serve: Ladle the risotto into bowls and serve immediately. Garnish with extra grated Parmesan cheese, if desired.

Bulgur Salad with Carrots and Almonds

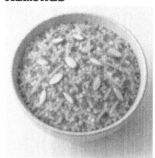

Ingredients:

- 1½ cups medium-grind bulgur, rinsed
- 1 cup water
- 6 tablespoons lemon juice (from about 2 lemons)
- Salt and freshly ground black pepper, to taste
- ⅓ cup extra-virgin olive oil
- ½ teaspoon ground cumin
- ⅛ teaspoon cayenne pepper
- 4 large carrots, peeled and shredded
- 3 scallions, thinly sliced
- ½ cup toasted sliced almonds
- ⅓ cup chopped fresh mint
- ⅓ cup chopped fresh cilantro

Instructions:

1. Prepare the Bulgur:
   o In a medium bowl, combine the rinsed bulgur, water, ¼ cup of the lemon juice, and ¼ teaspoon of salt.
   o Cover the bowl and let it sit at room temperature until the liquid is absorbed and the bulgur is softened, about 1½ hours.
2. Prepare the Dressing:

o In a large bowl, whisk together the remaining 2 tablespoons of lemon juice, olive oil, ground cumin, cayenne pepper, and ½ teaspoon of salt.
3. Assemble the Salad:
o Add the softened bulgur to the bowl with the dressing and toss to combine.
o Stir in the shredded carrots, sliced scallions, toasted almonds, chopped mint, and chopped cilantro.
o Gently toss the mixture until all ingredients are well combined.
o Season with additional salt and pepper to taste.
4. Serve:
o Transfer the salad to a serving dish or individual bowls.
o Serve immediately, or refrigerate until ready to serve.

Bulgur with Chickpeas, Spinach, and Za'atar

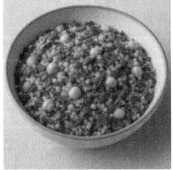

Ingredients:
- 3 tablespoons extra-virgin olive oil
- 1 onion, finely chopped
- 3 garlic cloves, minced
- 2 tablespoons za'atar
- 1 cup medium-grind bulgur, rinsed
- 1 (15-ounce) can chickpeas, rinsed and drained
- ¾ cup vegetable broth
- ¾ cup water
- 3 cups fresh spinach, chopped
- 1 tablespoon lemon juice

- Salt and pepper to taste

Instructions:
1. Sauté Aromatics: In a large saucepan, heat 2 tablespoons of olive oil over medium heat. Add the chopped onion and a pinch of salt, cooking until softened, about 5 minutes. Stir in the minced garlic and 1 tablespoon of za'atar, cooking until fragrant, about 30 seconds.

2. Cook Bulgur and Chickpeas: Add the rinsed bulgur, chickpeas, vegetable broth, and water to the saucepan. Bring to a simmer, reduce the heat to low, cover, and cook until the bulgur is tender and the liquid is absorbed, approximately 16 to 18 minutes.
3. Rest the Mixture: Remove the saucepan from heat, place a clean dish towel under the lid, and let the mixture sit for 10 minutes.
4. Incorporate Spinach and Seasonings: After resting, add the chopped spinach, lemon juice, the remaining 1 tablespoon of za'atar, and 1 tablespoon of olive oil to the bulgur mixture. Stir gently to combine, allowing the residual heat to wilt the spinach. Season with salt and pepper to taste.
5. Serve: Fluff the mixture with a fork and serve warm.

This dish pairs well with a side of pickled vegetables or a fresh cucumber salad. For a vegan variation, ensure the vegetable broth is used, and for added richness, a dollop of yogurt can be served alongside.

Tabbouleh

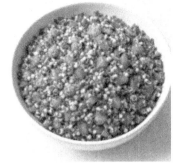

Ingredients:
- 3 tomatoes, cored and cut into ½-inch pieces
- ½ cup medium-grind bulgur, rinsed
- ¼ cup lemon juice (from 2 lemons)
- 6 tablespoons extra-virgin olive oil
- ⅛ teaspoon cayenne pepper
- 1½ cups minced fresh parsley
- ½ cup minced fresh mint
- 2 scallions, sliced thin
- Salt and pepper to taste

Instructions:
1. Prepare the Tomatoes: Place the chopped tomatoes in a fine-mesh strainer set over a bowl. Sprinkle with ¼ teaspoon salt and let them drain, tossing occasionally, for about 30 minutes. Reserve 2 tablespoons of the drained tomato juice.
2. Soak the Bulgur: In a bowl, combine the rinsed bulgur with the reserved tomato juice and 2 tablespoons of lemon juice. Toss to combine, cover, and let it sit until the grains begin to soften, approximately 30 to 40 minutes.
3. Prepare the Dressing: In a large bowl, whisk together the remaining 2 tablespoons of lemon juice, olive oil, cayenne pepper, and ¼ teaspoon salt.
4. Combine Ingredients: To the bowl with the dressing, add the drained tomatoes, soaked bulgur, parsley, mint, and scallions. Toss gently to combine.
5. Marinate: Cover the salad and let it sit at room temperature for about 1 hour to allow the flavors to meld. Before serving, toss the salad again and season with additional salt and pepper if needed.

Warm Farro with Lemon and Herbs

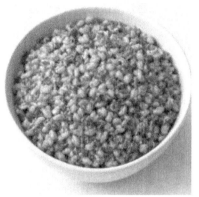

Ingredients:
- 1½ cups whole farro
- Salt and pepper to taste
- 3 tablespoons extra-virgin olive oil
- 1 onion, finely chopped
- 1 garlic clove, minced
- ¼ cup chopped fresh parsley
- ¼ cup chopped fresh mint
- 1 tablespoon lemon juice

Instructions:
1. Cook the Farro: Bring 4 quarts of water to a boil in a Dutch oven. Add the farro and 1 tablespoon of salt. Return to a boil, then reduce the heat and simmer until the grains are tender with a slight chew, about 15 to 30 minutes. Drain the farro and return it to the pot. Cover to keep warm.
2. Sauté Aromatics: Heat 2 tablespoons of olive oil in a 12-inch skillet over medium heat until shimmering. Add the chopped onion and ¼ teaspoon of salt. Cook until the onion is softened, about 5 minutes. Stir in the minced garlic and cook until fragrant, about 30 seconds.
3. Combine and Heat Through: Add the cooked farro to the skillet with the onion and garlic mixture. Stir in the remaining 1 tablespoon of olive oil. Cook, stirring frequently,

until the farro is heated through, about 2 minutes.

4. Finish the Dish: Off the heat, stir in the chopped parsley, mint, and lemon juice. Season with salt and pepper to taste. Serve warm.

Warm Farro with Fennel and Parmesan

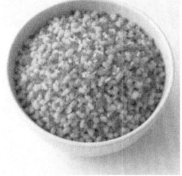

Ingredients:
- 1½ cups whole farro
- Salt and pepper, to taste
- 3 tablespoons extra-virgin olive oil
- 1 onion, finely chopped
- 1 small fennel bulb, stalks discarded, bulb halved, cored, and finely chopped
- 3 garlic cloves, minced
- 1 teaspoon fresh thyme, minced, or ¼ teaspoon dried
- 1 ounce Parmesan cheese, grated (about ½ cup)
- ¼ cup fresh parsley, minced
- 2 teaspoons sherry vinegar

Instructions:
1. Cook the Farro: Bring 4 quarts of water to a boil in a Dutch oven. Add the farro and 1 tablespoon of salt. Return to a boil, then reduce the heat and simmer until the grains are tender with a slight chew, approximately 15 to 30 minutes. Drain the farro and return it to the pot, covering it to keep warm.
2. Sauté the Vegetables: In a 12-inch skillet, heat 2 tablespoons of olive oil over medium heat until shimmering. Add the chopped onion, fennel, and a pinch of salt. Cook, stirring occasionally, until softened, about 8 to 10 minutes. Add the minced garlic and thyme, cooking for an additional 30 seconds until fragrant.
3. Combine and Heat Through: To the skillet with the sautéed vegetables, add the cooked farro and the remaining 1 tablespoon of olive oil. Cook, stirring frequently, until heated through, about 2 minutes.
4. Finish the Dish: Off the heat, stir in the grated Parmesan, minced parsley, and sherry vinegar. Season with salt and pepper to taste.
5. Serve: Transfer the mixture to a serving dish and serve warm.

This dish pairs wonderfully with a simple green salad or can be enjoyed on its own as a satisfying vegetarian main course.

Warm Wheat Berries with Zucchini, Red Pepper, and Oregano

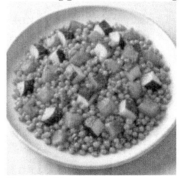

Ingredients:
- 1½ cups wheat berries
- Salt and pepper, to taste
- 2 tablespoons extra-virgin olive oil
- 3 tablespoons red wine vinegar
- 1 garlic clove, minced
- 1 tablespoon grated lemon zest
- 1 tablespoon minced fresh oregano
- 1 zucchini, cut into ½-inch pieces
- 1 red onion, chopped
- 1 red bell pepper, stemmed, seeded, and cut into ½-inch pieces

Instructions:

1. Cook the Wheat Berries: Bring 4 quarts of water to a boil in a Dutch oven. Add the wheat berries and 1½ teaspoons of salt. Return to a boil, then reduce the heat and simmer until the grains are tender but still chewy, about 60 to 70 minutes. Drain and transfer to a large bowl.
2. Prepare the Dressing: In a large bowl, whisk together the red wine vinegar, minced garlic, lemon zest, and minced oregano.
3. Sauté the Vegetables: Heat the olive oil in a large skillet over medium-high heat. Add the chopped red onion and cook, stirring occasionally, until softened, about 5 minutes. Add the red bell pepper and zucchini, season with salt and pepper, and continue to cook, stirring occasionally, until the vegetables are tender and slightly browned, about 8 to 10 minutes.
4. Combine and Serve: Add the warm wheat berries to the bowl with the dressing and toss to coat. Then, add the sautéed vegetables and toss gently to combine. Adjust seasoning with salt and pepper as needed. Serve warm.

This dish pairs well with a variety of main courses and can also be enjoyed as a hearty vegetarian main.

Penne with Roasted Cherry Tomatoes, Arugula, and Goat Cheese

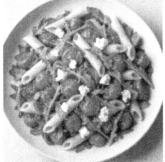

Ingredients:
- 1 shallot, thinly sliced
- ¼ cup extra-virgin olive oil
- 2 pounds cherry tomatoes, halved
- 3 large garlic cloves, thinly sliced
- 1 tablespoon sherry or red wine vinegar
- 1½ teaspoons sugar (adjust to taste)
- Salt and pepper to taste
- ¼ teaspoon red pepper flakes
- 1 pound penne pasta
- 4 ounces (about 4 cups) baby arugula
- 4 ounces goat cheese, crumbled (about 1 cup)

Instructions:
1. Roast the Tomatoes:
   o Preheat your oven to 350°F (175°C).
   o In a bowl, toss the sliced shallot with 1 teaspoon of olive oil.
   o In a separate bowl, gently toss the halved cherry tomatoes with the remaining olive oil, sliced garlic, vinegar, sugar, ½ teaspoon of salt, ¼ teaspoon of pepper, and red pepper flakes.
   o Spread the tomato mixture evenly on a rimmed baking sheet, scatter the shallot over the tomatoes, and roast for 35 to 40 minutes, until the shallot edges begin to brown and the tomato skins are slightly shriveled. Avoid stirring during roasting.
   o Let the roasted mixture cool for 5 to 10 minutes.
2. Cook the Pasta:
   o Bring 4 quarts of water to a boil in a large pot.
   o Add the penne and 1 tablespoon of salt. Cook, stirring often, until al dente.
   o Reserve ½ cup of the pasta cooking water, then drain the pasta and return it to the pot.

3. Combine and Serve:
   o Add the arugula to the drained pasta and toss until the arugula wilts.
   o Using a rubber spatula, scrape the roasted tomato and shallot mixture onto the pasta. Toss to combine.
   o Season with additional salt and pepper if needed. Adjust the consistency with the reserved pasta water as desired.
   o Serve the pasta topped with crumbled goat cheese.

Enjoy your meal!

Penne with Fresh Tomato Sauce, Spinach, and Feta

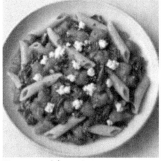

Ingredients:
- 1 pound penne pasta
- 3 tablespoons extra-virgin olive oil
- 2 cloves garlic, minced
- 3 pounds ripe tomatoes, cored, peeled, seeded, and cut into ½-inch pieces
- 5 ounces (about 5 cups) baby spinach
- 2 tablespoons chopped fresh mint or oregano
- 2 tablespoons lemon juice
- 4 ounces feta cheese, crumbled (about 1 cup)
- Salt and freshly ground black pepper, to taste
- Pinch of sugar (optional, to balance acidity)

Instructions:
1. Cook the Pasta:
   o Bring a large pot of salted water to a boil.
   o Add the penne and cook according to package instructions until al dente.
   o Reserve ½ cup of the pasta cooking water, then drain the pasta and return it to the pot.
2. Prepare the Sauce:
   o In a large skillet, heat 2 tablespoons of olive oil over medium heat.
   o Add the minced garlic and sauté until fragrant, about 1 minute.
   o Stir in the chopped tomatoes and cook until they begin to break down, about 8 minutes.
   o Add the spinach in batches, allowing it to wilt before adding more.
   o Season the mixture with salt, pepper, and a pinch of sugar if desired.
3. Combine and Serve:
   o Stir the chopped mint or oregano and lemon juice into the sauce.
   o Pour the sauce over the cooked penne, tossing to combine.
   o If the sauce appears dry, add some of the reserved pasta cooking water to reach the desired consistency.
   o Gently fold in the crumbled feta cheese.
   o Serve warm, garnished with additional feta if desired

Farfalle with Zucchini, Tomatoes, and Pine Nuts

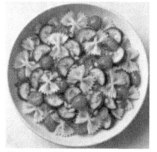

Ingredients:

- 2 pounds zucchini and/or summer squash, halved lengthwise and sliced ½ inch thick
- 1 tablespoon kosher salt
- 5 tablespoons extra-virgin olive oil, divided
- 3 garlic cloves, minced
- ½ teaspoon red pepper flakes
- 1 pound farfalle pasta
- 12 ounces grape tomatoes, halved
- ½ cup fresh basil, chopped
- ¼ cup toasted pine nuts
- 2 tablespoons balsamic vinegar
- Grated Parmesan cheese, for serving

Instructions:

1. Prepare the Zucchini:
   o Place the sliced zucchini in a colander, sprinkle with 1 tablespoon of kosher salt, and let it drain for 30 minutes. This process removes excess moisture and prevents the dish from becoming watery.
   o After 30 minutes, pat the zucchini dry with paper towels and gently wipe away any residual salt.
2. Cook the Zucchini:
   o Heat 1 tablespoon of olive oil in a 12-inch nonstick skillet over high heat until shimmering.
   o Add half of the zucchini slices and cook, stirring occasionally, until golden brown and slightly charred, about 5 to 7 minutes. Transfer this batch to a large plate.
   o Repeat the process with another tablespoon of olive oil and the remaining zucchini slices. Transfer to the plate once cooked.
3. Prepare the Sauce:
   o In the same skillet, heat the remaining 1 tablespoon of olive oil over medium heat until shimmering.

o Add the minced garlic and red pepper flakes, cooking until fragrant, about 30 seconds.
o Return all the cooked zucchini to the skillet, mixing to combine. Heat through for about 30 seconds.

4. Cook the Pasta:
   o Bring 4 quarts of water to a boil in a large pot.
   o Add the farfalle pasta and 1 tablespoon of salt. Cook, stirring occasionally, until al dente.
   o Reserve ½ cup of the pasta cooking water, then drain the pasta and return it to the pot.
5. Combine and Serve:
   o To the drained pasta, add the zucchini mixture, halved grape tomatoes, chopped basil, toasted pine nuts, balsamic vinegar, and the remaining 2 tablespoons of olive oil. Toss to combine.
   o Season with salt and pepper to taste. If the sauce appears too dry, add some of the reserved pasta cooking water to achieve the desired consistency.
   o Serve warm, topped with grated Parmesan cheese.

Spaghetti al Limone

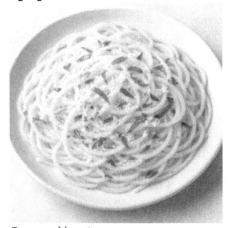

Ingredients:
- 1 pound (450g) spaghetti

- ½ cup (120ml) extra-virgin olive oil
- 2 teaspoons grated lemon zest (from about 2 lemons)
- ⅓ cup (80ml) fresh lemon juice (from about 2 lemons)
- 1 small garlic clove, minced to a paste
- 1 ounce (28g) Parmesan cheese, finely grated (about 1 cup)
- 6 tablespoons fresh basil, shredded
- Salt and freshly ground black pepper, to taste

Instructions:
1. Prepare the Pasta:
   o Bring a large pot of salted water to a boil.
   o Cook the spaghetti according to package instructions until al dente.
   o Reserve ½ cup of the pasta cooking water before draining.
   o Return the drained pasta to the pot.
2. Prepare the Sauce:
   o In a small bowl, whisk together the olive oil, lemon zest, lemon juice, minced garlic, and a pinch each of salt and pepper until well combined.
   o Stir in the grated Parmesan cheese until the mixture becomes a creamy consistency.
3. Combine Pasta and Sauce:
   o Pour the sauce over the warm pasta.
   o Add the shredded basil.
   o Toss everything together, adding reserved pasta water a little at a time if needed to achieve a silky, emulsified sauce that coats the spaghetti evenly.
4. Serve:
   o Divide the pasta among serving plates.
   o Garnish with additional Parmesan and basil if desired.
   o Serve immediately, enjoying the fresh, zesty flavors.

Tagliatelle with Artichokes and Parmesan

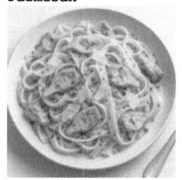

Ingredients:
- 4 cups jarred whole baby artichoke hearts packed in water
- ¼ cup extra-virgin olive oil, plus extra for serving
- 4 garlic cloves, minced
- 2 anchovy fillets, rinsed, patted dry, and minced
- 1 tablespoon minced fresh oregano or 1 teaspoon dried
- ⅛ teaspoon red pepper flakes
- ½ cup dry white wine
- 1 pound tagliatelle pasta
- 1 ounce Parmesan cheese, grated (½ cup), plus extra for serving
- ¼ cup minced fresh parsley
- 1½ teaspoons grated lemon zest
- Parmesan bread crumbs (optional, for topping)

Instructions:
1. Prepare the Artichokes:
   o Trim the tough outer leaves from the artichoke hearts, cut them in half, and pat them dry with paper towels. Place any discarded leaves in a bowl of water to prevent browning.
2. Sauté the Artichokes:
   o Heat 1 tablespoon of olive oil in a 12-inch nonstick skillet over medium-high heat until shimmering.
   o Add the artichoke hearts and a pinch of salt. Cook, stirring

frequently, until they develop a golden-brown color, approximately 7 to 9 minutes.
  - o Stir in the minced garlic, anchovy fillets, oregano, and red pepper flakes. Continue cooking, stirring constantly, until fragrant, about 30 seconds.
  - o Pour in the white wine, bring to a simmer, and let it reduce slightly. Remove the skillet from heat and set aside.
3. Cook the Pasta:
  - o Bring a large pot of salted water to a boil.
  - o Add the tagliatelle and cook according to package instructions until al dente. Reserve 1½ cups of the pasta cooking water before draining.
  - o Drain the pasta and return it to the pot.
4. Combine and Serve:
  - o To the pot with the drained pasta, add the artichoke mixture, grated Parmesan, minced parsley, lemon zest, and the remaining 3 tablespoons of olive oil.
  - o Toss everything together, adding reserved pasta water as needed to achieve a silky sauce that coats the pasta.
  - o Season with additional salt and pepper to taste.
  - o Serve the pasta in bowls, topping each serving with extra grated Parmesan and, if desired, a sprinkle of Parmesan bread crumbs.

Orecchiette with Broccoli Rabe and White Beans

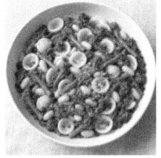

Ingredients:
- ¼ cup extra-virgin olive oil
- 1 shallot, minced
- 6 garlic cloves, minced
- 1 teaspoon minced fresh oregano (or ¼ teaspoon dried)
- ½ teaspoon fennel seeds, crushed
- ¼ teaspoon red pepper flakes
- 1 (15-ounce) can cannellini beans, rinsed
- 1 pound broccoli rabe, trimmed and cut into 1½-inch pieces
- Salt and pepper, to taste
- 1 pound orecchiette pasta
- 2 ounces Parmesan or Asiago cheese, grated (about 1 cup)

Instructions:
1. Prepare the Broccoli Rabe: Bring a large pot of salted water to a boil. Add the broccoli rabe and cook, stirring often, until crisp-tender, about 2 minutes. Using a slotted spoon, transfer the broccoli rabe to a bowl and set aside.
2. Sauté Aromatics: In a 12-inch skillet, heat the olive oil over medium heat until shimmering. Add the minced shallot and cook until softened, about 2 minutes. Stir in the minced garlic, oregano, fennel seeds, and red pepper flakes. Cook, stirring constantly, until fragrant, about 30 seconds.
3. Add Beans: Stir in the cannellini beans and cook until heated through, about 2 minutes. Season with salt and pepper to taste. Remove the

skillet from heat and set aside.

4. Cook the Pasta: In the same pot used for the broccoli rabe, bring water back to a boil. Add the orecchiette pasta and cook, stirring often, until al dente, about 9-11 minutes. Reserve 1 cup of the pasta cooking water, then drain the pasta and return it to the pot.

5. Combine and Serve: Add the sautéed broccoli rabe and bean mixture to the drained pasta. Stir in the grated Parmesan or Asiago cheese and toss to combine, adding reserved pasta water as needed to reach your desired sauce consistency. Adjust seasoning with salt and pepper if necessary. Serve warm.

Enjoy your meal!

Whole-Wheat Spaghetti with Greens, Beans, and Pancetta

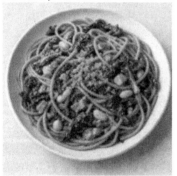

Ingredients:
- 1 tablespoon extra-virgin olive oil
- 3 ounces pancetta, cut into ½-inch pieces
- 1 onion, chopped finely
- 3 garlic cloves, minced
- ¼ to ½ teaspoon red pepper flakes (adjust to taste)
- 1½ pounds kale or collard greens, stemmed and cut into 1-inch pieces
- 1½ cups chicken broth
- Salt and pepper to taste
- 1 (15-ounce) can cannellini beans, rinsed and drained
- 1 pound whole-wheat spaghetti
- 4 ounces fontina cheese, shredded (about 1 cup)

- 1 cup Parmesan bread crumbs (optional, for topping)

Instructions:
1. Prepare the Greens: Heat the olive oil in a 12-inch straight-sided sauté pan over medium heat until shimmering. Add the pancetta and cook, stirring occasionally, until crisp, about 5 to 7 minutes. Using a slotted spoon, transfer the pancetta to a paper towel-lined plate.

2. Sauté Aromatics: In the same pan, add the chopped onion and cook over medium heat until softened and lightly browned, about 5 minutes. Stir in the minced garlic and red pepper flakes, cooking until fragrant, about 30 seconds.

3. Cook the Greens: Add half of the chopped greens to the pan, tossing until they start to wilt, about 2 minutes. Add the remaining greens, chicken broth, and ¾ teaspoon salt. Bring the mixture to a simmer, reduce the heat to medium-low, cover, and cook, tossing occasionally, until the greens are tender, about 15 minutes.

4. Combine Ingredients: Stir in the cannellini beans and the cooked pancetta. Remove the pan from heat.

5. Cook the Pasta: Bring a large pot of salted water to a boil. Add the whole-wheat spaghetti and cook, stirring often, until just shy of al dente. Reserve 1 cup of the cooking water, then drain the pasta and return it to the pot.

6. Combine Pasta and Sauce: Add the greens and bean mixture to the pasta, along with 1 cup of the reserved cooking water. Cook over medium heat, tossing to combine, until the pasta absorbs most of the liquid, about 2 minutes.

7. Finish the Dish: Stir in the shredded fontina cheese, allowing it to melt and create a creamy sauce. Season with

salt and pepper to taste. If desired, sprinkle individual servings with Parmesan bread crumbs for added texture and flavor.

Enjoy your meal!

Whole-Wheat Spaghetti with Greens, Beans, Tomatoes, and Garlic Chips

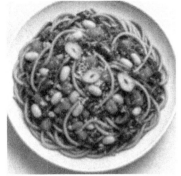

Ingredients:

- 3 tablespoons extra-virgin olive oil, plus extra for serving
- 8 garlic cloves, peeled (5 sliced thin lengthwise, 3 minced)
- Salt and pepper
- 1 onion, chopped fine
- ¼–½ teaspoon red pepper flakes
- 1¼ pounds curly-leaf spinach, stemmed and cut into 1-inch pieces
- ¾ cup vegetable broth
- 1 (14.5-ounce) can diced tomatoes, drained
- 1 (15-ounce) can cannellini beans, rinsed
- ¾ cup pitted kalamata olives, chopped coarse
- 1 pound whole-wheat spaghetti
- 2 ounces Parmesan cheese, grated (1 cup), plus extra for serving

Instructions:

1. Prepare the Garlic Chips:
   - Heat olive oil and sliced garlic in a 12-inch straight-sided sauté pan over medium heat.
   - Cook, stirring often, until garlic turns golden but not brown, about 3 minutes.
   - Using a slotted spoon, transfer garlic to a paper towel-lined plate and season lightly with salt.
2. Cook the Vegetables:
   - Add chopped onion to the same pan and cook over medium heat until softened and lightly browned, about 5 minutes.
   - Stir in minced garlic and red pepper flakes; cook until fragrant, about 30 seconds.
   - Add half of the spinach; toss occasionally until starting to wilt, about 2 minutes.
   - Add the remaining spinach, vegetable broth, diced tomatoes, and ¾ teaspoon salt.
   - Bring to a simmer, reduce heat to medium, cover, and cook, tossing occasionally, until spinach is completely wilted, about 10 minutes.
   - Stir in rinsed cannellini beans and chopped kalamata olives.
3. Cook the Pasta:
   - Meanwhile, bring 4 quarts of water to a boil in a large pot.
   - Add whole-wheat spaghetti and 1 tablespoon salt; cook, stirring often, until just shy of al dente.
   - Reserve ½ cup of cooking water, then drain pasta and return it to the pot.
4. Combine and Serve:
   - Add the vegetable and bean mixture to the pasta.
   - Cook over medium heat, tossing to combine, until pasta absorbs most of the liquid, about 2 minutes.
   - Off heat, stir in grated Parmesan cheese.
   - Season with salt and pepper to taste.
   - Serve immediately, drizzling individual

portions with extra olive oil and passing additional Parmesan separately.

Enjoy your meal!

Whole-Wheat Spaghetti with Lentils, Pancetta, and Escarole

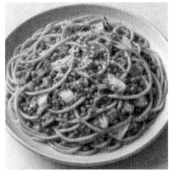

Ingredients:
- ¼ cup extra-virgin olive oil
- 4 ounces pancetta, cut into ¼-inch pieces
- 1 onion, chopped finely
- 2 carrots, peeled, halved lengthwise, and sliced ¼ inch thick
- 2 garlic cloves, minced
- ¾ cup lentilles du Puy (French green lentils), picked over and rinsed
- 2 cups chicken broth
- 1½ cups water
- ¼ cup dry white wine
- 1 head escarole (about 1 pound), trimmed and sliced ½ inch thick
- 1 pound whole-wheat spaghetti
- Salt and pepper to taste
- ¼ cup chopped fresh parsley
- Grated Parmesan cheese for serving

Instructions:
1. Prepare the Lentil Mixture:
   o In a large saucepan, heat 2 tablespoons of olive oil over medium heat. Add the pancetta and cook, stirring occasionally, until it begins to brown, about 3 to 5 minutes.
   o Add the chopped onion and sliced carrots to the pan. Cook until softened, about 5 to 7 minutes.
   o Stir in the minced garlic and cook until fragrant, about 30 seconds.
   o Add the lentils, chicken broth, and water. Bring the mixture to a simmer. Reduce the heat to medium-low, cover, and cook until the lentils are fully tender, about 30 to 40 minutes.
   o Stir in the white wine and let it simmer uncovered for 2 minutes.
   o Add the sliced escarole, a handful at a time, cooking until completely wilted, about 5 minutes.
2. Cook the Pasta:
   o Bring a large pot of salted water to a boil. Add the whole-wheat spaghetti and cook, stirring occasionally, until just shy of al dente. Reserve ¾ cup of the pasta cooking water, then drain the pasta and return it to the pot.
3. Combine and Serve:
   o Add the lentil and escarole mixture to the pasta, along with ½ cup of the reserved cooking water. Toss to combine.
   o Stir in the chopped parsley and season with salt and pepper to taste. Adjust the consistency with the remaining reserved cooking water if needed.
   o Serve the pasta in bowls, topped with grated Parmesan cheese.

No-Cook Fresh Tomato Sauce

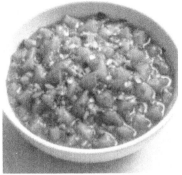

Ingredients:
- 2 pounds very ripe tomatoes, cored and cut into ½-inch pieces
- ¼ cup extra-virgin olive oil
- 2 teaspoons lemon juice, plus extra as needed
- 1 shallot, minced
- 1 garlic clove, minced
- Salt and pepper, to taste
- Pinch of sugar
- 3 tablespoons chopped fresh basil

Instructions:
1. Prepare the Tomatoes: In a large bowl, combine the diced tomatoes, shallot, and minced garlic.
2. Season the Sauce: Add the extra-virgin olive oil, lemon juice, salt, pepper, and a pinch of sugar to the tomato mixture. Stir well to combine all ingredients.
3. Marinate: Let the mixture sit at room temperature for about 30 minutes. This allows the flavors to meld and the tomatoes to release their juices, creating a flavorful base for your sauce.
4. Finish the Sauce: Just before serving, stir in the chopped fresh basil. Taste and adjust seasoning with additional salt, pepper, or lemon juice if needed.

Classic Marinara Sauce Recipe

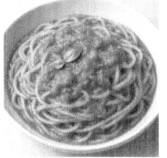

Ingredients:
- 2 tablespoons extra-virgin olive oil
- 1 small onion, finely chopped
- 2 cloves garlic, minced
- 1 (28-ounce) can whole peeled tomatoes
- 1 teaspoon dried oregano
- 1 teaspoon dried basil
- Salt and freshly ground black pepper, to taste
- A pinch of sugar (optional, to balance acidity)

Instructions:
1. Prepare the Tomatoes: Drain the canned tomatoes, reserving the juice. Crush the tomatoes by hand or with a spoon, removing and discarding any seeds.
2. Sauté Aromatics: In a large skillet or saucepan, heat the olive oil over medium heat. Add the chopped onion and sauté until softened and translucent, about 5 minutes. Add the minced garlic and cook for another minute until fragrant.
3. Add Tomatoes and Herbs: Stir in the crushed tomatoes, oregano, basil, salt, pepper, and a pinch of sugar if desired.
4. Simmer: Bring the sauce to a simmer. Reduce the heat to low and let it cook, uncovered, for about 15-20 minutes, stirring occasionally, until it thickens and the flavors meld.
5. Adjust Seasoning: Taste and adjust the seasoning with more salt, pepper, or herbs as needed.
6. Serve: Toss with your favorite pasta, such as spaghetti or penne. Garnish with fresh basil or grated Parmesan cheese if

desired.

Classic Basil Pesto Recipe

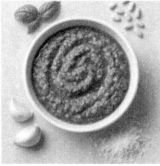

Ingredients:
- 2 cups fresh basil leaves, packed
- 2 cloves garlic, peeled
- 1/2 cup pine nuts, toasted
- 1 cup extra-virgin olive oil
- 1 cup freshly grated Parmesan cheese
- Salt and freshly ground black pepper, to taste

Instructions:
1. In a food processor, combine basil, garlic, and pine nuts. Pulse until coarsely chopped.
2. With the processor running, slowly drizzle in olive oil until the mixture is smooth.
3. Add Parmesan cheese and pulse to combine.
4. Season with salt and pepper to taste.

Note: If pine nuts are unavailable, walnuts or almonds can be used as substitutes.

Roasted Red Pepper Pesto

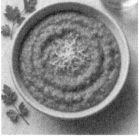

Ingredients:
- 2 roasted red bell peppers, peeled and chopped (1 cup)
- ¼ cup fresh parsley leaves
- 3 garlic cloves, toasted and minced
- 1 shallot, chopped
- 1 tablespoon fresh thyme leaves
- ½ cup extra-virgin olive oil
- ¼ cup grated Parmesan cheese

Instructions:
1. Prepare the Roasted Red Peppers:

If using homemade roasted red peppers, follow these steps:
Slice the peppers into flat slabs.
Roast at 450°F (230°C) until the skins are blistered and darkened, about 25-30 minutes.
Let them steam in a bowl covered with a plate for 10-20 minutes.
Peel off the skins, remove seeds and membranes, and chop.
If using jarred roasted red peppers, rinse and dry them well to reduce acidity.

2. Toast the Garlic:
   o In a dry skillet over medium heat, toast the unpeeled garlic cloves until their color darkens slightly.
   o Let them cool, then peel and mince.

3. Make the Pesto:
   o In a food processor, combine the roasted red peppers, parsley, minced toasted garlic, shallot, and thyme.
   o Process until smooth, scraping down the sides as needed.
   o With the processor running, slowly drizzle in the olive oil until fully incorporated.
   o Transfer the pesto to a bowl, stir in the Parmesan cheese, and season with salt and pepper to taste.

Pesto alla Trapanese

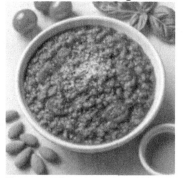

Ingredients:

- 1 pound (450g) ripe cherry or grape tomatoes, halved
- 1 cup (150g) toasted almonds
- 1 cup fresh basil leaves
- 2 cloves garlic, minced
- 1/2 cup extra-virgin olive oil
- 1 cup grated Pecorino Romano cheese
- Salt and pepper to taste

Instructions:

1. Prepare the Tomatoes: Place the halved cherry or grape tomatoes in a bowl and gently press them with a spoon to release some of their juices. This helps create a flavorful base for the pesto.
2. Toast the Almonds: If your almonds aren't already toasted, heat a dry skillet over medium heat. Add the almonds and toast them, stirring frequently, until they become fragrant and lightly browned. This process enhances their flavor.
3. Combine Ingredients: In a food processor, combine the minced garlic, toasted almonds, fresh basil leaves, and a pinch of salt. Pulse until the mixture reaches a coarse, crumbly consistency.
4. Incorporate Tomatoes: Add the prepared tomatoes to the food processor. Pulse a few times to combine, ensuring the tomatoes are broken down but not completely pureed.
5. Emulsify the Pesto: While the processor is running, slowly drizzle in the extra-virgin olive oil. Continue processing until the mixture forms a cohesive, slightly chunky paste.
6. Add Cheese: Transfer the pesto to a bowl and fold in the grated Pecorino Romano cheese. Stir until well combined.
7. Season: Taste the pesto and adjust the seasoning with salt and pepper as needed.
8. Serve: Toss the pesto with your choice of cooked pasta, adding a bit of pasta cooking water if necessary to achieve the desired consistency. Serve with additional grated cheese on top.

Spanish-Style Toasted Pasta with Shrimp

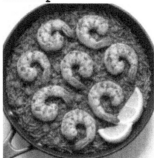

Serves: 4
Ingredients:
- For the Shrimp and Stock:
    - 3 tablespoons plus 2 teaspoons extra-virgin olive oil
    - 3 garlic cloves, minced
    - Salt and pepper
    - 1½ pounds extra-large shrimp (21 to 25 per pound), peeled and deveined, shells reserved
    - 2¾ cups water
    - 1 cup chicken broth
    - 1 bay leaf
- For the Pasta and Sauce:
    - 8 ounces vermicelli pasta or thin spaghetti, broken into 1- to 2-inch lengths
    - 1 onion, chopped fine
    - 1 (14.5-ounce) can diced tomatoes, drained and chopped fine
    - 1 teaspoon paprika
    - 1 teaspoon smoked paprika
    - ½ teaspoon anchovy paste
    - ¼ cup dry white wine
    - 1 tablespoon chopped fresh parsley
    - Lemon wedges (for serving)

Instructions:

1. Marinate the Shrimp: Combine 1 tablespoon oil, 1 teaspoon garlic, ¼ teaspoon salt, and ⅛ teaspoon pepper in a medium bowl. Add shrimp, toss to coat, and refrigerate until ready to use.
2. Make the Shrimp Stock: Place reserved shrimp shells, water, chicken broth, and bay

leaf in a medium bowl. Cover and microwave until liquid is hot and shells have turned pink (about 6 minutes). Set aside.

3. Toast the Pasta:
   Toss pasta with 2 teaspoons oil in a broiler-safe 12-inch skillet. Toast over medium-high heat, stirring often, until browned and nutty in aroma (pasta should resemble the color of peanut butter), about 6 to 10 minutes. Transfer pasta to a bowl and wipe out skillet.

4. Cook the Sofrito:
   Heat remaining 2 tablespoons oil in the skillet over medium-high heat. Add the onion and ¼ teaspoon salt, cooking until softened and starting to brown, about 4 to 6 minutes. Add tomatoes and cook until thick and dry, about 4 to 6 minutes. Reduce heat to medium, add garlic, paprika, smoked paprika, and anchovy paste, cooking for 1½ minutes until fragrant. Stir in pasta until well combined.

5. Simmer the Pasta and Shrimp:
   Pour shrimp stock through a fine-mesh strainer into the skillet (discard shells). Add wine, ¼ teaspoon salt, and ½ teaspoon pepper, stirring well. Bring to simmer over medium-high heat, cooking until the liquid is slightly thickened and pasta is tender, 8 to 10 minutes. Scatter shrimp over pasta, stirring to partially submerge them.

6. Broil the Dish:
   Transfer the skillet to the oven and broil until the shrimp are opaque and the pasta surface is crisp and browned (5 to 7 minutes). Remove from oven and let sit, uncovered, for 5 minutes.

7. Serve:
   Sprinkle with fresh parsley and serve immediately with lemon wedges.

Enjoy this quick and flavorful Spanish-inspired dish!

Rigatoni with Warm-Spiced Beef Ragu

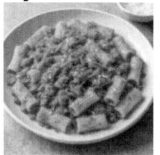

Serves: 6
Ingredients:
- 1½ lbs bone-in English-style short ribs, trimmed
- Salt and pepper
- 1 tbsp extra-virgin olive oil
- 1 onion, chopped fine
- 3 garlic cloves, minced
- 1 tsp minced fresh thyme (or ¼ tsp dried)
- ½ tsp ground cinnamon
- Pinch ground cloves
- ½ cup dry red wine
- 1 (28-ounce) can whole peeled tomatoes, drained and chopped fine, with juice reserved
- 1 lb rigatoni
- 2 tbsp minced fresh parsley
- Grated Parmesan cheese

Instructions:
1. Brown the Ribs:
   o Pat the ribs dry and season with salt and pepper. Heat oil in a 12-inch skillet over medium-high heat. Brown the ribs on all sides for 8-10 minutes, then transfer them to a plate.

2. Prepare the Sauce:
   o Pour off all but 1 teaspoon of fat from the skillet, then add onion and cook over medium heat for 5 minutes until softened. Stir in garlic, thyme, cinnamon, and cloves, and cook for 30 seconds until fragrant. Add wine, scraping up any browned bits, and simmer for 2 minutes until nearly evaporated.

3. Simmer the Ragu:
   o Stir in chopped tomatoes and reserved juice. Nestle the ribs into the sauce and bring to a simmer. Reduce heat to low, cover, and simmer for about 2 hours, turning ribs occasionally until the meat is tender and falls off the bone.
4. Shred the Meat:
   o Remove ribs from the sauce, let cool slightly, and shred the meat using two forks. Discard bones and excess fat. Skim the fat from the surface of the sauce, then stir in the shredded meat and any juices. Bring the sauce to a simmer and season with salt and pepper.
5. Cook the Pasta:
   o Bring 4 quarts of water to a boil in a large pot. Add pasta and 1 tablespoon of salt, cooking until al dente. Reserve ½ cup of cooking water, then drain and return the pasta to the pot. Add the sauce and parsley, tossing to combine. Adjust the consistency with the reserved pasta water as needed. Season with salt and pepper to taste.
6. Serve:
   o Serve the pasta with grated Parmesan cheese.

Orzo Salad with Arugula and Sun-Dried Tomatoes

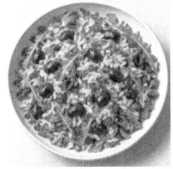

Serves: 4 to 6
VEG

Ingredients:
- 1¼ cups orzo
- Salt and pepper
- ¼ cup extra-virgin olive oil (plus extra for serving)
- 3 tbsp balsamic vinegar
- 2 garlic cloves, minced
- 2 oz (2 cups) baby arugula, chopped
- 1 oz Parmesan cheese, grated (½ cup)
- ½ cup oil-packed sun-dried tomatoes, minced
- ½ cup pitted Kalamata olives, halved
- ½ cup chopped fresh basil
- ¼ cup toasted pine nuts

Instructions:
1. Cook the Orzo:
   o Bring 2 quarts of water to a boil in a large pot. Add orzo and 1½ teaspoons salt. Cook, stirring often, until al dente. Drain orzo and transfer to a rimmed baking sheet. Toss with 1 tablespoon of olive oil and let cool completely for about 15 minutes.
2. Make the Vinaigrette:
   o Whisk the remaining 3 tablespoons olive oil, balsamic vinegar, garlic, ½ teaspoon salt, and ½ teaspoon pepper in a large bowl.
3. Combine the Ingredients:
   o Add arugula, Parmesan, sun-dried tomatoes, olives, basil, pine nuts, and the cooled orzo to the bowl. Gently toss to combine. Season with salt and pepper to taste.
4. Let it Rest:
   o Let the salad sit for about 30 minutes for the flavors to meld. Serve drizzled with extra olive oil. The salad can be refrigerated for up to 2 days.

Toasted Orzo with Fennel, Orange, and Olives

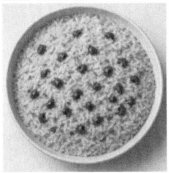

Serves: 6 to 8
VEG
Ingredients:
- 2 tbsp extra-virgin olive oil
- 1 fennel bulb, stalks discarded, bulb halved, cored, and chopped fine
- 1 onion, chopped fine
- Salt and pepper
- 2 garlic cloves, minced
- 1 tsp grated orange zest
- ¾ tsp fennel seeds
- Pinch red pepper flakes
- 2⅔ cups orzo
- 2 cups chicken or vegetable broth
- 1½ cups water
- ¾ cup dry white wine
- ½ cup pitted Kalamata olives, chopped
- 1½ oz Parmesan cheese, grated (¾ cup)
- Pinch ground nutmeg

Instructions:
1. Cook Aromatics:
   o Heat olive oil in a 12-inch nonstick skillet over medium heat. Add fennel, onion, and ¾ teaspoon salt, cooking until softened and lightly browned, about 5 to 7 minutes.
   o Stir in garlic, orange zest, fennel seeds, and red pepper flakes. Cook until fragrant, about 30 seconds.
2. Toast Orzo:
   o Add orzo to the skillet and cook, stirring frequently, until orzo is coated with oil and lightly browned, about 5 minutes.
3. Simmer:
   o Stir in broth, water, and wine, and bring to a boil. Cook, stirring occasionally, until all liquid has been absorbed and orzo is tender, about 10 to 15 minutes.
4. Finish the Pilaf:
   o Stir in chopped olives, Parmesan, and nutmeg. Season with salt and pepper to taste. Serve.

Orzo with Shrimp, Feta, and Lemon

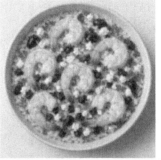

Serves: 4
Ingredients:
- 1 tbsp grated lemon zest plus 1 tbsp lemon juice
- Salt and pepper
- 1½ lbs extra-large shrimp (21 to 25 per pound), peeled and deveined
- 2 tbsp extra-virgin olive oil (plus extra for serving)
- 1 onion, chopped fine
- 2 garlic cloves, minced
- 2 cups orzo
- 2 cups chicken broth
- 2 cups water
- ½ cup pitted Kalamata olives, chopped coarse
- 2 oz feta cheese, crumbled (½ cup)
- 2 tbsp chopped fresh parsley

Instructions:
1. Prepare the Shrimp:
   o In a medium bowl, combine lemon zest, ½ teaspoon salt, and ½ teaspoon pepper. Add the shrimp and toss to coat. Refrigerate until ready to use.
2. Cook the Orzo:

- Heat 1 tablespoon of olive oil in a 12-inch nonstick skillet over medium-high heat. Add the onion and cook until softened, about 5 minutes. Stir in garlic and cook for about 30 seconds until fragrant.
- Add the orzo and cook, stirring frequently, until lightly browned and coated with oil, about 5 minutes.
- Stir in the broth and water, bringing it to a boil. Cook, stirring occasionally, until orzo is al dente, about 6 minutes.
- Stir in the olives, ¼ cup feta, and lemon juice. Season with salt and pepper to taste.

3. Cook the Shrimp:
   - Reduce heat to medium-low, nestle the shrimp into the orzo, cover, and cook until the shrimp are opaque throughout, about 5 minutes.
4. Serve:
   - Sprinkle with parsley and the remaining ¼ cup feta. Drizzle with extra olive oil and serve.

Orzo with Greek Sausage and Spiced Yogurt

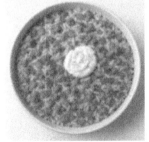

Serves: 4 to 6
Ingredients:
- 1½ cups orzo
- 1 tbsp extra-virgin olive oil
- 4 oz loukaniko sausage (chopped fine) (or substitute kielbasa or Italian sausage)
- 1 onion, chopped fine
- 1 red bell pepper, stemmed, seeded, and chopped fine
- 1 tbsp tomato paste
- 2 garlic cloves, minced
- 1 tsp paprika
- ¼ tsp ground cinnamon
- ⅛ tsp red pepper flakes
- ½ cup dry white wine
- 2½ cups chicken broth
- ¼ cup plain whole-milk Greek yogurt
- 1½ tsp grated lemon zest
- Salt and pepper
- ¼ cup chopped fresh mint

Instructions:
1. Toast the Orzo:
   - In a 12-inch skillet, toast the orzo over medium-high heat until lightly browned, 3 to 5 minutes. Transfer to a bowl.
2. Cook the Sausage and Vegetables:
   - Heat olive oil in the same skillet over medium heat. Add the sausage and cook until browned and the fat is rendered, about 4 to 6 minutes.
   - Stir in the onion and bell pepper, cooking until softened, 5 to 7 minutes. Add tomato paste, garlic, paprika, cinnamon, and red pepper flakes, cooking until fragrant, about 1 minute.
3. Simmer the Orzo:
   - Stir in the wine, scraping up any browned bits from the pan. Add the broth and toasted orzo. Bring to a simmer, reduce the heat to low, cover, and simmer until most of the liquid is absorbed, about 10 minutes, stirring once halfway through.
4. Finish the Dish:
   - Uncover and continue cooking, stirring occasionally, until the

orzo is al dente and creamy, about 4 minutes.
- o Off heat, stir in the yogurt and lemon zest. Season with salt and pepper to taste, and adjust the consistency with hot water if needed.
5. Serve:
- o Sprinkle with fresh mint and serve.

Baked Orzo with Eggplant and Tomatoes

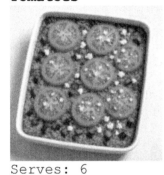

Serves: 6
VEG
Ingredients:
- 1 lb eggplant, cut into ½-inch pieces
- Salt and pepper
- 2 cups orzo
- 3 tbsp extra-virgin olive oil (plus extra for serving)
- 1 onion, chopped fine
- 3 garlic cloves, minced
- 4 tsp minced fresh oregano (or 1 tsp dried)
- 2 tsp tomato paste
- 2 anchovy fillets, rinsed, patted dry, and minced
- 1¼ cups chicken or vegetable broth
- 1¼ cups water
- 1 oz Parmesan cheese, grated (½ cup)
- 2 tbsp capers, rinsed and minced
- 4 tomatoes, cored and sliced ¼ inch thick
- 3 oz feta cheese, crumbled (¾ cup)

Instructions:
1. Prepare the Eggplant:
- o Adjust oven rack to the upper-middle position and preheat the oven to 400°F.
- o Line a large plate with a double layer of coffee filters and spray with vegetable oil spray.
- o Toss the eggplant with ½ teaspoon salt and spread it evenly on the coffee filters. Microwave the eggplant uncovered until dry to the touch and slightly shriveled, about 7 to 10 minutes, tossing halfway through.
2. Toast the Orzo:
- o Toast orzo in a 12-inch nonstick skillet over medium-high heat until lightly browned, 3 to 5 minutes. Transfer to a bowl.
- o Heat 1 tablespoon of oil in the same skillet over medium-high heat. Add the eggplant and cook, stirring occasionally, until well browned, 5 to 7 minutes. Transfer to a separate bowl.
3. Cook the Aromatics:
- o Heat the remaining 2 tablespoons of oil in the same skillet over medium heat. Add the onion and cook until softened and lightly browned, 5 to 7 minutes.
- o Stir in garlic, 1 tablespoon oregano, tomato paste, and anchovies. Cook for about 30 seconds until fragrant.
- o Off heat, stir in the orzo, eggplant, broth, water, Parmesan, capers, and ¼ teaspoon pepper. Transfer the mixture to a greased 13x9-inch baking dish and spread into an even layer.
4. Assemble and Bake:
- o Shingle the tomato slices attractively over the top

of the orzo and sprinkle with ¼ teaspoon salt.
- o Bake until all the liquid is absorbed and the orzo is tender, about 30 to 35 minutes.
- o Let cool for 5 minutes. Sprinkle with feta and the remaining 1 teaspoon oregano. Drizzle with extra olive oil.
5. Serve:
- o Serve warm.

Spiced Vegetable Couscous

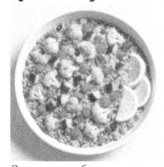

Serves: 6
VEG
Ingredients:
- 1 head cauliflower (2 pounds), cored and cut into 1-inch florets
- 6 tbsp extra-virgin olive oil (plus extra for serving)
- Salt and pepper
- 1½ cups couscous
- 1 zucchini, cut into ½-inch pieces
- 1 red bell pepper, stemmed, seeded, and cut into ½-inch pieces
- 4 garlic cloves, minced
- 2 tsp ras el hanout
- 1 tsp grated lemon zest (plus lemon wedges for serving)
- 1¾ cups chicken or vegetable broth
- 1 tbsp minced fresh marjoram

Instructions:
1. Cook the Cauliflower:
- o Toss cauliflower with 2 tablespoons olive oil, ¾ teaspoon salt, and ½ teaspoon pepper in a 12-inch nonstick skillet. Cover and cook over medium-high heat until

florets start to brown and edges become translucent, about 5 minutes.
- o Remove the lid and cook, stirring every 2 minutes, until the florets are golden brown in several spots, about 10 minutes. Transfer to a bowl and wipe the skillet clean.
2. Toast the Couscous:
- o Heat 2 tablespoons olive oil in the same skillet over medium-high heat. Add couscous and cook, stirring frequently, until the grains start to brown, about 3 to 5 minutes. Transfer to a separate bowl and wipe the skillet clean.
3. Sauté the Vegetables:
- o Heat the remaining 2 tablespoons olive oil in the skillet over medium-high heat. Add zucchini, bell pepper, and ½ teaspoon salt. Cook until tender, about 6 to 8 minutes.
- o Stir in garlic, ras el hanout, and lemon zest. Cook until fragrant, about 30 seconds. Stir in broth and bring to a simmer.
4. Combine with Couscous:
- o Stir in the couscous. Cover, remove the skillet from heat, and let sit until the couscous is tender, about 7 minutes. Add cauliflower and marjoram to the couscous and gently fluff with a fork to combine.
5. Serve:
- o Season with salt and pepper to taste, drizzle with extra olive oil, and serve with lemon wedges.

Moroccan-Style Couscous with Chickpeas

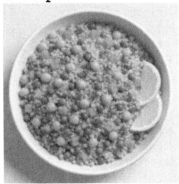

Serves: 6
FAST
  VEG
Ingredients:
- ¼ cup extra-virgin olive oil (plus extra for serving)
- 1½ cups couscous
- 2 carrots, peeled and chopped fine
- 1 onion, chopped fine
- Salt and pepper
- 3 garlic cloves, minced
- 1 tsp ground coriander
- 1 tsp ground ginger
- ¼ tsp ground anise seed
- 1¾ cups chicken or vegetable broth
- 1 (15-ounce) can chickpeas, rinsed
- 1½ cups frozen peas
- ½ cup chopped fresh parsley, cilantro, and/or mint
- Lemon wedges

Instructions:
1. Toast the Couscous:
    o Heat 2 tablespoons of olive oil in a 12-inch skillet over medium-high heat. Add the couscous and cook, stirring frequently, until the grains begin to brown, about 3 to 5 minutes. Transfer to a bowl and wipe the skillet clean.
2. Cook the Vegetables and Spices:
    o Heat the remaining 2 tablespoons of olive oil in the same skillet over medium heat. Add the carrots, onion, and 1 teaspoon of salt. Cook until softened and lightly browned, about 5 to 7 minutes.
    o Stir in garlic, coriander, ginger, and anise, and cook until fragrant, about 30 seconds. Add the broth and chickpeas, then bring to a simmer.
3. Combine the Couscous and Peas:
    o Stir in the peas and couscous. Cover, remove the skillet from heat, and let sit until the couscous is tender, about 7 minutes.
4. Finish the Dish:
    o Add parsley and gently fluff the couscous with a fork to combine. Season with salt and pepper to taste. Drizzle with extra olive oil and serve with lemon wedges.

Couscous with Lamb, Chickpeas, and Orange

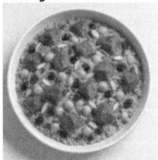

Serves: 6
Ingredients:
- 3 tbsp extra-virgin olive oil (plus extra for serving)
- 1½ cups couscous
- 1 lb lamb shoulder chops (blade or round bone), 1 to 1½ inches thick, trimmed and halved
- Salt and pepper
- 1 onion, chopped fine
- 10 (2-inch) strips orange zest (1 orange)
- 1 tsp grated fresh ginger
- 1 tsp ground coriander
- ¼ tsp ground cinnamon
- ⅛ tsp cayenne pepper
- ½ cup dry white wine
- 2½ cups chicken broth

- 1 (15-ounce) can chickpeas, rinsed
- ½ cup raisins
- ½ cup sliced almonds, toasted
- ⅓ cup minced fresh parsley

Instructions:

1. Toast the Couscous:
   o Adjust the oven rack to the lower-middle position and preheat the oven to 325°F.
   o Heat 2 tablespoons of oil in a Dutch oven over medium-high heat until shimmering. Add the couscous and cook, stirring frequently, until the grains begin to brown, 3 to 5 minutes. Transfer to a bowl and wipe the pot clean with paper towels.
2. Brown the Lamb:
   o Pat the lamb dry with paper towels and season with salt and pepper. Heat the remaining 1 tablespoon oil in the pot over medium-high heat until just smoking. Brown the lamb, about 4 minutes per side, then transfer to a plate.
3. Cook the Aromatics:
   o Add the chopped onion to the fat left in the pot and cook over medium heat until softened, about 5 minutes.
   o Stir in the orange zest, ginger, coriander, cinnamon, cayenne, and ⅛ teaspoon pepper. Cook until fragrant, about 30 seconds.
   o Stir in the wine, scraping up any browned bits from the pot.
4. Simmer the Broth:
   o Stir in the broth and chickpeas, then bring to a boil.

Simple Pearl Couscous

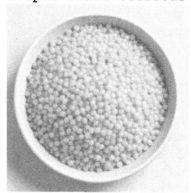

Serves: 6
FAST
VEG

Ingredients:

- 2 cups pearl couscous
- 1 tbsp extra-virgin olive oil
- 2½ cups water
- ½ tsp salt

Instructions:

1. Heat couscous and olive oil in a medium saucepan over medium heat, stirring frequently, until about half of the grains are golden brown, about 5 minutes.
2. Stir in water and salt, increase heat to high, and bring to a boil. Reduce heat to medium-low, cover, and simmer, stirring occasionally, until water is absorbed and couscous is tender, 9 to 12 minutes.
3. Off heat, let couscous sit, covered, for 3 minutes before serving.

Simple Pearl Couscous with Radishes and Watercress

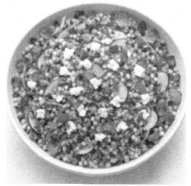

Serves: 6
VEG

Ingredients:

- ¼ cup extra-virgin olive oil

- 2 cups pearl couscous
- 2½ cups water
- Salt and pepper
- 3 tbsp sherry vinegar
- 1 tsp Dijon mustard
- 1 tsp smoked paprika
- ¼ tsp sugar
- 2 oz (2 cups) watercress, torn into bite-size pieces
- 6 scallions, sliced thin
- 6 radishes, trimmed and cut into matchsticks
- 1½ cups coarsely chopped parsley
- ½ cup walnuts, toasted and chopped coarse
- 4 oz goat cheese, crumbled (1 cup)

Instructions:
1. Cook the Couscous:
   o Heat 1 tablespoon of oil and couscous in a medium saucepan over medium heat, stirring frequently, until about half of the grains are golden brown, about 5 minutes.
   o Stir in water and ½ teaspoon salt, increase heat to high, and bring to a boil. Reduce heat to medium-low, cover, and simmer, stirring occasionally, until the water is absorbed and couscous is tender, 9 to 12 minutes.
   o Off heat, let couscous sit, covered, for 3 minutes. Transfer to a rimmed baking sheet and let cool completely, about 15 minutes.
2. Make the Dressing:
   o Whisk vinegar, mustard, paprika, sugar, ⅛ teaspoon salt, and the remaining 3 tablespoons of oil in a large bowl.
3. Assemble the Salad:
   o Add the couscous, watercress, scallions, radishes, parsley, and 6 tablespoons of walnuts to

the bowl. Gently toss to combine. Season with salt and pepper to taste, and transfer to a serving bowl. Let sit for 5 minutes.
4. Finish and Serve:
   o Sprinkle with goat cheese and the remaining 2 tablespoons of walnuts. Serve.

Simple Pearl Couscous with Peas, Feta, and Pickled Shallots

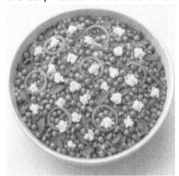

Serves: 6
VEG
Ingredients:
- ¼ cup extra-virgin olive oil
- 2 cups pearl couscous
- 2½ cups water
- Salt and pepper
- ⅓ cup red wine vinegar
- 2 tbsp sugar
- 2 shallots, sliced thin
- 3 tbsp lemon juice
- 1 tsp Dijon mustard
- ⅛ tsp red pepper flakes
- 4 oz (4 cups) baby arugula, coarsely chopped
- 1 cup fresh mint leaves, torn
- ½ cup frozen peas, thawed
- ½ cup shelled pistachios, toasted and chopped
- 3 oz feta cheese, crumbled (¾ cup)

Instructions:
1. Cook the Couscous:
   o Heat 1 tablespoon of olive oil and couscous in a medium saucepan over medium heat, stirring frequently, until about half of the grains are golden brown, about 5 minutes.

- Stir in water and ½ teaspoon salt, increase heat to high, and bring to a boil. Reduce heat to medium-low, cover, and simmer, stirring occasionally, until the water is absorbed and couscous is tender, 9 to 12 minutes.
- Off heat, let couscous sit, covered, for 3 minutes. Transfer to a rimmed baking sheet and let cool completely, about 15 minutes.

2. Pickle the Shallots:
- While the couscous cools, bring vinegar, sugar, and a pinch of salt to a simmer in a small saucepan over medium-high heat, stirring occasionally, until the sugar dissolves.
- Add shallots, stir to combine, and remove from heat. Cover and let cool completely for about 30 minutes. Drain and discard the liquid.

3. Make the Dressing:
- Whisk the remaining 3 tablespoons of olive oil, lemon juice, mustard, red pepper flakes, and ⅛ teaspoon salt together in a large bowl.

4. Assemble the Salad:
- Add the cooled couscous, arugula, mint, peas, 6 tablespoons of pistachios, ½ cup of feta, and pickled shallots to the dressing. Gently toss to combine.
- Season with salt and pepper to taste, and transfer to a serving bowl. Let sit for 5 minutes.

5. Serve:
- Sprinkle with the remaining ¼ cup of feta and remaining 2 tablespoons of

pistachios. Serve.

Hearty Pearl Couscous with Eggplant, Spinach, and Beans

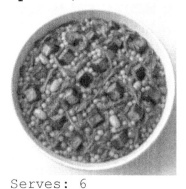

Serves: 6
VEG
Ingredients:
- 1 tsp ground sumac
- 1 tsp ground fenugreek
- Salt and pepper
- ¼ tsp ground cardamom
- 1 lb eggplant, cut into ½-inch pieces
- 1½ cups pearl couscous
- 5 tbsp extra-virgin olive oil (plus extra for serving)
- 1 onion, chopped
- 3 garlic cloves, minced
- 1 tbsp tomato paste
- 2 cups chicken or vegetable broth
- 1 (15-ounce) can great Northern beans, rinsed
- 3 oz (3 cups) baby spinach

Instructions:
1. Prepare the Eggplant:
- Combine sumac, fenugreek, ½ teaspoon salt, ½ teaspoon pepper, and cardamom in a small bowl.
- Line a large plate with a double layer of coffee filters and spray with vegetable oil spray.
- Toss the eggplant with ½ teaspoon of the spice mixture and spread evenly on the coffee filters. Microwave the eggplant uncovered until dry to the touch and slightly shriveled, about 7 to 10 minutes, tossing halfway through.

2. Toast the Couscous:

- o Heat couscous and 2 tablespoons of oil in a 12-inch nonstick skillet over medium heat, stirring frequently, until about half of the grains are golden brown, about 5 minutes. Transfer to a bowl and wipe the skillet clean.
3. Cook the Eggplant:
   - o Toss the eggplant with 1 teaspoon of the spice mixture. Heat 1 tablespoon of oil in the skillet over medium-high heat until shimmering. Add the eggplant and cook, stirring occasionally, until well browned, about 5 to 7 minutes. Transfer to a separate bowl.
4. Prepare the Broth Base:
   - o Heat the remaining 2 tablespoons of oil in the skillet over medium heat until shimmering. Add the onion and cook until softened and lightly browned, about 5 to 7 minutes.
   - o Stir in the garlic, tomato paste, and the remaining spice mixture. Cook until fragrant, about 1 minute.
5. Cook the Couscous:
   - o Stir in the broth, beans, and couscous, then bring to a simmer. Reduce heat to medium-low, cover, and simmer, stirring occasionally, until the broth is absorbed and the couscous is tender, 9 to 12 minutes.
   - o Off heat, stir in the spinach and eggplant, cover, and let sit for 3 minutes.
6. Serve:
   - o Season with salt and pepper to taste and drizzle with extra olive oil. Serve warm.

French Lentils with Carrots and Parsley

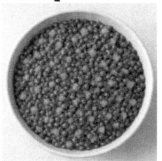

Serves: 4 to 6
VEG
Ingredients:
- 2 carrots, peeled and chopped fine
- 1 onion, chopped fine
- 1 celery rib, chopped fine
- 2 tbsp extra-virgin olive oil
- Salt and pepper
- 2 garlic cloves, minced
- 1 tsp minced fresh thyme (or ¼ tsp dried)
- 2½ cups water
- 1 cup lentilles du Puy (French green lentils), picked over and rinsed
- 2 tbsp minced fresh parsley
- 2 tsp lemon juice

Instructions:
1. Cook the Vegetables:
   - o Combine carrots, onion, celery, 1 tablespoon of oil, and ½ teaspoon salt in a large saucepan. Cover and cook over medium-low heat, stirring occasionally, until vegetables are softened, about 8 to 10 minutes.
   - o Stir in garlic and thyme, cooking until fragrant, about 30 seconds.
2. Cook the Lentils:
   - o Stir in water and lentils, then bring to a simmer. Reduce heat to low, cover, and simmer gently, stirring occasionally, until lentils are mostly tender, about 40 to 50 minutes.

3. Finish Cooking:
   o Uncover and continue cooking, stirring occasionally, until lentils are completely tender, about 8 minutes.
   o Stir in the remaining 1 tablespoon of oil, parsley, and lemon juice. Season with salt and pepper to taste, and serve.

Lentils with Spinach and Garlic Chips

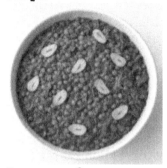

Serves: 6
VEG
Ingredients:
- 2 tbsp extra-virgin olive oil
- 4 garlic cloves, sliced thin
- Salt and pepper
- 1 onion, chopped fine
- 1 tsp ground coriander
- 1 tsp ground cumin
- 2½ cups water
- 1 cup green or brown lentils, picked over and rinsed
- 8 oz curly-leaf spinach, stemmed and chopped coarse
- 1 tbsp red wine vinegar

Instructions:
1. Fry the Garlic:
   o Heat the olive oil and garlic in a large saucepan over medium-low heat, stirring often, until the garlic turns crisp and golden but not brown, about 5 minutes.
   o Use a slotted spoon to transfer the garlic to a paper towel-lined plate, season lightly with salt, and set aside.
2. Cook the Onion and Spices:
   o Add the chopped onion and ½ teaspoon salt to the oil left in the saucepan. Cook over medium heat until softened and lightly browned, about 5 to 7 minutes.
   o Stir in the ground coriander and cumin, cooking until fragrant, about 30 seconds.
3. Cook the Lentils:
   o Stir in the water and lentils, then bring to a simmer. Reduce heat to low, cover, and simmer gently, stirring occasionally, until the lentils are mostly tender but still intact, about 45 to 55 minutes.
4. Add the Spinach:
   o Stir in the spinach, one handful at a time. Cook uncovered, stirring occasionally, until the spinach is wilted and the lentils are completely tender, about 8 minutes.
5. Finish and Serve:
   o Stir in the red wine vinegar and season with salt and pepper to taste. Transfer to a serving dish, sprinkle with the toasted garlic chips, and serve.

Lentil Salad with Olives, Mint, and Feta

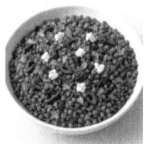

Serves: 4 to 6
Vegetarian

Ingredients:
- Salt and pepper
- 1 cup lentilles du Puy, picked over and rinsed

- 5 garlic cloves, lightly crushed and peeled
- 1 bay leaf
- 5 tablespoons extra-virgin olive oil
- 3 tablespoons white wine vinegar
- ½ cup pitted kalamata olives, coarsely chopped
- ½ cup chopped fresh mint
- 1 large shallot, minced
- 1 ounce feta cheese, crumbled (about ¼ cup)

Instructions:
1. In a bowl, mix 1 teaspoon salt with 4 cups warm water (around 110°F). Add lentils and let them soak at room temp for 1 hour. Drain well.
2. Set your oven rack in the middle and preheat to 325°F. In a medium oven-safe saucepan, mix lentils, 4 cups fresh water, garlic, bay leaf, and ½ teaspoon salt. Cover and bake until the lentils are tender but still holding their shape, 40-60 minutes.
3. Drain the lentils, tossing out the garlic and bay leaf. In a large bowl, whisk together the olive oil and vinegar. Add the warm lentils, olives, mint, and shallot. Toss everything together and season with salt and pepper to taste. Move to a serving dish and sprinkle with crumbled feta. Serve warm or at room temperature.

Chickpeas with Garlic and Parsley

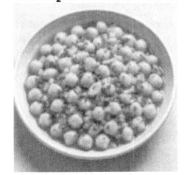

Serves: 4 to 6
Quick • Vegetarian

Ingredients:
- ¼ cup extra-virgin olive oil
- 4 garlic cloves, thinly sliced
- ⅛ teaspoon red pepper flakes
- 1 onion, finely chopped
- Salt and pepper
- 2 (15-ounce) cans chickpeas, rinsed
- 1 cup chicken or vegetable broth
- 2 tablespoons fresh parsley, minced
- 2 teaspoons lemon juice

Instructions:
1. In a large skillet (12-inch), heat 3 tablespoons of the olive oil over medium. Add garlic and red pepper flakes. Stir often and cook until the garlic turns golden—about 3 minutes.
2. Stir in the chopped onion and about ¼ teaspoon of salt. Cook until the onion softens and starts to brown a bit, 5-7 minutes.
3. Add chickpeas and broth. Bring it all to a simmer, then lower the heat to medium-low. Cover and cook for about 7 minutes, until everything's warmed through and the flavors have come together.
4. Take off the lid, turn the heat to high, and cook for another 3 minutes or so, until most of the liquid has cooked off.
5. Turn off the heat, stir in the parsley and lemon juice, then season with salt and pepper. Drizzle with the remaining tablespoon of olive oil and serve.

Chickpeas with Spinach, Chorizo, and Smoked Paprika

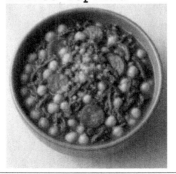

Serves: 4 to 6
Quick

Ingredients:
- Pinch of saffron threads, crumbled
- 2 teaspoons extra-virgin olive oil
- 8 ounces curly-leaf spinach, stems removed
- 3 ounces Spanish-style chorizo, finely chopped
- 5 garlic cloves, thinly sliced
- 1 tablespoon smoked paprika
- 1 teaspoon ground cumin
- Salt and pepper
- 2 (15-ounce) cans chickpeas
- 1 cup water
- 1 recipe Picada (see below)
- 1 tablespoon sherry vinegar

Instructions:
1. In a small bowl, combine saffron and 2 tablespoons of boiling water. Let it steep for 5 minutes.
2. Heat 1 teaspoon of oil in a Dutch oven over medium. Add the spinach and 2 tablespoons water, cover, and cook, stirring occasionally, for about 1 minute until wilted but still bright green. Transfer to a colander, press gently to release excess water, then chop coarsely. Return to the colander and press again to remove more liquid.
3. In the same pot, heat the remaining 1 teaspoon oil. Add the chorizo and cook until lightly browned, about 5 minutes. Stir in garlic, paprika, cumin, and ¼ teaspoon pepper. Cook until fragrant, about 30 seconds.
4. Add the chickpeas with their liquid, 1 cup water, and the saffron mixture. Bring to a simmer and cook, stirring now and then, until the chickpeas are tender and the broth thickens slightly, about 10-15 minutes.

5. Off heat, stir in the picada, spinach, and vinegar. Let sit for 2 minutes to warm through. If needed, adjust the thickness with a splash of hot water. Season to taste and serve.

Stewed Chickpeas with Eggplant and Tomatoes

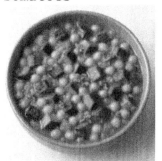

Serves: 6
Vegetarian

Ingredients:
- ¼ cup extra-virgin olive oil
- 2 onions, chopped
- 1 green bell pepper, finely chopped
- Salt and pepper
- 3 garlic cloves, minced
- 1 tablespoon fresh oregano (or 1 teaspoon dried), plus 2 teaspoons more for finishing
- 2 bay leaves
- 1 pound eggplant, cut into 1-inch pieces
- 1 (28-ounce) can whole peeled tomatoes, drained and chopped, juices reserved
- 2 (15-ounce) cans chickpeas, drained, with 1 cup liquid reserved

Instructions:
1. Preheat oven to 400°F and set rack to the lower-middle position. Heat oil in a Dutch oven over medium. Add onions, bell pepper, ½ teaspoon salt, and ¼ teaspoon pepper. Cook about 5 minutes, until softened.
2. Stir in garlic, 1 teaspoon oregano, and bay leaves. Cook for about 30 seconds, until fragrant.

3. Add eggplant, chopped tomatoes with their juice, chickpeas, and reserved chickpea liquid. Bring everything to a boil.
4. Transfer the pot to the oven, uncovered, and bake for 45 to 60 minutes, stirring twice, until the eggplant is very tender and the stew has thickened.
5. Remove bay leaves. Stir in the remaining 2 teaspoons of oregano, and season with more salt and pepper if needed. Serve warm, at room temp, or cold.

Spicy Chickpeas with Turnips

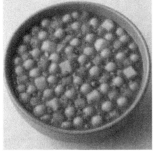

Serves: 4 to 6
Vegetarian

Ingredients:
- 2 tablespoons extra-virgin olive oil
- 2 onions, chopped
- 2 red bell peppers, chopped
- Salt and pepper
- ¼ cup tomato paste
- 1 jalapeño pepper, seeded and minced
- 5 garlic cloves, minced
- ¾ teaspoon ground cumin
- ¼ teaspoon cayenne pepper
- 2 (15-ounce) cans chickpeas, including liquid
- 12 ounces turnips, peeled and cut into ½-inch pieces
- ¾ cup water (plus more if needed)
- ¼ cup fresh parsley, chopped
- 2 tablespoons lemon juice (plus more to taste)

Instructions:
1. Heat the olive oil in a Dutch oven over medium heat. Add the

onions, bell peppers, ½ teaspoon salt, and ¼ teaspoon pepper. Cook for 5-7 minutes, until softened and lightly browned.
2. Stir in the tomato paste, jalapeño, garlic, cumin, and cayenne. Cook for about 30 seconds until fragrant.
3. Add the chickpeas with their liquid, the turnips, and ¾ cup water. Bring it all to a simmer and cook for 25-35 minutes, until the turnips are tender and the sauce has thickened up.
4. Stir in the parsley and lemon juice. Taste and adjust with more salt, pepper, or lemon juice if needed. If the sauce seems too thick, add a splash of hot water to loosen it up. Serve warm.

Chickpea Salad with Carrots, Arugula, and Olives

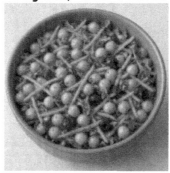

Serves: 6
Quick • Vegetarian

Ingredients:
- 2 (15-ounce) cans chickpeas, rinsed
- ¼ cup extra-virgin olive oil
- 2 tablespoons lemon juice
- Salt and pepper
- Pinch of cayenne pepper
- 3 carrots, peeled and shredded
- 1 cup baby arugula, roughly chopped
- ½ cup pitted kalamata olives, coarsely chopped

Instructions:
1. Place the chickpeas in a medium bowl and microwave until hot, about 2 minutes. Stir in the olive oil, lemon juice, ¾

teaspoon salt, ½ teaspoon pepper, and cayenne. Let sit for 30 minutes.
2. Add the shredded carrots, arugula, and olives. Toss well to combine. Taste and adjust seasoning with more salt and pepper if needed. Serve.

Falafel

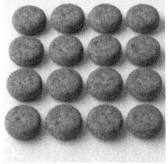

Makes: About 24
Vegetarian

Ingredients:
- Salt and pepper
- 12 ounces (2 cups) dried chickpeas, picked over and rinsed
- 10 scallions, chopped
- 1 cup fresh parsley leaves
- 1 cup fresh cilantro leaves
- 6 garlic cloves, minced
- ½ teaspoon ground cumin
- ⅛ teaspoon ground cinnamon
- 2 cups vegetable oil

Instructions:
1. In a large container, dissolve 3 tablespoons salt in 4 quarts of cold water. Add chickpeas and soak at room temp for 8 to 24 hours. Drain and rinse well.
2. In a food processor, blend the soaked chickpeas, scallions, parsley, cilantro, garlic, 1 teaspoon salt, 1 teaspoon pepper, cumin, and cinnamon. Process for about a minute until mostly smooth, scraping the bowl as needed.
3. Shape the mixture into small disks, about 2 tablespoons each, roughly 1½ inches wide and 1 inch thick. Place them on a parchment-lined baking sheet.

(You can refrigerate them for up to 2 hours at this point.)
4. Heat oven to 200°F and set a wire rack in a baking sheet. In a 12-inch skillet, heat oil over medium-high until it hits 375°F. Fry half the falafel at a time, 2-3 minutes per side, until deep golden brown. Adjust the heat as needed to keep the oil hot. Transfer cooked falafel to the rack and keep warm in the oven. Repeat with the rest.
5. Serve warm with your favorite sauce and toppings.

Making Falafel — Step-by-Step

1. Soak Chickpeas
Dissolve 3 tablespoons of salt in 4 quarts of water. Add the dried chickpeas and let them soak at room temperature for at least 8 hours (or overnight).

2. Process
In a food processor, blend the soaked chickpeas with fresh herbs, spices, and aromatics. Process until the mixture is smooth and well combined.

3. Shape
Scoop out about 2 tablespoons of the mixture and shape into disks roughly 1½ inches wide and 1 inch thick.

4. Fry
Heat oil to 375°F in a skillet. Fry half of the falafel at a time until they're deep golden brown on both sides, about 2-3 minutes per side. Keep them warm in a 200°F oven while you fry the rest.

Pink Pickled Turnips

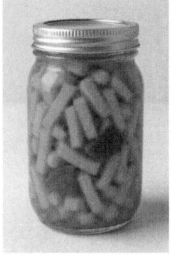

Makes: 4 cups
  Vegetarian

Ingredients:
- 1¼ cups white wine vinegar
- 1¼ cups water
- 2½ tablespoons sugar
- 1½ tablespoons canning/pickling salt
- 3 garlic cloves, smashed and peeled
- ¾ teaspoon whole allspice berries
- ¾ teaspoon black peppercorns
- 1 pound turnips, peeled and cut into 2-inch by ½-inch sticks
- 1 small beet, peeled and cut into 1-inch pieces

Instructions:
1. In a medium saucepan, bring the vinegar, water, sugar, salt, garlic, allspice, and peppercorns to a boil. Remove from heat, cover, and let steep for 10 minutes. Strain the brine and return it to the saucepan.
2. Run two 1-pint jars under hot water for 1-2 minutes to warm them. Shake dry. Pack the turnip sticks vertically into the jars, adding beet pieces evenly throughout.
3. Bring the strained brine back to a quick boil. Using a funnel, pour the hot brine over the vegetables to fully cover them. Let the jars cool to room temperature, then cover with lids and refrigerate for at least 2 days before serving.

Note: These can be stored in the fridge for up to 1 month. The turnips will soften a bit over time.

Black-Eyed Peas with Walnuts and Pomegranate

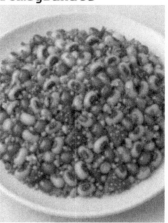

Serves: 4 to 6
  Quick • Vegetarian

Ingredients:
- 3 tablespoons extra-virgin olive oil
- 3 tablespoons dukkah (homemade or store-bought)
- 2 tablespoons lemon juice
- 2 tablespoons pomegranate molasses
- Salt and pepper
- 2 (15-ounce) cans black-eyed peas, rinsed
- ½ cup toasted walnuts, chopped
- ½ cup pomegranate seeds
- ½ cup minced fresh parsley
- 4 scallions, thinly sliced

Instructions:
1. In a large bowl, whisk together the olive oil, 2 tablespoons dukkah, lemon juice, pomegranate molasses, ¼ teaspoon salt, and ⅛ teaspoon pepper until smooth.
2. Add the black-eyed peas, walnuts, pomegranate seeds, parsley, and scallions. Toss everything gently to combine.
3. Taste and season with more salt and pepper if needed. Sprinkle the remaining tablespoon of

dukkah on top just before serving.

Cranberry Beans with Warm Spices

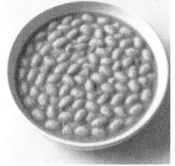

Serves: 6 to 8
Vegetarian

Ingredients:
- Salt and pepper
- 1 pound (2½ cups) dried cranberry beans, picked over and rinsed
- ¼ cup extra-virgin olive oil
- 1 onion, finely chopped
- 2 carrots, peeled and finely chopped
- 4 garlic cloves, thinly sliced
- 1 tablespoon tomato paste
- ½ teaspoon ground cinnamon
- ½ cup dry white wine
- 4 cups chicken or vegetable broth
- 2 tablespoons lemon juice, plus more to taste
- 2 tablespoons fresh mint, minced

Instructions:
1. Dissolve 3 tablespoons salt in 4 quarts cold water in a large bowl or container. Add the beans and soak at room temperature for 8 to 24 hours. Drain and rinse well.
2. Preheat oven to 350°F and set a rack in the lower-middle position. In a Dutch oven, heat the olive oil over medium. Add the onion and carrots and cook until softened, about 5 minutes.
3. Stir in garlic, tomato paste, cinnamon, and ¼ teaspoon pepper. Cook for about 1 minute, until fragrant. Add the

wine and scrape up any bits stuck to the bottom of the pot.
4. Stir in the broth, ½ cup water, and the drained beans. Bring to a boil. Cover the pot and transfer to the oven. Cook for about 1½ hours, stirring every 30 minutes, until the beans are tender.
5. Remove from the oven and stir in the lemon juice and mint. Taste and season with more salt, pepper, or lemon juice as needed. If the mixture is too thick, stir in a little hot water to loosen it up. Serve warm.

Cranberry Beans with Fennel, Grapes, and Pine Nuts

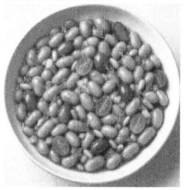

Serves: 6 to 8
Vegetarian

Ingredients:
- Salt and pepper
- 1 pound (2½ cups) dried cranberry beans, picked over and rinsed
- 3 tablespoons extra-virgin olive oil
- ½ fennel bulb, chopped (save 2 tablespoons fronds, discard stalks, core bulb)
- 1 cup + 2 tablespoons red wine vinegar
- ½ cup sugar
- 1 teaspoon fennel seeds
- 6 ounces seedless red grapes, halved (about 1 cup)
- ½ cup toasted pine nuts

Instructions:
1. Dissolve 3 tablespoons salt in 4 quarts of cold water in a

large bowl or container. Add beans and soak at room temp for 8 to 24 hours. Drain and rinse well.
2. In a Dutch oven, bring soaked beans, 4 quarts water, and 1 teaspoon salt to a boil. Reduce to a simmer and cook until beans are tender, 1 to 1½ hours. Drain and set aside.
3. Wipe out the pot. Heat olive oil over medium heat. Add chopped fennel, ¼ teaspoon salt, and ¼ teaspoon pepper. Cook about 5 minutes, until softened.
4. Stir in 1 cup red wine vinegar, sugar, and fennel seeds. Cook at a simmer until the mixture thickens into a syrupy glaze and the fennel edges begin to brown, about 10 minutes.
5. Add the beans to the glaze and toss to coat. Transfer to a large bowl and let cool to room temperature.
6. Once cool, stir in the grapes, pine nuts, fennel fronds, and remaining 2 tablespoons vinegar. Season with salt and pepper to taste. Serve.

Mashed Fava Beans with Cumin and Garlic (Ful Medames)

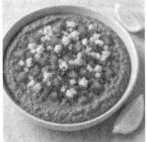

Serves: 4 to 6
Quick • Vegetarian

Ingredients:
- 4 garlic cloves, minced
- 1 tablespoon extra-virgin olive oil, plus more for drizzling
- 1 teaspoon ground cumin
- 2 (15-ounce) cans fava beans (with liquid)
- 3 tablespoons tahini
- 2 tablespoons lemon juice, plus lemon wedges for serving

- Salt and pepper
- 1 tomato, cored and diced
- 1 small onion, finely chopped
- 2 tablespoons fresh parsley, minced
- 2 hard-cooked eggs, chopped (optional)

Instructions:
1. In a medium saucepan, cook the garlic, olive oil, and cumin over medium heat until fragrant, about 2 minutes.
2. Stir in the fava beans with their liquid and the tahini. Bring to a simmer and cook until slightly thickened, 8-10 minutes.
3. Remove from heat. Mash the beans with a potato masher until they're the texture of refried beans—mostly smooth but a bit chunky. Add lemon juice and 1 teaspoon pepper. Season to taste with salt and more pepper if needed.
4. Transfer to a serving dish and top with tomato, onion, parsley, and eggs (if using). Drizzle with extra olive oil and serve with lemon wedges.

Mashed Fava Beans with Sautéed Escarole and Parmesan

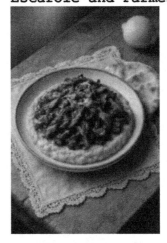

Serves: 4
Vegetarian

Ingredients:
- 2½ cups chicken or vegetable broth

- 2½ cups water (plus more if needed)
- 8 ounces (1½ cups) dried split fava beans
- 1 Yukon Gold potato, peeled and cut into 1-inch pieces
- 3 tablespoons extra-virgin olive oil, plus more for drizzling
- Salt and pepper
- 3 garlic cloves, minced
- ¼ teaspoon red pepper flakes
- 1 head escarole (about 1 pound), cored and chopped into 1-inch pieces
- 1 tablespoon grated lemon zest
- 1 ounce Parmesan cheese, shaved

Instructions:
1. In a large saucepan, bring the broth, water, and fava beans to a boil. Lower heat and simmer for about 15 minutes, until the beans begin to break down. Add the potato and continue simmering for 25-30 minutes, until tender and most of the liquid is absorbed.
2. Pass the bean and potato mixture through a food mill or ricer into a bowl. Stir in 2 tablespoons olive oil and season with salt and pepper. If it's too thick, add a little hot water to reach a thin mashed potato consistency. Cover to keep warm.
3. Meanwhile, heat the remaining 1 tablespoon olive oil in a large skillet over medium heat. Add garlic, red pepper flakes, and ¼ teaspoon salt. Cook for about 30 seconds until fragrant. Add escarole, cover, and cook 3-5 minutes until wilted. Stir in lemon zest and season with salt and pepper to taste.
4. Spread the warm fava bean mash onto a serving platter. Top with sautéed escarole, sprinkle with shaved Parmesan, and drizzle with a little extra olive oil. Serve warm.

Gigante Beans with Spinach and Feta

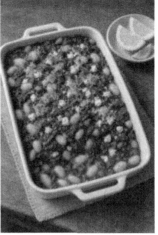

Serves: 6 to 8
Vegetarian

Ingredients:
- Salt and pepper
- 8 ounces (1½ cups) dried gigante beans, picked over and rinsed
- 6 tablespoons extra-virgin olive oil
- 2 onions, finely chopped
- 3 garlic cloves, minced
- 20 ounces curly-leaf spinach, stems removed
- 2 (14.5-ounce) cans diced tomatoes, drained
- ¼ cup minced fresh dill
- 2 slices hearty white sandwich bread, torn into pieces
- 6 ounces feta cheese, crumbled (about 1½ cups)
- Lemon wedges, for serving

Instructions:
1. Dissolve 3 tablespoons salt in 4 quarts of cold water in a large bowl or container. Add the beans and soak at room temperature for 8 to 24 hours. Drain and rinse.
2. In a Dutch oven, bring beans and 2 quarts water to a boil. Reduce to a simmer and cook, stirring occasionally, until beans are tender, about 1 to 1½ hours. Drain and set aside.
3. Wipe out the Dutch oven. Heat 2 tablespoons olive oil over medium heat. Add onions and ½ teaspoon salt and cook until

softened, about 5 minutes. Add garlic and cook until fragrant, about 30 seconds.

4. Stir in half the spinach, cover, and cook until just wilted, about 2 minutes. Add the remaining spinach, cover, and cook another 2 minutes. Turn off the heat and gently stir in the cooked beans, drained tomatoes, dill, and 2 more tablespoons oil. Season with salt and pepper to taste.

5. Preheat oven to 400°F. In a food processor, pulse bread and the remaining 2 tablespoons oil into coarse crumbs (about 5 pulses).

6. Transfer the bean mixture to a 13x9-inch baking dish. Top with crumbled feta and then sprinkle evenly with breadcrumbs. Bake until the top is golden and the edges are bubbling, about 20 minutes.

7. Serve warm with lemon wedges on the side.

Turkish Pinto Bean Salad with Tomatoes, Eggs, and Parsley

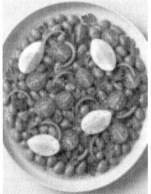

Serves: 4 to 6
Quick • Vegetarian

Ingredients:
- ¼ cup extra-virgin olive oil
- 3 garlic cloves, lightly crushed and peeled
- 2 (15-ounce) cans pinto beans, rinsed
- Salt and pepper
- ¼ cup tahini
- 3 tablespoons lemon juice
- 1 tablespoon ground Aleppo pepper (or ¾ tsp paprika + ¾ tsp crushed red pepper flakes)
- 8 ounces cherry tomatoes, halved
- ¼ red onion, thinly sliced
- ½ cup fresh parsley leaves
- 2 hard-cooked large eggs, quartered
- 1 tablespoon toasted sesame seeds

Instructions:
1. In a medium saucepan, heat 1 tablespoon of olive oil with the garlic over medium. Cook, stirring often, until the garlic is golden, about 3 minutes.

2. Add the pinto beans, 2 cups of water, and 1 teaspoon salt. Bring to a simmer, then remove from heat, cover, and let sit for 20 minutes.

3. Drain the beans and discard the garlic. In a large bowl, whisk together the remaining 3 tablespoons olive oil, tahini, lemon juice, Aleppo pepper, 1 tablespoon water, and ¼ teaspoon salt until smooth.

4. Add the warm beans, cherry tomatoes, red onion, and parsley to the dressing and toss gently to combine. Season with salt and pepper to taste.

5. Transfer to a serving platter, top with the quartered eggs, and sprinkle with sesame seeds and extra Aleppo pepper if desired. Serve warm or at room temperature.

Easy-Peel Hard-Cooked Eggs

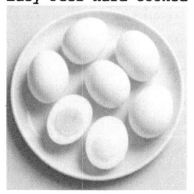

Makes: 6 eggs
Vegetarian

Ingredients:
- 6 large eggs (cold, no cracks)

Instructions:
1. In a medium saucepan, bring 1 inch of water to a rolling boil over high heat. Place the eggs in a steamer basket and lower into the pan. (If you don't have a basket, gently lower the eggs into the water using a spoon or tongs.)
2. Cover the pot, reduce the heat to medium-low, and steam the eggs for 13 minutes.
3. While the eggs cook, prepare an ice bath by combining 2 cups ice and 2 cups cold water in a medium bowl.
4. Once the eggs are done, transfer them to the ice bath and let them chill for 15 minutes.
5. Peel and use as needed, or store unpeeled in the fridge until ready to use.

Moroccan Braised White Beans with Lamb (Loubia)

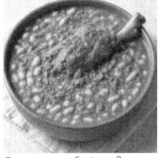

Serves: 6 to 8

Ingredients:
- Salt and pepper
- 1 pound (2½ cups) dried great Northern beans, picked over and rinsed
- 1 (12- to 16-ounce) lamb shank
- 1 tablespoon extra-virgin olive oil, plus more for serving
- 1 onion, chopped
- 1 red bell pepper, finely chopped
- 2 tablespoons tomato paste
- 3 garlic cloves, minced
- 2 teaspoons paprika
- 2 teaspoons ground cumin
- 1½ teaspoons ground ginger
- ¼ teaspoon cayenne pepper
- ½ cup dry white wine
- 4 cups chicken broth
- 2 tablespoons fresh parsley, minced

Instructions:
1. Soak the Beans:
   Dissolve 3 tablespoons salt in 4 quarts cold water in a large container. Add the beans and soak at room temperature for 8 to 24 hours. Drain and rinse well.
2. Brown the Lamb:
   Preheat oven to 350°F and set a rack in the lower-middle position. Pat lamb dry and season with salt and pepper. In a Dutch oven, heat 1 tablespoon oil over medium-high until just smoking. Brown the lamb on all sides, 10-15 minutes. Transfer to a plate and pour off all but 2 tablespoons of fat.
3. Build the Flavor Base:
   Add the onion and bell pepper to the pot and cook over medium heat until softened and lightly browned, about 5-7 minutes. Stir in tomato paste, garlic, paprika, cumin, ginger, cayenne, and ⅛ teaspoon pepper; cook about 30 seconds until fragrant. Add wine, scraping up any browned bits. Stir in the broth, 1 cup water, and the soaked beans. Bring to a boil.
4. Braise:
   Nestle the lamb back into the pot with its juices. Cover and transfer to the oven. Cook for 1½ to 1¾ hours, stirring every 30 minutes, until the lamb is fork-tender and the beans are creamy.
5. Finish the Dish:
   Remove lamb and let cool slightly. Shred with two forks, discarding fat and bone. Stir the lamb and parsley into the beans. Taste and season with

salt and pepper. Add hot water if the beans are too thick. Drizzle with a little olive oil before serving.

Sicilian White Beans and Escarole

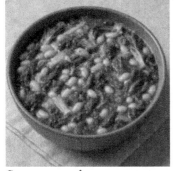

Serves: 4
Quick • Vegetarian

Ingredients:
- 1 tablespoon extra-virgin olive oil, plus more for drizzling
- 2 onions, finely chopped
- Salt and pepper
- 4 garlic cloves, minced
- ⅛ teaspoon red pepper flakes
- 1 head escarole (about 1 pound), trimmed and sliced into 1-inch strips
- 1 (15-ounce) can cannellini beans, rinsed
- 1 cup chicken or vegetable broth
- 1 cup water
- 2 teaspoons lemon juice

Instructions:
1. In a Dutch oven, heat 1 tablespoon olive oil over medium heat. Add onions and ½ teaspoon salt. Cook for 5-7 minutes, stirring occasionally, until softened and lightly browned.
2. Stir in garlic and red pepper flakes; cook for about 30 seconds until fragrant.
3. Add escarole, cannellini beans, broth, and water. Bring to a simmer and cook, stirring occasionally, until the escarole is wilted—about 5 minutes.

4. Increase the heat to high and cook until most of the liquid evaporates, 10 to 15 minutes.
5. Off heat, stir in lemon juice. Season with salt and pepper to taste, then drizzle with extra olive oil. Serve warm.

White Bean Salad

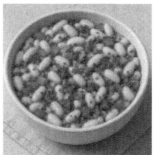

Serves: 6 to 8
Vegetarian

Ingredients:
- ¼ cup extra-virgin olive oil
- 3 garlic cloves, peeled and smashed
- 2 (15-ounce) cans cannellini beans, rinsed
- Salt and pepper
- 2 teaspoons sherry vinegar
- 1 small shallot, minced
- 1 red bell pepper, diced (¼-inch pieces)
- ¼ cup chopped fresh parsley
- 2 teaspoons chopped fresh chives

Instructions:
1. In a medium saucepan, heat 1 tablespoon olive oil with the garlic over medium. Cook, stirring often, until garlic is golden but not browned—about 3 minutes.
2. Add beans, 2 cups water, and 1 teaspoon salt. Bring to a simmer, then remove from heat, cover, and let sit for 20 minutes.
3. Meanwhile, in a large bowl, combine the sherry vinegar and minced shallot. Let sit while the beans steep.
4. Drain the beans and discard the garlic. Add the beans to the shallot mixture, along with the remaining 3 tablespoons olive

oil, bell pepper, parsley, and chives. Toss gently to combine.
5. Season with salt and pepper to taste. Let sit for another 20 minutes before serving.

White Bean Salad with Sautéed Squid and Pepperoncini

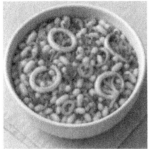

Serves: 4 to 6

Ingredients:
- 1 tablespoon baking soda
- Salt and pepper
- 1 pound small squid (bodies sliced into ½-inch rings, tentacles halved)
- 6 tablespoons extra-virgin olive oil
- 1 red onion, finely chopped
- 3 garlic cloves, minced
- 2 (15-ounce) cans cannellini beans, rinsed
- ⅓ cup pepperoncini, sliced into ¼-inch rings, plus 2 tablespoons brine
- 2 tablespoons sherry vinegar
- ½ cup fresh parsley leaves
- 3 scallions, green parts only, thinly sliced

Instructions:
1. In a medium bowl, dissolve the baking soda and 1 tablespoon salt in 3 cups cold water. Add squid, cover, and refrigerate for 15 minutes. Rinse and dry thoroughly with paper towels. Toss squid with 1 tablespoon olive oil.
2. In a medium saucepan, heat 1 tablespoon oil over medium. Add the onion and ¼ teaspoon salt. Cook, stirring occasionally, until soft and lightly browned, 5-7 minutes. Stir in garlic and cook until fragrant, about 30 seconds. Add the beans and ¼

cup water. Bring to a simmer, cover, and cook on low for 2-3 minutes. Set aside.
3. Heat 1 tablespoon oil in a 12-inch nonstick skillet over high heat until just smoking. Add half of the squid in a single layer. Cook without stirring for about 3 minutes until browned, then flip and cook another 2 minutes. Transfer to a bowl. Wipe out the skillet and repeat with 1 tablespoon oil and the remaining squid.
4. In a large bowl, whisk the remaining 2 tablespoons oil with the pepperoncini brine and vinegar. Add the warm beans (with any cooking liquid), squid, parsley, scallions, and pepperoncini. Toss to combine and season with salt and pepper to taste.
5. Serve warm or at room temperature.

North African Vegetable and Bean Stew

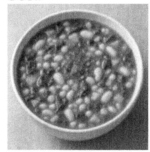

Serves: 6 to 8
Vegetarian

Ingredients:
- 1 tablespoon extra-virgin olive oil
- 1 onion, finely chopped
- 8 ounces Swiss chard, stems chopped, leaves cut into ½-inch pieces
- 4 garlic cloves, minced
- 1 teaspoon ground cumin
- ½ teaspoon paprika
- ½ teaspoon ground coriander
- ¼ teaspoon ground cinnamon
- 2 tablespoons tomato paste
- 2 tablespoons all-purpose flour
- 7 cups vegetable broth

- 2 carrots, peeled and cut into ½-inch pieces
- 1 (15-ounce) can chickpeas, rinsed
- 1 (15-ounce) can butter beans (or frozen baby lima beans), rinsed
- ½ cup small pasta (ditalini, tubettini, or elbow macaroni)
- ⅓ cup minced fresh parsley
- 6 tablespoons harissa (store-bought or homemade)
- Salt and pepper

Instructions:
1. In a Dutch oven, heat olive oil over medium. Add the onion and chard stems and cook until softened, about 5 minutes.
2. Stir in garlic, cumin, paprika, coriander, and cinnamon. Cook until fragrant, about 30 seconds. Add tomato paste and flour and cook, stirring, for 1 minute.
3. Gradually add the broth and carrots, scraping the pot to loosen any browned bits and smooth out any lumps. Bring to a boil, then reduce to a gentle simmer. Cook for 10 minutes.
4. Stir in chard leaves, chickpeas, butter beans, and pasta. Simmer until vegetables and pasta are tender, 10 to 15 minutes.
5. Stir in parsley and ¼ cup harissa. Season with salt and pepper to taste. Serve hot, passing the remaining harissa at the table.

Vegetables

Roasted Artichokes with Lemon Vinaigrette

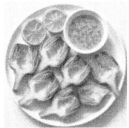

Serves: 4
Vegetarian

Ingredients:
- 3 lemons
- 4 artichokes (8 to 10 ounces each)
- 9 tablespoons extra-virgin olive oil
- Salt and pepper
- ½ teaspoon garlic, minced to a paste
- ½ teaspoon Dijon mustard
- 2 teaspoons chopped fresh parsley

Instructions:
1. Preheat oven to 475°F and adjust oven rack to lower-middle position. Fill a bowl with 2 quarts of water. Cut 1 lemon in half, squeeze juice into the water, and drop in the lemon halves.
2. Prep each artichoke: Trim the stem to about ¾ inch, cut off the top quarter, and remove 3-4 rows of tough outer leaves. Use a paring knife to trim the stem and base, removing dark green parts. Halve the artichoke lengthwise, scoop out the fuzzy choke and any inner purple leaves. Submerge each in the lemon water as you go.
3. Coat the bottom of a 13x9-inch baking dish with 1 tablespoon oil. Remove artichokes from the water and shake off excess (leave some moisture clinging). Toss with 2 tablespoons oil, ¾ teaspoon salt, and a pinch of pepper, rubbing the oil between the leaves. Arrange cut side down in the dish.
4. Trim ends off the remaining 2 lemons, halve them crosswise, and place cut side up in the dish. Cover tightly with foil and roast for 25-30 minutes, until artichokes are tender and starting to brown on the cut sides.
5. Transfer artichokes to a serving platter. Let roasted lemons cool slightly, then squeeze juice through a fine-mesh strainer to yield about 1½ tablespoons. Whisk in garlic, mustard, and ½ teaspoon salt. Slowly whisk in remaining 6 tablespoons oil until emulsified. Stir in parsley and adjust seasoning.
6. Serve artichokes with vinaigrette spooned over or on the side for dipping.

Making Roasted Artichokes — Step-by-Step

1. Prep
Trim the artichokes, cut them in half, and scoop out the fuzzy chokes. Drop them into a bowl of lemon water right after trimming to keep them from browning.

2. Season
Take the artichokes out of the lemon water, leaving some water clinging to the leaves. Toss them with olive oil, salt, and pepper, making sure to work the seasoning between the leaves. Arrange them cut side down in a baking dish.

3. Roast
Trim and halve a couple of lemons and place them cut side up in the dish with the artichokes. Cover the whole dish tightly with foil and roast until the artichokes are tender and just starting to brown.

4. Make Dressing
Let the lemons cool slightly, then squeeze the juice through a strainer into a bowl. Whisk in garlic, Dijon,

and salt, then slowly whisk in olive oil until smooth. Stir in chopped parsley and serve with the artichokes.

Braised Artichokes with Tomatoes and Thyme

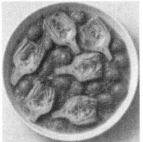

Serves: 4 to 6

Ingredients:
- 1 lemon
- 4 artichokes (8 to 10 ounces each)
- 2 tablespoons extra-virgin olive oil
- 1 onion, finely chopped
- Salt and pepper
- 3 garlic cloves, minced
- 2 anchovy fillets, rinsed, dried, and minced
- 1 teaspoon minced fresh thyme (or ¼ teaspoon dried)
- ½ cup dry white wine
- 1 cup chicken broth
- 6 ounces cherry tomatoes, halved
- 2 tablespoons chopped fresh parsley

Instructions:
1. Fill a large bowl with 2 quarts water. Squeeze in the juice of a lemon and drop in the spent halves.
2. Working one at a time, trim the stem of each artichoke to about ¾ inch and cut off the top quarter. Peel away 3-4 rows of tough outer leaves. Trim the stem and base with a paring knife to remove any dark green parts. Halve lengthwise, scoop out the fuzzy choke and any small purple leaves, then cut each half into thick wedges. Drop into the lemon water as you go.
3. In a 12-inch skillet, heat olive oil over medium. Add onion, ¾ teaspoon salt, and ¼ teaspoon pepper. Cook, stirring, until the onion softens and browns slightly, about 5-7 minutes. Stir in garlic, anchovies, and thyme; cook for 30 seconds until fragrant.
4. Add the wine and simmer until nearly evaporated, about 1 minute. Stir in the broth and bring to a simmer.
5. Drain artichokes and add to the skillet. Cover, reduce heat to medium-low, and simmer until tender, 20-25 minutes.
6. Stir in cherry tomatoes and cook uncovered for 3-5 minutes, just until they begin to soften.
7. Off heat, stir in parsley. Season with salt and pepper to taste. Serve warm.

Artichoke, Pepper, and Chickpea Tagine

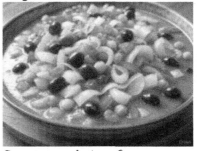

Serves: 4 to 6
Vegetarian

Ingredients:
- ¼ cup extra-virgin olive oil, plus more for serving
- 3 cups jarred whole baby artichoke hearts (rinsed, patted dry, quartered)
- 2 red or yellow bell peppers, cut into ½-inch-wide strips
- 1 onion, halved and sliced ¼ inch thick
- 4 (2-inch) strips lemon zest, plus 1 teaspoon grated zest (from 2 lemons)
- 8 garlic cloves, minced
- 1 tablespoon paprika
- ½ teaspoon ground cumin

- ¼ teaspoon ground ginger
- ¼ teaspoon ground coriander
- ¼ teaspoon ground cinnamon
- ⅛ teaspoon cayenne pepper
- 2 tablespoons all-purpose flour
- 3 cups vegetable broth
- 2 (15-ounce) cans chickpeas, rinsed
- ½ cup pitted kalamata olives, halved
- ½ cup golden raisins
- 2 tablespoons honey
- ½ cup plain whole-milk Greek yogurt
- ½ cup minced fresh cilantro
- Salt and pepper

Instructions:
1. In a Dutch oven, heat 1 tablespoon olive oil over medium heat. Add the artichoke hearts and cook, turning occasionally, until golden brown, about 5 to 7 minutes. Transfer to a bowl.
2. Add the bell peppers, onion, lemon zest strips, and 1 tablespoon more oil. Cook over medium until softened and lightly browned, about 5 to 7 minutes.
3. Stir in two-thirds of the garlic, all the spices, and cayenne. Cook until fragrant, about 30 seconds. Add the flour and cook for 1 minute, stirring constantly.
4. Slowly whisk in the broth, scraping up any browned bits and smoothing out any lumps. Add the artichokes back to the pot along with chickpeas, olives, raisins, and honey. Bring to a simmer, cover, and cook on low until vegetables are tender, about 15 minutes.
5. Remove from heat and discard the lemon zest strips. Temper the yogurt by mixing ¼ cup of the hot broth with the yogurt in a small bowl, then stir it into the pot.
6. Stir in the remaining 2 tablespoons oil, the rest of the garlic, chopped cilantro,

and grated lemon zest. Season with salt and pepper to taste.
7. Serve warm, drizzled with a little extra olive oil. Pairs well with couscous.

Pan-Roasted Asparagus with Cherry Tomatoes and Kalamata Olives

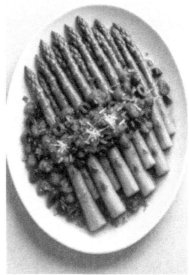

Serves: 6
Quick • Vegetarian

Ingredients:
- 2 tablespoons extra-virgin olive oil
- 2 garlic cloves, minced
- 12 ounces cherry tomatoes, halved
- ½ cup pitted kalamata olives, coarsely chopped
- 2 pounds thick asparagus, trimmed
- 2 tablespoons fresh basil, shredded
- ¼ cup grated Parmesan cheese
- Salt and pepper

Instructions:
1. In a 12-inch skillet, heat 1 tablespoon olive oil over medium. Add garlic and cook, stirring often, until golden but not brown—about 3 minutes.
2. Add tomatoes and olives and cook until the tomatoes begin to soften and break down, about 3 minutes. Transfer mixture to a bowl.
3. In the now-empty skillet, heat the remaining 1 tablespoon oil

over medium-high. Add the asparagus, arranging half with tips in one direction and the rest in the opposite. Shake the pan gently to distribute evenly. Add 1 teaspoon water, cover, and cook for about 5 minutes, until bright green and crisp.

4. Uncover, increase heat to high, and cook 5-7 minutes more, turning occasionally with tongs, until browned on one side and just tender.
5. Season with salt and pepper, then transfer asparagus to a serving platter. Spoon tomato mixture over top, sprinkle with basil and Parmesan, and serve warm.

Roasted Asparagus

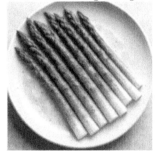

Serves: 4 to 6
Quick • Vegetarian

Ingredients:
- 2 pounds thick asparagus, trimmed
- 2 tablespoons plus 2 teaspoons extra-virgin olive oil
- ½ teaspoon salt
- ¼ teaspoon pepper

Instructions:
1. Place a rimmed baking sheet on the lowest oven rack and heat oven to 500°F. Peel the bottom halves of the asparagus to expose the white flesh.
2. Toss the spears with 2 tablespoons of olive oil, salt, and pepper.
3. Carefully spread the asparagus in a single layer on the hot baking sheet. Roast—without moving them—until browned underneath and bright green on

top, and a paring knife slides easily into the base of the largest spear, about 8-10 minutes.

4. Transfer to a serving platter and drizzle with the remaining 2 teaspoons olive oil. Serve as is, or with a gremolata topping (see below).

Braised Asparagus, Peas, and Radishes with Tarragon

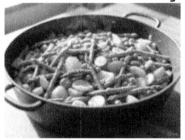

Serves: 4 to 6
Quick • Vegetarian

Ingredients:
- ¼ cup extra-virgin olive oil
- 1 shallot, thinly sliced into rounds
- 2 garlic cloves, thinly sliced
- 3 fresh thyme sprigs
- Pinch of red pepper flakes
- 10 radishes, trimmed and quartered lengthwise
- 1¼ cups water
- 2 teaspoons grated lemon zest
- 2 teaspoons grated orange zest
- 1 bay leaf
- Salt and pepper
- 1 pound asparagus, trimmed and cut into 2-inch pieces
- 2 cups frozen peas
- 4 teaspoons chopped fresh tarragon

Instructions:
1. In a Dutch oven, heat olive oil over medium. Add shallot, garlic, thyme, and red pepper flakes. Cook for about 2 minutes, until shallot softens.
2. Stir in radishes, water, lemon and orange zest, bay leaf, and 1 teaspoon salt. Bring to a simmer, then reduce heat to medium-low, cover, and cook for

3-5 minutes, until radishes are tender.

3. Stir in asparagus, cover, and cook for another 3-5 minutes, until just tender.

4. Off heat, add frozen peas, cover, and let sit for 5 minutes to warm through.

5. Remove thyme sprigs and bay leaf. Stir in tarragon, season with salt and pepper to taste, and serve warm.

Stuffed Bell Peppers with Spiced Beef, Currants, and Feta

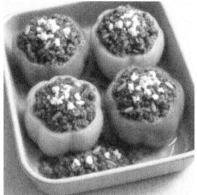

Serves: 4

Ingredients:
- 4 red, yellow, or orange bell peppers, tops trimmed and seeds removed
- Salt and pepper
- ½ cup long-grain white rice
- 1 tablespoon extra-virgin olive oil, plus more for serving
- 1 onion, finely chopped
- 3 garlic cloves, minced
- 2 teaspoons grated fresh ginger
- 2 teaspoons ground cumin
- ¾ teaspoon ground cardamom
- ½ teaspoon red pepper flakes
- ¼ teaspoon ground cinnamon
- 10 ounces 90% lean ground beef
- 1 (14.5-ounce) can diced tomatoes, drained, 2 tablespoons juice reserved
- ¼ cup currants
- 2 teaspoons chopped fresh oregano (or ½ teaspoon dried)
- 2 ounces feta cheese, crumbled (½ cup)
- ¼ cup slivered almonds, toasted and chopped

Instructions:
1. Prep the Peppers and Rice:
   Bring 4 quarts water to a boil in a large pot. Add 1 tablespoon salt and the bell peppers. Boil for 3-5 minutes until just beginning to soften. Remove with tongs and place cut side up on paper towels. In the same water, boil the rice until tender, about 13 minutes. Drain and transfer to a large bowl.

2. Make the Filling:
   Preheat oven to 350°F. In a 12-inch skillet, heat 1 tablespoon oil over medium-high heat. Add onion and ¼ teaspoon salt. Cook until softened and lightly browned, 5-7 minutes. Stir in garlic, ginger, cumin, cardamom, red pepper flakes, and cinnamon. Cook for about 30 seconds, until fragrant.

3. Add the ground beef and cook, breaking it up with a spoon, until no longer pink, about 4 minutes. Remove from heat and stir in tomatoes, reserved juice, currants, and oregano. Scrape up any browned bits. Transfer mixture to the bowl with the rice. Stir in ¼ cup feta and almonds. Season with salt and pepper.

4. Stuff and Bake:
   Place peppers cut side up in an 8-inch square baking dish. Pack the filling into each pepper, mounding it slightly. Bake until heated through, about 30 minutes.

5. Finish and Serve:
   Sprinkle with remaining ¼ cup feta and drizzle with a bit more olive oil. Serve warm.

Broccoli Rabe with Garlic and Red Pepper Flakes

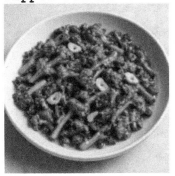

Serves: 4
Quick • Vegetarian

Ingredients:
- 14 ounces broccoli rabe, trimmed and cut into 1-inch pieces
- Salt and pepper
- 2 tablespoons extra-virgin olive oil
- 3 garlic cloves, minced
- ¼ teaspoon red pepper flakes

Instructions:
1. Bring 3 quarts of water to a boil in a large saucepan. Fill a large bowl halfway with ice water.
2. Add broccoli rabe and 2 teaspoons salt to the boiling water. Cook until wilted and just tender, about 2½ minutes. Drain and transfer to the ice bath to cool. Drain again and pat very dry.
3. In a 10-inch skillet, heat olive oil, garlic, and red pepper flakes over medium. Stir often until garlic begins to sizzle, about 2 minutes.
4. Increase heat to medium-high, add the broccoli rabe, and cook, stirring, until heated through—about 1 minute. Season with salt and pepper to taste and serve.

Sautéed Cabbage with Parsley and Lemon

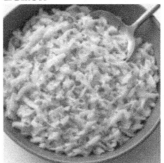

Serves: 4 to 6
Quick • Vegetarian

Ingredients:
- 1 small head green cabbage (about 1¼ pounds), cored and thinly sliced
- 2 tablespoons extra-virgin olive oil
- 1 onion, halved and thinly sliced
- Salt and pepper
- ¼ cup chopped fresh parsley
- 1½ teaspoons lemon juice

Instructions:
1. Place sliced cabbage in a large bowl, cover with cold water, and let soak for 3 minutes. Drain well.
2. In a 12-inch nonstick skillet, heat 1 tablespoon olive oil over medium-high heat until shimmering. Add onion and ¼ teaspoon salt; cook, stirring occasionally, until softened and lightly browned, 5 to 7 minutes. Transfer to a bowl.
3. Add the remaining 1 tablespoon oil to the empty skillet and heat over medium-high. Add cabbage, sprinkle with ½ teaspoon salt and ¼ teaspoon pepper, and cover. Cook without stirring for 3 minutes, until wilted and browned on the bottom.
4. Uncover and stir. Continue to cook, uncovered, stirring once halfway through, until cabbage is crisp-tender and lightly browned in spots, about 4 more minutes.

5. Off heat, stir in the cooked onion, parsley, and lemon juice. Season with salt and pepper to taste and serve warm.

Spicy Roasted Carrots with Cilantro

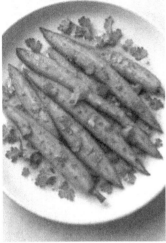

Serves: 4 to 6
Quick • Vegetarian

Ingredients:
- 2 tablespoons extra-virgin olive oil
- 1 tablespoon packed dark brown sugar
- Salt and pepper
- 1½ pounds carrots, peeled
- ¼ cup chopped fresh cilantro
- 2 tablespoons orange juice
- ½ teaspoon ground Aleppo pepper (or substitute ⅛ tsp paprika + ⅛ tsp finely chopped red pepper flakes)
- ¼ teaspoon ground cumin
- ⅛ teaspoon ground cinnamon

Instructions:
1. Preheat oven to 450°F and adjust rack to middle position. In a large bowl, whisk together olive oil, brown sugar, ½ teaspoon salt, and ½ teaspoon pepper.
2. Cut carrots in half crosswise, then slice lengthwise into halves or quarters to make even pieces. Toss carrots in the oil mixture to coat.
3. Spread carrots in a single layer on a foil-lined rimmed baking sheet. Cover tightly with foil and roast for 12 minutes.
4. Remove foil and continue roasting for 16–22 minutes, stirring once halfway through, until carrots are well browned and tender.
5. In a large bowl, whisk together orange juice, Aleppo pepper, cumin, and cinnamon. Add roasted carrots and cilantro; toss gently to combine. Season with salt and pepper to taste. Serve warm or at room temperature.

Cutting Carrots for Roasting – Step-by-Step

1. Cut Crosswise
Start by slicing each carrot in half across the middle. This gives you more manageable pieces to work with.

2. Cut Lengthwise
Take each half and slice it lengthwise into halves or quarters, depending on the thickness. The goal is to create pieces that are similar in size so they cook evenly and roast up beautifully.

Slow-Cooked Whole Carrots

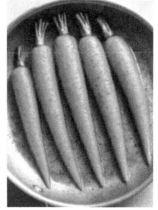

Serves: 4 to 6
Vegetarian

Ingredients:
- 1 tablespoon extra-virgin olive oil
- ½ teaspoon salt
- 1½ pounds carrots, peeled (¾ to 1¼ inches thick at the top)

Instructions:
1. Cut a piece of parchment paper into an 11-inch circle and cut a 1-inch hole in the center. Fold paper to size as needed.
2. In a 12-inch skillet, bring 3 cups water, olive oil, and salt to a simmer over high heat. Turn off the heat, add carrots, cover with the parchment round, and cover the skillet with a lid. Let sit for 20 minutes.
3. Remove the lid but leave the parchment in place. Bring to a simmer over high heat, then reduce heat to medium-low and cook until most of the water has evaporated and carrots are very tender, about 45 minutes.
4. Discard parchment, increase heat to medium-high, and cook, shaking the skillet often, until any remaining water is gone and the carrots are lightly glazed, 2 to 4 minutes.
5. Serve as is or with one of the relishes below.

Skillet-Roasted Cauliflower

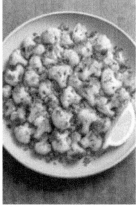

Serves: 4 to 6
Quick • Vegetarian

Ingredients:
- 1 head cauliflower (2 pounds)
- 1 slice hearty white sandwich bread, torn into 1-inch pieces
- 5 tablespoons extra-virgin olive oil
- Salt and pepper
- 1 garlic clove, minced
- 1 teaspoon grated lemon zest, plus lemon wedges for serving
- ¼ cup chopped fresh parsley

Instructions:
1. Prep the Cauliflower:
   Trim outer leaves and cut stem flush with base. Slice cauliflower into ¾-inch-thick slabs. Cut around the core to remove the florets, then cut larger ones into roughly 1½-inch pieces. Save any small pieces that break off.
2. Make the Breadcrumbs:
   Pulse bread in a food processor to make coarse crumbs (about 10 pulses). In a 12-inch nonstick skillet, heat 1 tablespoon oil over medium with the breadcrumbs, a pinch of salt, and a pinch of pepper. Stir often until golden brown, 3-5 minutes. Transfer to a bowl and wipe skillet clean.
3. Steam and Sear the Cauliflower:
   Combine cauliflower, 2 tablespoons oil, 1 teaspoon salt, and ½ teaspoon pepper in the same skillet. Cover and cook over medium-high for 5 minutes—do not lift the lid.
4. Brown and Finish:
   Uncover and cook, stirring every 2 minutes, until deeply browned in spots, about 12 minutes. Push cauliflower to the sides of the pan. In the center, add remaining 2 tablespoons oil, garlic, and lemon zest. Cook until fragrant, about 30 seconds, then mix into cauliflower.
5. Add Final Touches:
   Cook 2-3 more minutes until just tender. Off heat, stir in parsley. Season with salt and pepper. Transfer to a serving platter, top with breadcrumbs, and serve with lemon wedges.

Braised Cauliflower with Garlic and White Wine

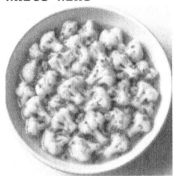

Serves: 4 to 6
  Quick • Vegetarian

Ingredients:
* 3 tablespoons plus 1 teaspoon extra-virgin olive oil
* 3 garlic cloves, minced
* ⅛ teaspoon red pepper flakes
* 1 head cauliflower (2 pounds), cored and cut into 1½-inch florets
* Salt and pepper
* ⅓ cup chicken or vegetable broth
* ⅓ cup dry white wine
* 2 tablespoons minced fresh parsley

Instructions:
1. In a small bowl, mix 1 teaspoon olive oil, garlic, and red pepper flakes.
   In a 12-inch skillet, heat the remaining 3 tablespoons olive oil over medium-high. Add cauliflower and ¼ teaspoon salt. Cook, stirring occasionally, until nicely browned, 7 to 9 minutes.
2. Push cauliflower to the sides of the skillet. Add the garlic mixture to the center and mash it into the skillet with your spoon. Cook until fragrant, about 30 seconds, then stir into the cauliflower.
3. Add broth and wine, bring to a simmer, then reduce heat to medium-low. Cover and cook until cauliflower is crisp-tender, 4 to 6 minutes.
4. Remove from heat. Stir in parsley and season with salt

and pepper to taste. Serve warm.

Skillet-Roasted Cauliflower

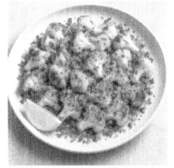

Serves: 4 to 6
  Quick • Vegetarian

Ingredients:
* 1 head cauliflower (2 pounds)
* 1 slice hearty white sandwich bread, torn into 1-inch pieces
* 5 tablespoons extra-virgin olive oil
* Salt and pepper
* 1 garlic clove, minced
* 1 teaspoon grated lemon zest, plus lemon wedges for serving
* ¼ cup chopped fresh parsley

Instructions:
1. Prep Cauliflower:
   Trim off outer leaves and cut stem flush with the bottom. Place cauliflower stem side down and slice into ¾-inch-thick slabs. Cut around the core to separate florets; discard core. Cut larger florets into 1½-inch pieces.
2. Make Breadcrumbs:
   Pulse bread in a food processor into coarse crumbs (about 10 pulses). Toast in a 12-inch nonstick skillet with 1 tablespoon oil, a pinch of salt, and a pinch of pepper over medium heat, stirring frequently, until golden brown (3-5 minutes). Transfer to a bowl and wipe out skillet.
3. Cook Cauliflower:
   In the clean skillet, combine cauliflower with 2 tablespoons oil, 1 teaspoon salt, and ½ teaspoon pepper. Cover and cook over medium-high heat for 5

minutes without lifting the lid—this steams the florets.

4. Brown and Finish:
   Remove lid and cook, stirring every 2 minutes, until florets are deeply browned in spots (about 12 minutes). Push cauliflower to the sides, add remaining 2 tablespoons oil, garlic, and lemon zest to the center, and cook until fragrant (about 30 seconds). Stir everything together and cook 3 more minutes, until just tender.

5. Garnish and Serve:
   Remove from heat. Stir in parsley, season with salt and pepper, and transfer to serving platter. Sprinkle with breadcrumbs and serve with lemon wedges.

Braised Cauliflower with Garlic and White Wine

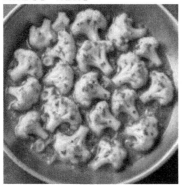

Serves: 4 to 6
Quick • Vegetarian

Ingredients:
- 3 tablespoons plus 1 teaspoon extra-virgin olive oil
- 3 garlic cloves, minced
- ⅛ teaspoon red pepper flakes
- 1 head cauliflower (2 pounds), cored and cut into 1½-inch florets
- Salt and pepper
- ⅓ cup chicken or vegetable broth
- ⅓ cup dry white wine
- 2 tablespoons minced fresh parsley

Instructions:

1. In a small bowl, mix 1 teaspoon olive oil, garlic, and red pepper flakes.
   In a 12-inch skillet, heat the remaining 3 tablespoons olive oil over medium-high heat. Add cauliflower and ¼ teaspoon salt. Cook, stirring occasionally, until florets are golden brown, about 7 to 9 minutes.

2. Push cauliflower to the edges of the skillet. Add the garlic mixture to the center and mash it into the pan. Cook until fragrant, about 30 seconds. Stir it through the cauliflower.

3. Add broth and wine. Bring to a simmer, then reduce heat to medium-low. Cover and cook until the cauliflower is just tender, about 4 to 6 minutes.

4. Remove from heat. Stir in parsley and season with salt and pepper to taste. Serve warm.

Cauliflower Cakes

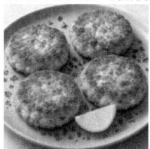

Serves: 4
Vegetarian

Ingredients:
- 1 head cauliflower (2 pounds), cored and cut into 1-inch florets
- ¼ cup extra-virgin olive oil
- 1 teaspoon ground turmeric
- 1 teaspoon ground coriander
- 1 teaspoon salt
- ½ teaspoon ground ginger
- ¼ teaspoon pepper
- 4 ounces goat cheese, softened
- 2 scallions, sliced thin
- 1 large egg, lightly beaten
- 2 garlic cloves, minced

- 1 teaspoon grated lemon zest, plus lemon wedges for serving
- ¼ cup all-purpose flour

Instructions:

1. Roast the Cauliflower:
   Preheat oven to 450°F and place rack in the middle. Toss cauliflower with 1 tablespoon oil, turmeric, coriander, salt, ginger, and pepper. Spread on a foil-lined baking sheet and roast until browned and tender, about 25 minutes. Let cool slightly, then transfer to a large bowl.
2. Make the Mixture:
   Line a clean baking sheet with parchment. Coarsely mash the roasted cauliflower with a potato masher. Stir in goat cheese, scallions, egg, garlic, and lemon zest. Sprinkle in flour and stir to combine. With wet hands, form into 4 equal cakes, about ¾ inch thick. Place on prepared sheet and refrigerate for 30 minutes to firm up.
3. Cook the Cakes:
   Line a plate with paper towels. Heat remaining 3 tablespoons oil in a 12-inch nonstick skillet over medium heat until shimmering. Carefully add the cakes and cook until deep golden brown and crisp, 5 to 7 minutes per side. Transfer to the paper towel-lined plate to drain.
4. Serve:
   Plate the cakes and serve with lemon wedges. Great with Cucumber-Yogurt Sauce or Yogurt-Herb Sauce if you have them!

Roasted Celery Root with Yogurt and Sesame Seeds

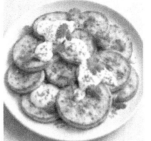

Serves: 6
Vegetarian

Ingredients:
- 3 celery roots (2½ pounds), peeled, halved, and sliced ½ inch thick
- 3 tablespoons extra-virgin olive oil
- Salt and pepper
- ¼ cup plain yogurt
- ¼ teaspoon grated lemon zest + 1 teaspoon lemon juice
- 1 teaspoon sesame seeds, toasted
- 1 teaspoon coriander seeds, toasted and crushed
- ¼ teaspoon dried thyme
- ¼ cup fresh cilantro leaves

Instructions:

1. Roast the Celery Root:
   Preheat oven to 425°F and adjust rack to the lowest position. Toss sliced celery root with olive oil, ½ teaspoon salt, and ¼ teaspoon pepper. Arrange in a single layer on a rimmed baking sheet.
   Roast for 25-30 minutes, until the undersides (especially those at the back of the oven) are well browned. Rotate the pan and roast for another 6-10 minutes until more slices are browned.
2. Flip and Finish Roasting:
   Use a metal spatula to flip each slice. Roast another 10-15 minutes, until the second sides are nicely browned and the slices are very tender.
3. Make the Toppings:
   In a small bowl, mix yogurt, lemon zest, lemon juice, and a

pinch of salt. In another bowl, mix sesame seeds, crushed coriander, thyme, and a pinch of salt.

4. Serve:
   Arrange the roasted celery root on a platter. Drizzle with the yogurt sauce, sprinkle with the seed mixture, and top with fresh cilantro leaves. Serve warm or at room temperature.

Peeling Celery Root – Step-by-Step

1. Trim the Ends
Start by slicing off about ½ inch from both the root end and the opposite end using a sharp chef's knife. This gives you a stable base to work from.

2. Peel with Knife
Stand the celery root on one of the flat ends. Using your knife, slice from top to bottom to remove the thick, rough skin in wide strips. Rotate the root as you go to peel all around, making sure to cut deep enough to remove all the nubby outer layer.

Marinated Eggplant with Capers and Mint

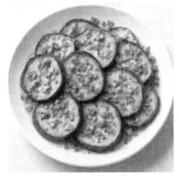

Serves: 4 to 6
Vegetarian

Ingredients:
- 1½ pounds Italian eggplant, sliced into 1-inch-thick rounds
- Kosher salt and pepper
- ¼ cup extra-virgin olive oil
- 4 teaspoons red wine vinegar
- 1 tablespoon capers, rinsed and minced
- 1 garlic clove, minced
- ½ teaspoon grated lemon zest
- ½ teaspoon minced fresh oregano
- 3 tablespoons minced fresh mint

Instructions:
1. Salt the Eggplant:
   Lay eggplant slices on a paper towel-lined baking sheet. Sprinkle both sides with ½ teaspoon kosher salt and let sit for 30 minutes to draw out moisture.
2. Broil:
   Adjust oven rack to 4 inches from the broiler and heat the broiler. Pat eggplant dry thoroughly. Arrange on a foil-lined rimmed baking sheet in a single layer and brush both sides with 1 tablespoon of the oil. Broil until deeply browned and lightly charred, 6-8 minutes per side.
3. Marinate:
   In a large bowl, whisk together the remaining 3 tablespoons oil, red wine vinegar, capers, garlic, lemon zest, oregano, and ¼ teaspoon pepper. Add the warm eggplant and mint, and gently toss to coat.
4. Rest and Serve:
   Let the eggplant sit for about 1 hour at room temperature to absorb the marinade. Taste and adjust seasoning with more pepper if needed. Serve as part of an appetizer platter or alongside grilled meats or seafood.

Broiled Eggplant with Basil

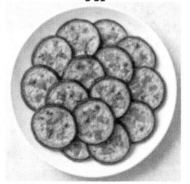

Serves: 4 to 6
Quick • Vegetarian

Ingredients:
- 1½ pounds eggplant, sliced into ¼-inch-thick rounds
- Kosher salt and pepper
- 3 tablespoons extra-virgin olive oil
- 2 tablespoons chopped fresh basil

Instructions:
1. Salt the Eggplant:
   Lay the eggplant slices on a paper towel-lined baking sheet. Sprinkle both sides with 1½ teaspoons kosher salt. Let sit for 30 minutes to release moisture.
2. Broil:
   Adjust oven rack to 4 inches below the broiler and heat the broiler. Pat eggplant dry with paper towels. Arrange slices in a single layer on a foil-lined baking sheet and brush both sides with olive oil.
3. Cook:
   Broil eggplant until deeply browned and lightly charred, about 4 minutes per side.z
4. Serve:
   Transfer to a serving platter, season with pepper, and sprinkle with fresh basil. Serve warm or at room temp.

Stuffed Eggplant with Bulgur

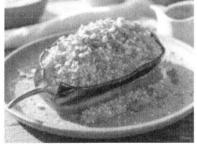

Serves: 4
Vegetarian

Ingredients:
- 4 (10-ounce) Italian eggplants, halved lengthwise
- 2 tablespoons extra-virgin olive oil
- Salt and pepper
- ½ cup medium-grind bulgur, rinsed
- ¼ cup water
- 1 onion, finely chopped
- 3 garlic cloves, minced
- 2 teaspoons minced fresh oregano (or ½ teaspoon dried)
- ¼ teaspoon ground cinnamon
- Pinch cayenne pepper
- 1 pound plum tomatoes, cored, seeded, and chopped
- 2 ounces Pecorino Romano cheese, grated (1 cup)
- 2 tablespoons pine nuts, toasted
- 2 teaspoons red wine vinegar
- 2 tablespoons minced fresh parsley

Instructions:
1. Roast the Eggplant:
   Preheat oven to 400°F. Place a parchment-lined baking sheet on the lowest oven rack to preheat.
   Score the cut side of each eggplant half in a 1-inch-deep diamond pattern. Brush with 1 tablespoon olive oil and season with salt and pepper. Place cut side down on the hot sheet and roast until tender, 40-50 minutes. Transfer to a paper towel-lined sheet, cut side down, to drain.
2. Soften the Bulgur:
   In a bowl, combine rinsed bulgur with ¼ cup water and let sit until softened and water is absorbed, 20-40 minutes.
3. Make the Filling:
   Heat remaining tablespoon oil in a skillet over medium heat. Add onion and cook until soft, about 5 minutes. Stir in garlic, oregano, cinnamon, cayenne, and ½ teaspoon salt; cook until fragrant, about 30 seconds.
   Off heat, stir in softened bulgur, chopped tomatoes, ¾ cup Pecorino, pine nuts, and vinegar. Let sit for 1 minute until heated through. Adjust seasoning with salt and pepper.
4. Stuff and Bake:
   Turn eggplants cut side up on a baking sheet. Use two forks

to gently push flesh to the sides to create space for filling. Spoon in the bulgur mixture, pressing lightly to fill. Top with remaining ¼ cup Pecorino.

Bake on the upper oven rack until cheese melts, 5-10 minutes.

5. Finish and Serve:
Sprinkle with fresh parsley and serve warm.

Making Stuffed Eggplant – Step by Step

1. Prepare Eggplant
Score the flesh of each eggplant half with a 1-inch diamond pattern, about 1 inch deep. Brush with olive oil, season with salt and pepper, and place cut side down on a hot, preheated baking sheet. Roast until tender and lightly browned.

2. Make Stuffing
While the eggplant roasts, soak bulgur in water until soft. Sauté onion, garlic, oregano, and spices in olive oil. Off the heat, stir in bulgur, chopped tomatoes, Pecorino, pine nuts, and vinegar.

3. Stuff Eggplant
Turn roasted eggplant halves cut side up. Use two forks to gently push the flesh aside and create space for the filling. Spoon in the bulgur mixture and press it down lightly.

4. Bake and Serve
Top each stuffed eggplant with the remaining cheese and bake just until the Pecorino melts. Finish with fresh parsley and serve warm.

Braised Fennel with Radicchio and Parmesan

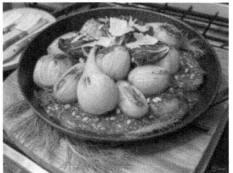

Serves: 6
Vegetarian

Ingredients:
- 3 tablespoons extra-virgin olive oil
- 3 fennel bulbs (about 12 oz each), stalks discarded, bulbs cut into ½-inch-thick slabs, 2 tablespoons fronds minced
- ½ teaspoon grated lemon zest, plus 2 teaspoons lemon juice
- Salt and pepper
- ½ cup dry white wine
- 1 head radicchio (about 10 oz), cored and thinly sliced
- ¼ cup water
- 2 teaspoons honey
- 2 tablespoons pine nuts, toasted and chopped
- Shaved Parmesan cheese, for serving

Instructions:
1. Cook the Fennel:
In a 12-inch skillet, heat oil over medium heat. Add fennel slabs, lemon zest, ½ tsp salt, and ¼ tsp pepper. Pour wine over fennel. (Skillet may be crowded at first.) Cover, reduce heat to medium-low, and cook until fennel is just tender, about 20 minutes.
2. Brown the Fennel:
Increase heat to medium. Flip fennel and cook uncovered until the first side is deeply browned and most liquid has evaporated, 5-8 minutes. Flip again and brown the other side, 2-4 minutes. Transfer fennel to a platter and tent with foil.

3. Cook the Radicchio:
   Add radicchio, water, honey, and a pinch of salt to the empty skillet. Cook over low heat, scraping up any browned bits, until wilted, 3-5 minutes. Off heat, stir in lemon juice and adjust seasoning with salt and pepper.
4. Finish and Serve:
   Spoon radicchio over fennel. Sprinkle with pine nuts, fennel fronds, and shaved Parmesan. Serve warm.

Slicing Fennel for Braising - Step-by-Step Guide

1. Trim the Fennel
   - Slice off the stalks and fronds at the top.
   - Cut a very thin slice from the base to level it.
   - Peel off any outer layers that look tough or blemished.

2. Slice into Slabs
   - Stand the fennel bulb upright on the trimmed base.
   - Cut straight down vertically to create ½-inch-thick slabs.

These thick slices hold up well during braising and develop a lovely golden crust as they cook.

Fava Beans with Artichokes, Asparagus, and Peas

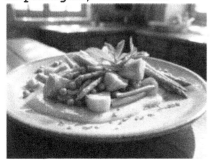

Serves 6 | Vegetarian

Ingredients
- 2 tsp grated lemon zest, plus 1 lemon
- 4 baby artichokes (about 3 oz each)
- 1 tsp baking soda
- 1 lb fresh fava beans, shelled (1 cup)
- 1 tbsp extra-virgin olive oil, plus more for serving
- 1 leek (white/light green only), halved, thinly sliced, and washed
- Salt and pepper
- 3 garlic cloves, minced
- 1 cup chicken or vegetable broth
- 1 lb asparagus, trimmed and cut into 2-inch pieces on a bias
- 1 lb fresh peas, shelled (1¼ cups) (or use frozen, thawed)
- 2 tbsp shredded fresh basil
- 1 tbsp chopped fresh mint

Instructions
1. Prep Artichokes:
   Squeeze the lemon into 2 quarts of water and toss in the lemon halves. Trim artichokes: remove stems, tough outer leaves, and top quarter. Slice into quarters and place in lemon water to prevent browning.
2. Cook Favas:
   Boil 2 cups water with baking soda. Add fava beans and boil for 1-2 minutes, until their edges start to darken. Drain and rinse thoroughly with cold water.
3. Sauté Leek & Garlic:
   Heat 1 tbsp oil in a large skillet over medium. Add leek, 1 tbsp water, and 1 tsp salt. Cook until softened, about 3 minutes. Stir in garlic and cook for 30 seconds.
4. Braise Veggies:
   Remove artichokes from lemon water, shake off excess, and add to skillet. Stir in broth and bring to a simmer. Cover, reduce heat, and cook for 6-8 minutes until almost tender. Add asparagus and peas, cover, and cook for 5-7 minutes. Stir in fava beans and cook for 2 more minutes, just to heat through.
5. Finish and Serve:
   Off heat, stir in basil, mint,

and lemon zest. Season to taste with salt and pepper. Drizzle with olive oil and serve warm.

Roasted Green Beans with Pecorino and Pine Nuts

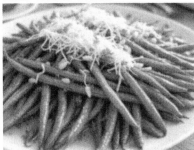

Serves 4 to 6 | Vegetarian | Fast
Ingredients
- 1½ lbs green beans, trimmed
- ¼ cup extra-virgin olive oil
- ¾ tsp sugar
- Salt and pepper
- 2 garlic cloves, minced
- 1 tsp grated lemon zest + 1 tbsp lemon juice
- 1 tsp Dijon mustard
- 2 tbsp chopped fresh basil
- ¼ cup shredded Pecorino Romano
- 2 tbsp pine nuts, toasted

Instructions
1. Roast the Beans:
   Preheat oven to 475°F and adjust rack to the lowest position.
   Toss green beans with 1 tbsp oil, sugar, ¼ tsp salt, and ½ tsp pepper.
   Spread them out on a rimmed baking sheet, cover tightly with foil, and roast for 10 minutes.
2. Uncover and Brown:
   Remove the foil and roast for another 10 minutes, stirring halfway, until spotty brown.
3. Make the Dressing:
   While the beans roast, combine garlic, lemon zest, and remaining 3 tbsp oil in a bowl.
   Microwave until bubbling, about 1 minute.
   Let it sit for a minute, then whisk in lemon juice, mustard, ⅛ tsp salt, and ¼ tsp pepper.
4. Finish and Serve:
   Toss roasted beans with the

dressing and basil.
   Transfer to a platter and top with Pecorino and pine nuts. Serve warm.

Braised Green Beans with Potatoes and Basil

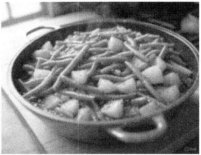

Serves 6 | Vegetarian
Ingredients
- 5 tbsp extra-virgin olive oil
- 1 onion, finely chopped
- 2 tbsp minced fresh oregano (or 2 tsp dried)
- 4 garlic cloves, minced
- 1½ cups water
- 1½ lbs green beans, trimmed and cut into 2-inch pieces
- 1 lb Yukon Gold potatoes, peeled and cut into 1-inch chunks
- ½ tsp baking soda
- 1 (14.5-oz) can diced tomatoes, drained and chopped (juice reserved)
- 1 tbsp tomato paste
- Salt and pepper
- 3 tbsp chopped fresh basil
- Lemon juice

Instructions
1. Preheat Oven:
   Set oven rack to lower-middle position and heat to 275°F.
2. Sauté Aromatics:
   Heat 3 tbsp olive oil in a Dutch oven over medium heat.
   Add onion and cook until soft, about 5 minutes.
   Stir in oregano and garlic, cook for 30 seconds until fragrant.
3. Start Braise:
   Add water, green beans, potatoes, and baking soda.
   Bring to a simmer, stirring

occasionally, and cook for 10 minutes.
4. Add Tomatoes:
   Stir in tomatoes, their reserved juice, tomato paste, 2 tsp salt, and ¼ tsp pepper.
   Cover and transfer to oven. Braise until beans are very tender, 40-50 minutes.
5. Finish and Serve:
   Stir in basil, adjust seasoning with salt, pepper, and lemon juice.
   Drizzle with remaining 2 tbsp oil. Serve warm.

Garlicky Braised Kale

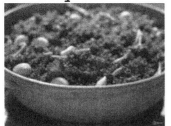

Serves 8 | Vegetarian

Ingredients
- 6 tbsp extra-virgin olive oil
- 1 large onion, finely chopped
- 10 garlic cloves, minced
- ¼ tsp red pepper flakes
- 2 cups chicken or vegetable broth
- 1 cup water
- Salt and pepper
- 4 lbs kale, stemmed and cut into 3-inch pieces
- 1 tbsp lemon juice, plus more to taste

Instructions
1. Sauté Base:
   Heat 3 tbsp oil in a Dutch oven over medium heat.
   Add onion and cook until softened and lightly browned, about 5-7 minutes.
   Stir in garlic and red pepper flakes and cook for 1 minute, until fragrant.
2. Braise the Kale:
   Add broth, water, and ½ tsp salt; bring to a simmer.
   Add one-third of the kale, cover, and cook until wilted,

2-4 minutes.
   Repeat twice with remaining kale, letting each batch wilt before adding the next.
   Cover and cook until kale is tender, 13-15 minutes.
3. Finish and Serve:
   Uncover, raise heat to medium-high, and cook until most of the liquid evaporates and greens sizzle slightly, about 10-12 minutes.
   Off heat, stir in remaining 3 tbsp oil and lemon juice.
   Season with salt, pepper, and more lemon juice to taste. Serve warm.

Making Garlicky Braised Kale

1. Cook Aromatics
Start by sautéing the onion in a Dutch oven until it softens. Stir in the garlic and red pepper flakes and cook just until fragrant.

2. Add Liquid and Kale
Pour in the broth, water, and salt. Bring it to a simmer. Add the kale in batches, letting each handful wilt before adding more. Cover and cook until all the kale is tender.

3. Uncover and Evaporate
Take off the lid and turn up the heat to medium-high. Let the remaining liquid cook off until the kale starts to sizzle.

4. Season and Serve
Off the heat, stir in the remaining olive oil and lemon juice. Taste and adjust with salt, pepper, and extra lemon juice if needed. Serve warm.

Roasted Mushrooms with Parmesan and Pine Nuts

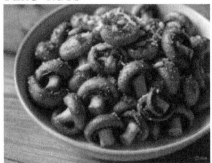

Serves 4 | Vegetarian
Ingredients:
- Salt and pepper
- 1½ lbs cremini mushrooms (whole, halved, or quartered depending on size)
- 1 lb shiitake mushrooms, stems removed (halve caps if larger than 3")
- 3 tbsp extra-virgin olive oil
- 1 tsp lemon juice
- 1 oz Parmesan cheese, grated (½ cup)
- 2 tbsp pine nuts, toasted
- 2 tbsp chopped fresh parsley

Instructions:
1. Preheat oven to 450°F and set rack to lowest position. In a large container, dissolve 5 tsp salt in 2 quarts room-temp water. Add mushrooms and submerge with a plate. Soak 10 minutes.
2. Drain mushrooms and pat dry with paper towels. Toss with 2 tbsp olive oil and spread in a single layer on a rimmed baking sheet. Roast until the moisture cooks off, about 35–45 minutes.
3. Carefully stir mushrooms with a spatula. Roast another 5–10 minutes until deeply browned.
4. In a large bowl, whisk the remaining 1 tbsp oil with lemon juice. Toss mushrooms in the mixture. Add Parmesan, pine nuts, and parsley. Season with salt and pepper. Serve warm.

Grilled Portobello Mushrooms and Shallots with Rosemary-Dijon Vinaigrette

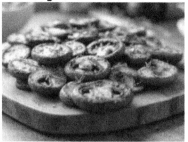

Serves 4 to 6 | Vegetarian | Fast
Ingredients:
- 6 tbsp extra-virgin olive oil
- 1 small garlic clove, minced
- 2 tsp lemon juice
- 1 tsp Dijon mustard
- 1 tsp minced fresh rosemary
- Salt and pepper
- 8 shallots, peeled
- 6 portobello mushroom caps (4-5 inches wide)

Instructions:
1. Make the Vinaigrette:
   In a small bowl, whisk together 2 tbsp oil, garlic, lemon juice, mustard, rosemary, and ¼ tsp salt. Season with pepper to taste and set aside.
2. Prep the Veggies:
   Thread shallots onto two 12-inch metal skewers, piercing through root and stem ends. Score the tops of each mushroom cap with a shallow ½-inch crosshatch pattern. Brush both mushrooms and shallots with remaining ¼ cup oil and season with salt and pepper.

3A. For a Charcoal Grill:
 Open bottom vent, light a chimney starter with 3 quarts of coals. When coals are ashed over, spread evenly in grill. Set grate, cover, open lid vent, and heat grill for 5 minutes.
3B. For a Gas Grill:
 Turn all burners to high, cover, and heat for about 15 minutes. Reduce to medium.
4.   Grill the Veggies:
 Clean and oil the grate. Place mushrooms gill side up, and shallots on the grill. Cook (covered if using gas) for about 8 minutes until

charred and mushrooms release liquid. Flip everything and cook another 8 minutes until nicely charred and tender.
Finish and Serve:
 Transfer mushrooms and shallots to a platter. Remove shallots from skewers and peel off any burnt outer layers. Whisk vinaigrette again and drizzle over warm veggies. Serve.

Greek-Style Garlic-Lemon Potatoes

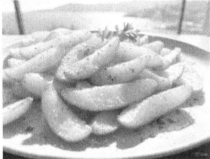

Serves 4 to 6 | Vegetarian | Fast
Ingredients:
- 3 tbsp extra-virgin olive oil
- 1½ lbs Yukon Gold potatoes, peeled and cut into ¾-inch wedges
- 1½ tbsp minced fresh oregano
- 3 garlic cloves, minced
- 2 tsp grated lemon zest + 1½ tbsp lemon juice
- Salt and pepper
- 1½ tbsp minced fresh parsley

Instructions:
1. Brown the Potatoes:
   Heat 2 tbsp oil in a 12-inch nonstick skillet over medium-high until shimmering. Add potatoes in a single layer, cut side down. Cook for about 6 minutes until golden. Flip to the other cut side and cook another 5 minutes.
2. Steam to Finish:
   Lower heat to medium-low, cover skillet, and cook until potatoes are fork-tender, about 8-12 minutes.
3. Add Flavor:
   While potatoes cook, mix remaining 1 tbsp oil, oregano, garlic, lemon zest and juice, ½ tsp salt, and ½ tsp pepper in a small bowl.

4. Combine and Serve:
   Once potatoes are tender, uncover and stir in the garlic-lemon mixture. Cook for about 2 minutes until fragrant. Off heat, mix in parsley. Season to taste and serve.

Roasted Root Vegetables with Lemon-Caper Sauce

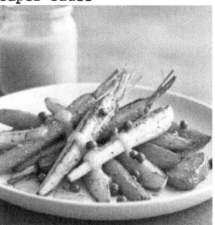

Serves: 4 to 6
 Vegetarian | Fast
Ingredients
- 1 lb Brussels sprouts, trimmed and halved
- 1 lb red potatoes, unpeeled, cut into 1-inch pieces
- 8 shallots, peeled and halved
- 4 carrots, peeled and cut into 2-inch lengths (halve thick ends)
- 6 garlic cloves, peeled
- 3 tbsp extra-virgin olive oil
- 2 tsp minced fresh thyme
- 1 tsp minced fresh rosemary
- 1 tsp sugar
- Salt and pepper
- 2 tbsp minced fresh parsley
- 1½ tbsp capers, rinsed and minced
- 1 tbsp lemon juice, plus more to taste

Instructions
1. Preheat oven to 450°F.
   Toss Brussels sprouts, potatoes, shallots, carrots, and garlic with 1 tbsp oil, thyme, rosemary, sugar, ¾ tsp salt, and ¼ tsp pepper.
2. Roast the vegetables:
   Spread in a single layer on a

rimmed baking sheet. Place Brussels sprouts cut side down in the center. Roast for 30-35 minutes, rotating the sheet halfway, until everything is browned and tender.
3. Make the sauce:
    In a large bowl, whisk together parsley, capers, lemon juice, and remaining 2 tbsp oil. Add roasted veggies and toss to coat. Season with more salt, pepper, and lemon juice if needed. Serve warm.

Grilled Radicchio with Garlic and Rosemary Oil

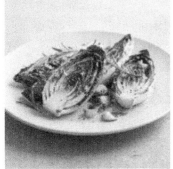

Serves: 4 to 6 | Fast | Vegetarian
Ingredients
* 6 tbsp extra-virgin olive oil
* 1 garlic clove, minced
* 1 tsp minced fresh rosemary
* 3 heads radicchio (about 10 oz each), quartered through the core
* Salt and pepper

Instructions
1. Infuse the oil:
    Microwave the oil, garlic, and rosemary in a bowl until it's bubbling—about 1 minute. Let it sit for 1 more minute to steep.
2. Prep the radicchio:
    Brush the radicchio quarters all over with ¼ cup of the garlic-rosemary oil. Season with salt and pepper.
3. Grill setup:
    o Charcoal Grill: Light a chimney with 3 quarts of briquettes. When ashed over, spread evenly and heat the grate for 5 minutes.

    o Gas Grill: Turn all burners to high, heat for 15 minutes with lid closed, then reduce to medium.
4. Grill the radicchio:
    Clean and oil the grate. Place radicchio quarters directly on the grill. Cook, flipping as needed, until softened and lightly charred on both sides—about 3 to 5 minutes total. Cover grill if using gas.
5. Finish and serve:
    Transfer to a platter and drizzle with the rest of the infused oil. Serve warm or at room temp.

How to Cut Radicchio for Grilling
1. Halve it through the core:
    Start by slicing the whole head of radicchio in half lengthwise, making sure to cut through the core so the leaves stay together.
2. Quarter it:
    Take each half and slice it again, still cutting through the core. This gives you sturdy quarters that won't fall apart on the grill.

Sautéed Spinach with Yogurt and Dukkah

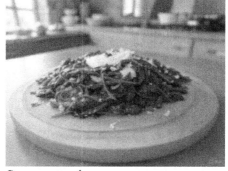

Serves: 4
Time: Fast
Vegetarian
Ingredients:
* ½ cup plain yogurt
* 1½ tsp lemon zest + 1 tsp lemon juice
* 3 tbsp extra-virgin olive oil
* 20 oz curly-leaf spinach, stemmed
* 2 garlic cloves, minced
* Salt and pepper

- ¼ cup dukkah

Directions:
1. Make the yogurt sauce:
   In a bowl, mix the yogurt with lemon zest and juice. Set aside.
2. Cook the spinach:
   Heat 1 tbsp oil in a Dutch oven over high heat. Add the spinach a handful at a time, stirring to wilt before adding more. Cook until all the spinach is wilted, about 1 minute total. Transfer to a colander and squeeze out excess liquid using tongs.
3. Sauté garlic and finish:
   Wipe the pot dry. Add the remaining 2 tbsp oil and garlic. Cook over medium heat until fragrant, about 30 seconds. Add the spinach back in and toss to coat. Season with salt and pepper.
4. Serve:
   Transfer to a platter, drizzle with yogurt sauce, and sprinkle with dukkah. Serve immediately.

Sautéed Swiss Chard with Garlic

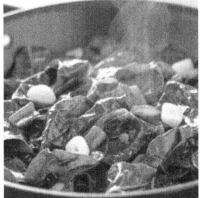

Serves 4 - Fast - Vegetarian

Ingredients:
- 2 tbsp extra-virgin olive oil
- 3 garlic cloves, thinly sliced
- 1½ lbs Swiss chard (stems sliced ¼" thick on the bias, leaves cut into ½" strips)
- Salt and pepper
- 2 tsp lemon juice

Instructions:
1. Sauté stems and garlic:
   Heat oil in a large nonstick skillet over medium-high until shimmering. Add garlic and cook, stirring constantly, until lightly browned, about 30-60 seconds. Stir in chard stems and ⅛ tsp salt. Cook, stirring occasionally, until they're spotty brown and crisp-tender, about 6 minutes.
2. Add leaves:
   Add two-thirds of the chard leaves and toss until they start to wilt, 30-60 seconds. Add the rest and cook, stirring often, until all leaves are tender, about 3 more minutes.
3. Finish and serve:
   Off heat, stir in lemon juice and season with salt and pepper to taste. Serve warm.

Roasted Winter Squash with Tahini and Feta

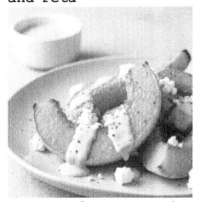

Serves 6 - Vegetarian

Ingredients:
- 3 lbs butternut squash
- 3 tbsp extra-virgin olive oil
- Salt and pepper
- 1 tbsp tahini
- 1½ tsp lemon juice
- 1 tsp honey
- 1 oz feta, crumbled (¼ cup)
- ¼ cup shelled pistachios, toasted and chopped
- 2 tbsp chopped fresh mint

Instructions:
1. Prep the squash:
   Heat oven to 425°F and position a rack at the bottom. Peel the squash thoroughly, removing all white fibrous flesh beneath the skin. Halve lengthwise, scoop out seeds,

then slice crosswise into ½-inch-thick pieces.

2. Roast:
   Toss squash with 2 tbsp oil, ½ tsp salt, and ½ tsp pepper. Arrange on a rimmed baking sheet in a single layer. Roast for 25-30 minutes. Rotate the pan and roast another 6-10 minutes until sides are browned.

3. Flip and finish:
   Flip each piece with a spatula. Roast until squash is tender and other side is browned, 10-15 minutes more.

4. Dress and serve:
   Whisk tahini, lemon juice, honey, remaining 1 tbsp oil, and a pinch of salt. Drizzle over the roasted squash. Top with feta, pistachios, and mint. Serve warm or at room temp.

Roasted Tomatoes

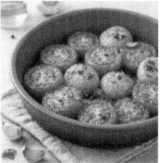

Serves: 4 | Vegetarian
Why This Recipe Works
Ingredients:
- 3 pounds large tomatoes, cored, bottom ⅛ inch trimmed, and sliced into ¾-inch thick rounds
- 2 garlic cloves, peeled and smashed
- ¼ teaspoon dried oregano
- Kosher salt and freshly ground black pepper, to taste
- ¾ cup extra-virgin olive oil

Instructions:
1. Preheat Oven:
   Adjust the oven rack to the middle position and preheat the oven to 425°F. Line a rimmed baking sheet with aluminum foil. Arrange the tomato slices in a single, even layer on the baking sheet, placing the larger slices around the edges and the smaller ones in the center. Place the smashed garlic cloves on top of the tomatoes. Sprinkle with oregano, season with ¼ teaspoon of salt, and add pepper to taste. Drizzle the olive oil evenly over the tomatoes.

2. Roast and Flip:
   Bake the tomatoes for 30 minutes, rotating the baking sheet halfway through. Once done, remove the sheet from the oven, reduce the temperature to 300°F, and prop open the oven door with a wooden spoon to let it cool slightly. Carefully flip the tomatoes using a thin spatula.

3. Finish Roasting:
   Return the tomatoes to the oven, close the door, and continue roasting until the tomatoes are lightly browned, their skins are blistered, and they've shrunk to about ¼ to ½ inch thick—this should take 1 to 2 hours. Once done, remove the sheet from the oven and let the tomatoes cool completely for about 30 minutes. Discard the garlic and transfer the tomatoes along with the oil into an airtight container.

Storage:
   These tomatoes can be refrigerated for up to 5 days or frozen for up to 2 months.

Sautéed Cherry Tomatoes

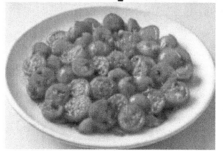

Serves: 4 to 6 | Quick | Vegetarian
Ingredients:
- 1 tablespoon extra-virgin olive oil

- 1½ pounds cherry tomatoes, halved
- 2 teaspoons sugar (optional, to taste)
- Salt and freshly ground black pepper
- 1 garlic clove, minced
- 2 tablespoons fresh basil, chopped

Instructions:
1. Heat Oil:
   Heat the olive oil in a 12-inch skillet over medium-high heat until shimmering.
2. Cook Tomatoes:
   Toss the halved tomatoes with sugar and ¼ teaspoon salt, then add them to the hot skillet. Cook, stirring often, for 1 minute.
3. Add Garlic and Basil:
   Stir in the minced garlic and cook for another 30 seconds until fragrant. Remove the skillet from the heat and stir in the fresh basil. Season with salt and pepper to taste, then serve.

Stuffed Tomatoes with Couscous, Olives, and Orange

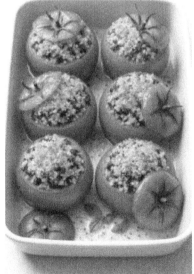

Serves: 6 | Vegetarian
Ingredients:
- 6 large ripe tomatoes (8 to 10 ounces each)
- 1 tablespoon sugar

- Kosher salt and pepper, to taste
- 4½ tablespoons extra-virgin olive oil
- ¼ cup panko bread crumbs
- 3 ounces Manchego cheese, shredded (¾ cup)
- 1 onion, halved and thinly sliced
- 2 garlic cloves, minced
- ⅛ teaspoon red pepper flakes
- 8 ounces (8 cups) baby spinach, chopped
- 1 cup couscous
- ½ teaspoon grated orange zest
- ¼ cup pitted kalamata olives, chopped
- 1 tablespoon red wine vinegar

Instructions:
1. Prepare Tomatoes:
   Preheat the oven to 375°F (190°C) and adjust the rack to the middle position. Cut off the top ½ inch of the tomatoes and set them aside. Using a melon baller or teaspoon, scoop out the tomato pulp, transferring it to a fine-mesh strainer over a bowl. Press down on the pulp to extract the juice, then set the juice aside. Discard the pulp. You should have about ⅔ cup of tomato juice; if not, add water to make up the difference.
2. Drain Tomatoes:
   In a small bowl, combine the sugar and 1 tablespoon of salt. Sprinkle 1 teaspoon of this mixture into the cavity of each tomato. Turn the tomatoes upside down on a plate and let them drain for 30 minutes.
3. Toast Panko:
   In a 10-inch skillet, heat 1½ teaspoons of oil over medium-high heat. Add the panko and toast, stirring frequently, until golden brown, about 3 minutes. Transfer the toasted panko to a bowl and let it cool for 10 minutes. Stir in ¼ cup of Manchego cheese.
4. Prepare Couscous Filling:
   In the same skillet, heat 2

tablespoons of olive oil over medium heat until shimmering. Add the sliced onion and ½ teaspoon of salt. Cook, stirring occasionally, until softened, about 5 minutes. Stir in the minced garlic and red pepper flakes, and cook for 30 seconds until fragrant. Add the spinach, one handful at a time, cooking until wilted, about 3 minutes. Stir in the couscous, orange zest, and reserved tomato juice. Cover the skillet, remove it from the heat, and let it sit for about 7 minutes, until the couscous is tender. Stir in the chopped olives and remaining ½ cup of Manchego. Gently fluff the mixture with a fork, and season with salt and pepper to taste.

5. Stuff the Tomatoes:
   Coat the bottom of a 13 x 9-inch baking dish with the remaining 2 tablespoons of olive oil. Pat the hollowed-out tomatoes dry with paper towels and season with salt and pepper. Stuff each tomato with about ½ cup of the couscous mixture, mounding the excess. Top each stuffed tomato with 1 heaping tablespoon of the panko mixture. Place the tomatoes in the prepared baking dish. Season the reserved tops with salt and pepper and place them in the empty spaces in the dish.

6. Bake and Serve:
   Bake the tomatoes, uncovered, for about 20 minutes, until the tomatoes have softened but still hold their shape. Using a slotted spoon, transfer the stuffed tomatoes to a serving platter. Whisk the red wine vinegar into the remaining oil in the baking dish and drizzle it over the tomatoes. Place the tops back on the tomatoes and serve.

Sautéed Zucchini Ribbons

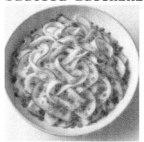

Serves: 4 to 6 | Quick | Vegetarian
Ingredients:
- 1 small garlic clove, minced
- 1 teaspoon grated lemon zest, plus 1 tablespoon lemon juice
- 4 (6 to 8 ounces each) zucchini or yellow summer squash, trimmed
- 2 tablespoons plus 1 teaspoon extra-virgin olive oil
- Salt and pepper, to taste
- 1½ tablespoons chopped fresh parsley

Instructions:
1. Prepare the Garlic and Lemon Juice:
   Combine the minced garlic and lemon juice in a large bowl. Set aside for at least 10 minutes to allow the garlic to mellow in the lemon juice.

2. Slice the Squash:
   Using a vegetable peeler, peel 3 ribbons from one side of each squash. Turn the squash 90 degrees and peel 3 more ribbons. Continue turning and peeling the squash until you reach the seeds. Discard the core with the seeds and repeat with the remaining squash.

3. Make the Dressing:
   Whisk 2 tablespoons of olive oil, ¼ teaspoon salt, ⅛ teaspoon pepper, and lemon zest into the garlic and lemon juice mixture.

4. Cook the Squash:
   Heat the remaining 1 teaspoon of olive oil in a 12-inch nonstick skillet over medium-high heat until it just starts to smoke. Add the squash ribbons and cook, tossing occasionally with tongs, for 3 to 4 minutes until the squash is tender and translucent.

5. Combine and Serve:
   Transfer the cooked squash to the bowl with the dressing. Add the chopped parsley and gently toss to coat. Season with additional salt and pepper to taste, then serve immediately.

Zucchini and Feta Fritters

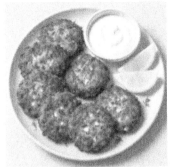

Serves: 4 to 6 | Vegetarian
Ingredients:
- 1 pound zucchini, shredded
- Salt and freshly ground pepper
- 4 ounces feta cheese, crumbled (about 1 cup)
- 2 scallions, minced
- 2 large eggs, lightly beaten
- 2 tablespoons fresh dill, minced
- 1 garlic clove, minced
- ¼ cup all-purpose flour
- 6 tablespoons extra-virgin olive oil
- Lemon wedges, for serving

Instructions:
1. Prepare Zucchini:
   Preheat the oven to 200°F (95°C) and adjust the rack to the middle position. Place the shredded zucchini in a fine-mesh strainer and toss with 1 teaspoon of salt. Let the zucchini drain for 10 minutes.
2. Squeeze Zucchini:
   After 10 minutes, wrap the zucchini in a clean dish towel and squeeze out as much excess liquid as possible. Transfer the dried zucchini to a large bowl.
3. Make the Fritter Batter:
   To the zucchini, add the crumbled feta, minced scallions, beaten eggs, dill, garlic, and ¼ teaspoon of pepper. Sprinkle the flour over the mixture and stir until fully combined.
4. Fry the Fritters:
   Heat 3 tablespoons of olive oil in a 12-inch nonstick skillet over medium heat until shimmering. Drop 2-tablespoon-sized portions of batter into the skillet, pressing each portion with the back of a spoon to form 2-inch-wide fritters. Fry the fritters for about 3 minutes per side, or until golden brown. Depending on the size of your skillet, you should be able to cook about 6 fritters at a time.
5. Keep Warm:
   Once golden and crisp, transfer the fritters to a paper towel-lined baking sheet and keep warm in the oven. Wipe the skillet clean with paper towels and repeat the process with the remaining 3 tablespoons of oil and batter.
6. Serve:
   Serve the fritters warm or at room temperature with lemon wedges on the side. For extra flavor, pair with Cucumber-Yogurt Sauce or Yogurt-Herb Sauce.

Squeezing Zucchini Dry
1. Shred the Zucchini:
   Use the large holes of a box grater to shred the zucchini.
2. Remove Excess Moisture:
   Place the shredded zucchini in a clean dish towel or between several layers of paper towels. Squeeze until the zucchini is completely dry.

Easy Meredith Sauces

Tahini Sauce

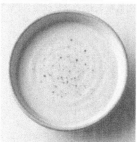

Makes: About 1¼ cups | Quick |
Vegetarian
Ingredients:

- ½ cup tahini
- ½ cup water
- ¼ cup lemon juice (about 2 lemons)
- 2 garlic cloves, minced
- Salt and pepper, to taste

Instructions:
1. Whisk together tahini, water, lemon juice, and minced garlic in a bowl until well combined.
2. Season with salt and pepper to taste.
3. Let the sauce sit for about 30 minutes to allow the flavors to meld.
4. Storage: Refrigerate for up to 4 days.

Yogurt-Herb Sauce

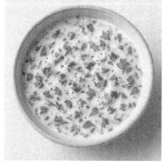

Makes: About 1 cup | Quick |
Vegetarian
Ingredients:

- 1 cup plain yogurt
- 2 tablespoons fresh cilantro, minced
- 2 tablespoons fresh mint, minced
- 1 garlic clove, minced
- Salt and pepper, to taste

Instructions:

1. Whisk together yogurt, cilantro, mint, and garlic in a bowl until well combined.
2. Season with salt and pepper to taste.
3. Let the sauce sit for about 30 minutes for the flavors to meld.
4. Storage: Refrigerate for up to 2 days.

Lemon-Yogurt Sauce

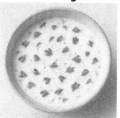

Makes: About 1 cup | Quick |
Vegetarian
Ingredients:

- 1 cup plain yogurt
- 1 tablespoon fresh mint, minced
- 1 teaspoon grated lemon zest
- 2 tablespoons lemon juice
- 1 garlic clove, minced
- Salt and pepper, to taste

Instructions:
1. Whisk together yogurt, mint, lemon zest, lemon juice, and garlic in a bowl until well combined.
2. Season with salt and pepper to taste.
3. Let the sauce sit for about 30 minutes for the flavors to meld.
4. Storage: Refrigerate for up to 2 days.

Cucumber-Yogurt Sauce

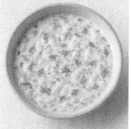

Makes: About 2½ cups | Quick |
Vegetarian
Ingredients:

- 1 cup plain Greek yogurt
- 2 tablespoons extra-virgin olive oil

- 2 tablespoons fresh dill, minced
- 1 garlic clove, minced
- 1 cucumber, peeled, halved lengthwise, seeded, and shredded
- Salt and pepper, to taste

Instructions:
1. Whisk together the yogurt, olive oil, dill, and garlic in a medium bowl until well combined.
2. Stir in the shredded cucumber and season with salt and pepper to taste.
3. Let the sauce sit for about 30 minutes to allow the flavors to meld.
4. Storage: Refrigerate for up to 1 day.

Garlic Aïoli

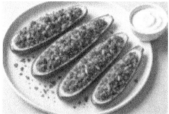

Makes: About 1¼ cups | Quick | Vegetarian

Ingredients:
- 2 large egg yolks
- 2 teaspoons Dijon mustard
- 2 teaspoons lemon juice
- 1 garlic clove, minced
- ¾ cup vegetable oil
- 1 tablespoon water
- Salt and pepper, to taste
- ¼ cup extra-virgin olive oil

Instructions:
1. In a food processor, combine the egg yolks, mustard, lemon juice, and minced garlic. Process for about 10 seconds until mixed.
2. With the processor running, slowly drizzle in the vegetable oil, about 1 minute, until emulsified.
3. Transfer the mixture to a medium bowl. Whisk in the water, ½ teaspoon salt, and ¼ teaspoon pepper.

4. While whisking constantly, slowly drizzle in the olive oil until the aïoli is fully emulsified.
5. Storage: Refrigerate for up to 4 days.

Stuffed Zucchini with Spiced Lamb, Dried Apricots, and Pine Nuts

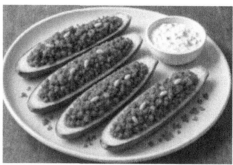

Serves: 4

Ingredients:
- 4 zucchini (about 8 ounces each), halved lengthwise and seeded
- 2 tablespoons plus 1 teaspoon extra-virgin olive oil
- Salt and pepper, to taste
- 8 ounces ground lamb
- 1 onion, finely chopped
- 4 garlic cloves, minced
- 2 teaspoons ras el hanout (North African spice blend)
- ⅔ cup chicken broth
- ½ cup medium-grind bulgur, rinsed
- ¼ cup dried apricots, finely chopped
- 2 tablespoons pine nuts, toasted
- 2 tablespoons fresh parsley, minced

Instructions:
1. Preheat the Oven:
   Adjust the oven racks to the upper-middle and lowest positions. Place a rimmed baking sheet on the lower rack and preheat the oven to 400°F (200°C).
2. Prepare the Zucchini:
   Brush the cut sides of the zucchini with 2 tablespoons of olive oil and season with salt and pepper. Lay the zucchini cut-side down on the hot baking

sheet and roast until slightly softened and the skins are wrinkled, about 8 to 10 minutes. Remove from the oven and flip the zucchini to place cut-side up; set aside.

3. Cook the Lamb:
   While the zucchini roasts, heat the remaining 1 teaspoon of olive oil in a large saucepan over medium-high heat until shimmering. Add the lamb, ½ teaspoon of salt, and ¼ teaspoon of pepper, and cook, breaking the meat apart with a wooden spoon, until browned, 3 to 5 minutes. Use a slotted spoon to transfer the lamb to a paper towel-lined plate.

4. Prepare the Filling:
   Pour off all but 1 tablespoon of fat from the saucepan. Add the onion to the fat remaining in the pan and cook over medium heat until softened, about 5 minutes. Stir in the garlic and ras el hanout and cook until fragrant, about 30 seconds. Add the chicken broth, bulgur, and chopped apricots, then bring to a simmer. Reduce the heat to low, cover, and cook gently until the bulgur is tender, about 16 to 18 minutes.

5. Finish the Pilaf:
   Once the pilaf is cooked, remove the pan from the heat. Lay a clean dish towel underneath the lid and let it sit for 10 minutes. Stir in the toasted pine nuts and fresh parsley, and fluff the pilaf with a fork to combine. Season with salt and pepper to taste.

6. Stuff the Zucchini:
   Fill each zucchini half with about ½ cup of the bulgur-lamb mixture, mounding the filling on top. Place the zucchini on the upper rack of the oven and bake for about 6 minutes, until the zucchini is heated through.

7. Serve:
   Serve the stuffed zucchini immediately, and enjoy!

Greek Stewed Zucchini
Serves: 6 to 8 | Vegetarian

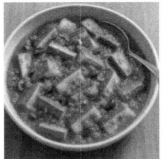

Why This Recipe Works
Ingredients:
- 1 (28-ounce) can whole peeled tomatoes
- 3 tablespoons extra-virgin olive oil, divided
- 5 zucchini (8 ounces each), trimmed, quartered lengthwise, seeded, and cut into 2-inch lengths
- 1 onion, finely chopped
- Salt and pepper, to taste
- 3 garlic cloves, minced
- 1 teaspoon fresh oregano (or ¼ teaspoon dried oregano)
- ¼ teaspoon red pepper flakes
- 2 tablespoons chopped pitted kalamata olives
d adjust the rack to the lower-middle position. Process the whole peeled tomatoes and their juice in a food processor until completely smooth, about 1 minute. Set aside.

1. Brown the Zucchini:
   Heat 2 teaspoons of olive oil in a Dutch oven over medium-high heat until shimmering. Brown one-third of the zucchini for about 3 minutes per side, then transfer to a bowl. Repeat the process with the remaining zucchini in two batches, using 4 teaspoons of oil total.

2. Cook the Onion and Build the Sauce:
   Add the remaining 1 tablespoon of olive oil to the Dutch oven, then stir in the chopped onion and ¾ teaspoon of salt. Cook over medium

1. Bake the Gratin:
   Bake the gratin until the vegetables are tender and the

tomatoes are starting to brown on the edges, about 40 to 45 minutes.

2. Finish and Serve:
   After baking, remove the dish from the oven and increase the oven temperature to 450°F (230°C). Sprinkle the bread crumb mixture evenly over the top and continue baking until the gratin is bubbling and the cheese is lightly browned, about 5 to 10 minutes. Let the gratin cool for 10 minutes, then sprinkle with fresh basil. Serve warm.

Assembling a Summer Vegetable Gratin

1. Arrange Vegetables:
   Place the zucchini and yellow squash in a greased baking dish.
2. Add Caramelized Onions:
   Evenly sprinkle the caramelized onions over the vegetables.
3. Layer Tomatoes:
   Arrange the tomato slices on top of the onions, slightly overlapping, then spoon the remaining garlic-oil mixture over the tomatoes.
4. Bake and Add Topping:
   Bake the gratin until the vegetables are tender and the tomatoes start to brown on the edges. Then, sprinkle the bread crumb mixture evenly over the top and bake for an additional 5 to 10 minutes, until the cheese is lightly browned.

Grilled Vegetable Kebabs with Grilled Lemon Dressing

Serves: 4 to 6 | Quick | Vegetarian

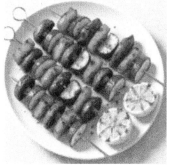

Ingredients:

- ¼ cup extra-virgin olive oil
- 1 teaspoon Dijon mustard
- 1 teaspoon fresh rosemary, minced
- 1 garlic clove, minced
- Salt and pepper, to taste
- 6 portobello mushroom caps (4 to 5 inches in diameter), quartered
- 2 zucchini, halved lengthwise and sliced into ¾-inch thick pieces
- 2 red bell peppers, stemmed, seeded, and cut into 1½-inch pieces
- 2 lemons, quartered

Instructions:

1. Prepare the Dressing:
   In a large bowl, whisk together the olive oil, Dijon mustard, minced rosemary, garlic, ½ teaspoon salt, and ¼ teaspoon pepper. Reserve half of the dressing for serving.
2. Prepare the Vegetables:
   Toss the portobello mushrooms, zucchini, and bell peppers with the remaining half of the dressing until evenly coated. Thread the vegetables onto eight 12-inch metal skewers, alternating the vegetables as you go.
3. Prepare the Grill:
   o For Charcoal Grill: Open the bottom vent completely. Light a large chimney starter filled halfway with charcoal briquettes (about 3 quarts). Once the top coals are partially covered with ash, spread them evenly over the grill. Place the cooking grate on top, cover the grill, and open the lid vent completely. Heat the grill for about 5 minutes.
   o For Gas Grill: Turn all burners to high, cover the grill, and heat for about 15 minutes. Once the grill is hot, turn all burners to medium.

4. Grill the Kebabs:
   Clean and oil the cooking grate. Place the kebabs and lemon quarters on the grill. Cook (covered if using gas), turning the kebabs as needed, until the vegetables are tender and well browned and the lemons are slightly charred and juicy, about 16 to 18 minutes.
5. Prepare and Serve:
   Transfer the kebabs and lemon quarters to a serving platter and remove the skewers. Juice 2 of the grilled lemon quarters and whisk the juice into the reserved dressing. Drizzle the dressing over the grilled vegetables and serve with the remaining lemon quarters on the side.

Mechouia
Serves: 4 to 6 | Vegetarian

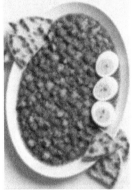

Ingredients:
For the Dressing:
- 2 teaspoons coriander seeds
- 1½ teaspoons caraway seeds
- 1 teaspoon cumin seeds
- 5 tablespoons extra-virgin olive oil
- ½ teaspoon paprika
- ⅛ teaspoon cayenne pepper
- 3 garlic cloves, minced
- ¼ cup chopped fresh parsley
- ¼ cup chopped fresh cilantro
- 2 tablespoons chopped fresh mint
- 1 teaspoon grated lemon zest
- 2 tablespoons lemon juice
- Salt, to taste

For the Vegetables:
- 2 red or green bell peppers, tops and bottoms trimmed, stemmed and seeded, and flattened
- 1 small eggplant, halved lengthwise and scored on the cut side
- 1 zucchini (8 to 10 ounces), halved lengthwise and scored on the cut side
- 4 plum tomatoes, cored and halved lengthwise
- Salt and pepper, to taste
- 2 shallots, unpeeled

Instructions:
1. Prepare the Dressing:
   o Grind the coriander seeds, caraway seeds, and cumin seeds in a spice grinder until finely ground.
   o Whisk the ground spices, olive oil, paprika, and cayenne pepper together in a bowl.
   o Reserve 3 tablespoons of the oil mixture for brushing the vegetables before grilling.
   o Heat the remaining oil mixture and garlic in an 8-inch skillet over low heat, stirring occasionally, until fragrant and small bubbles appear, about 8 to 10 minutes.
   o Transfer the oil mixture to a large bowl and let it cool for 10 minutes. Then whisk in the parsley, cilantro, mint, lemon zest, lemon juice, and season with salt to taste. Set aside for serving.
2. Prepare the Vegetables:
   o Brush the interior of the bell peppers and the cut sides of the eggplant, zucchini, and tomatoes with the reserved oil mixture. Season with salt.
3. Grill the Vegetables:
   o For Charcoal Grill: Open the bottom vent completely. Light a large

chimney starter, filled three-quarters with charcoal briquettes (about 4½ quarts). Once the top coals are partially covered with ash, spread them evenly over the grill. Place the cooking grate in place, cover, and open the lid vent completely. Heat the grill for about 5 minutes.

- o For Gas Grill: Turn all burners to high, cover, and heat the grill for about 15 minutes. Then, turn all burners to medium-high.

4. Grill the Vegetables:
   - o Clean and oil the cooking grate. Place the bell peppers, eggplant, zucchini, tomatoes, and shallots cut side down on the grill. Cook, turning as needed, until tender and slightly charred, about 8 to 16 minutes.
   - o Transfer the eggplant, zucchini, tomatoes, and shallots to a baking sheet as they finish cooking. Place the bell peppers in a bowl, cover with plastic wrap, and let them steam to loosen their skins.

5. Finish the Dish:
   - o Let the vegetables cool slightly. Peel the bell peppers, tomatoes, and shallots.
   - o Chop all the vegetables into ½-inch pieces, then toss gently with the dressing in a bowl. Season with salt and pepper to taste.
   - o Serve warm or at room temperature.

Prepping Vegetables for Mechouia
1. Flatten the Bell Pepper:
   Trim off the top and bottom of the bell pepper. Remove the stem and seeds, then cut

through one side of the pepper. Press the pepper flat and trim away any remaining ribs.

2. Score the Zucchini and Eggplant:
   Using the tip of a chef's knife (or a paring knife), score the cut sides of the zucchini and eggplant in a ½-inch diamond pattern. Be sure to cut down to, but not through, the skin.

Ratatouille
Serves: 4 to 6 | Vegetarian

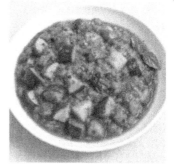

Ingredients:
- ⅓ cup plus 1 tablespoon extra-virgin olive oil, divided
- 2 large onions, cut into 1-inch pieces
- 8 large garlic cloves, peeled and smashed
- Salt and pepper, to taste
- 1½ teaspoons herbes de Provence
- ¼ teaspoon red pepper flakes
- 1 bay leaf
- 1½ pounds eggplant, peeled and cut into 1-inch pieces
- 2 pounds plum tomatoes, peeled, cored, and chopped coarse
- 2 small zucchini, halved lengthwise and cut into 1-inch pieces
- 1 red bell pepper, stemmed, seeded, and cut into 1-inch pieces
- 1 yellow bell pepper, stemmed, seeded, and cut into 1-inch pieces
- 2 tablespoons chopped fresh basil, plus more for garnish
- 1 tablespoon minced fresh parsley
- 1 tablespoon sherry vinegar

Instructions:

1. Preheat the Oven:
   Adjust the oven rack to the middle position and preheat the oven to 400°F (200°C).
2. Cook the Aromatics:
   Heat ⅓ cup of olive oil in a Dutch oven over medium-high heat until shimmering. Add the onions, garlic, 1 teaspoon of salt, and ¼ teaspoon of pepper. Cook, stirring occasionally, until the onions are translucent and starting to soften, about 10 minutes. Stir in the herbes de Provence, red pepper flakes, and bay leaf. Cook, stirring frequently, for 1 minute.
3. Roast the Eggplant and Tomatoes:
   Stir in the eggplant and chopped tomatoes, then sprinkle with ½ teaspoon of salt and ¼ teaspoon of pepper. Stir to combine, then transfer the pot to the oven and cook, uncovered, until the vegetables are very tender and lightly browned, about 40 to 45 minutes.
4. Mash the Eggplant Mixture:
   Remove the pot from the oven. Use a potato masher or heavy wooden spoon to smash and stir the eggplant mixture until it reaches a sauce-like consistency. Stir in the zucchini, bell peppers, ¼ teaspoon of salt, and ¼ teaspoon of pepper, and return the pot to the oven. Cook, uncovered, until the zucchini and bell peppers are just tender, about 20 to 25 minutes.
5. Finish the Dish:
   Remove the pot from the oven, cover, and let it sit for 10 to 15 minutes until the zucchini is translucent and easily pierced with the tip of a paring knife. Use a wooden spoon to scrape any browned bits from the sides of the pot and stir them back into the ratatouille. Discard the bay leaf.
6. Season and Serve:
   Stir in the basil, parsley, and sherry vinegar. Taste and adjust seasoning with salt and pepper as needed. Transfer the ratatouille to a serving platter, drizzle with the remaining 1 tablespoon of olive oil, and sprinkle with the remaining basil. Serve warm, at room temperature, or chilled.

Ciambotta
Serves: 6 | Vegetarian

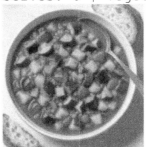

Ingredients:
For the Pesto:
- ⅓ cup chopped fresh basil
- ⅓ cup fresh oregano leaves
- 6 garlic cloves, minced
- 2 tablespoons extra-virgin olive oil
- ¼ teaspoon red pepper flakes

For the Stew:
- 12 ounces eggplant, peeled and cut into ½-inch pieces
- Salt, to taste
- ¼ cup extra-virgin olive oil, divided
- 1 large onion, chopped
- 1 pound russet potatoes, peeled and cut into ½-inch pieces
- 2 tablespoons tomato paste
- 2¼ cups water
- 1 (28-ounce) can whole peeled tomatoes, drained with juice reserved and chopped coarse
- 2 zucchini, halved lengthwise, seeded, and cut into ½-inch pieces
- 2 red or yellow bell peppers, stemmed, seeded, and cut into ½-inch pieces
- 1 cup shredded fresh basil

Instructions:
1. Make the Pesto:

- Combine all pesto ingredients in a food processor and process until finely ground, about 1 minute. Set aside.
2. Prepare the Eggplant:
   - Line a large plate with a double layer of coffee filters and spray them lightly with vegetable oil spray. Toss the eggplant with 1½ teaspoons of salt and spread it evenly over the coffee filters. Microwave the eggplant, uncovered, until it is dry to the touch and slightly shriveled, about 8 to 12 minutes, tossing halfway through.
3. Cook the Stew Base:
   - Heat 2 tablespoons of olive oil in a Dutch oven over high heat until shimmering. Add the eggplant, onion, and potatoes, cooking and stirring frequently until the eggplant is browned, about 2 minutes.
4. Develop the Flavor Base:
   - Push the vegetables to the sides of the pot. Add 1 tablespoon of oil and the tomato paste to the center, cooking until the paste begins to brown and a fond develops on the bottom of the pot, about 2 minutes. Stir in 2 cups of water and the tomatoes with their juice, scraping up any browned bits from the bottom. Bring to a simmer, reduce the heat to medium-low, cover, and simmer gently for 20 to 25 minutes, until the eggplant has broken down and the potatoes are tender.
5. Cook the Zucchini and Peppers:
   - While the stew simmers, heat the remaining 1 tablespoon of oil in a 12-inch skillet over high heat until just smoking. Add the zucchini, bell peppers, and ½ teaspoon salt. Cook, stirring occasionally, until the vegetables are browned and tender, about 10 to 12 minutes. Push the vegetables to the sides of the skillet and add the pesto to the center, cooking for 1 minute until fragrant. Stir the pesto into the vegetables and transfer the mixture to a bowl. Off heat, add the remaining ¼ cup of water to the skillet and scrape up any browned bits.
6. Combine the Vegetables:
   - Off heat, stir the vegetable mixture and water from the skillet into the pot with the eggplant and potatoes. Cover and let sit for about 20 minutes to allow the flavors to meld. Stir in the shredded basil and season with salt to taste.
7. Serve:
   - Serve the ciambotta warm with crusty bread on the side.

Seafood

Broiled Grape Leaf-Wrapped Grouper
Serves 4

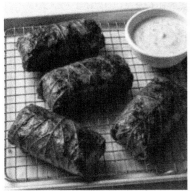

You'll Need:
- 3 tbsp extra-virgin olive oil, plus more for brushing
- 2 tbsp chopped fresh parsley
- 1 tbsp capers, rinsed and minced
- 1 tsp lemon zest
- ½ tsp salt
- ½ tsp pepper
- 4 skinless grouper fillets (4 to 6 oz each, ¾ to 1 inch thick)
- 1 (16-ounce) jar grape leaves
- ½ cup Tahini-Lemon Dressing

How to Make It:
1. In a medium bowl, mix the oil, parsley, capers, lemon zest, salt, and pepper. Add the grouper and gently toss to coat. Cover and stick it in the fridge while you prep the grape leaves.
2. Pull out 24 whole grape leaves (about 6 inches across). Bring 8 cups of water to a boil, then add the leaves and cook for 5 minutes. Drain them, toss them in a bowl of cold water to cool, then drain again.
3. Move your oven rack so it's 8 inches from the broiler and turn the broiler on. Set a wire rack in a rimmed baking sheet and spray it with cooking spray. On the counter, lay out 5 grape leaves (smooth side down) in a circle about 9 inches wide, with the stems pointing in. Lay a 6th leaf in the center to cover any gaps.
4. Put a piece of fish in the middle of your leaf circle. Spoon some of the leftover marinade on top. Fold the sides in, then roll it up tightly like a burrito. Place it seam-side down on the wire rack. Do the same with the rest of the fish and leaves.
5. Pat the tops dry and brush with olive oil. Broil for 12-18 minutes, rotating the sheet halfway through, until the grape leaves are crisp and a bit charred and the fish hits 140°F inside.
6. Serve with the tahini-lemon sauce on the side.

Lemon-Herb Hake Fillets with Garlic Potatoes
Serves 4 | Quick Weeknight Meal

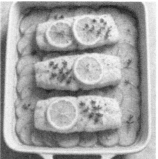

Here's What You Need:
- 1½ lbs russet potatoes, unpeeled and sliced into ¼-inch rounds
- ¼ cup extra-virgin olive oil
- 3 garlic cloves, minced
- Salt and pepper
- 4 skinless hake fillets (4 to 6 oz each, 1 to 1½ inches thick)
- 4 sprigs fresh thyme
- 1 lemon, thinly sliced

How to Make It:
1. Move your oven rack to the lower-middle spot and heat the oven to 425°F.
2. Toss the potato slices with 2 tablespoons of oil, garlic, salt, and pepper in a bowl. Microwave uncovered for 12-14 minutes, stirring halfway through, until they're just tender.

3. Spread the potatoes out in a 13x9-inch baking dish in an even layer.
4. Pat the hake dry with paper towels, season with salt and pepper, and lay them skinned-side down on top of the potatoes.
5. Drizzle the fish with the remaining 2 tablespoons of oil, then lay a few thyme sprigs and lemon slices on each fillet.
6. Bake for 15-18 minutes, or until the fish flakes easily and reaches 140°F inside.
7. Use a spatula to scoop up the potatoes and fish together and transfer to plates. Serve it up hot.

Hake in Saffron Broth with Chorizo and Potatoes
Serves 4

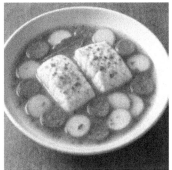

You'll Need:
- 1 tbsp extra-virgin olive oil, plus more for serving
- 1 onion, finely chopped
- 3 oz Spanish-style chorizo, sliced ¼-inch thick
- 4 garlic cloves, minced
- ¼ tsp saffron threads, crumbled
- 1 (8-oz) bottle clam juice
- ¾ cup water
- ½ cup dry white wine
- 4 oz small red potatoes, sliced ¼-inch thick
- 1 bay leaf
- 4 skinless hake fillets (4 to 6 oz each, 1 to 1½ inches thick)
- Salt and pepper
- 1 tsp lemon juice
- 2 tbsp chopped fresh parsley

How to Make It:

1. Heat 1 tablespoon oil in a large skillet over medium. Add onion and chorizo, and cook for 5-7 minutes, until the onion softens and begins to brown. Stir in garlic and saffron, cooking for about 30 seconds.
2. Pour in the clam juice, water, wine, potatoes, and bay leaf. Bring it all to a simmer. Lower the heat, cover, and cook for about 10 minutes, until the potatoes are almost tender.
3. Pat the hake fillets dry, season with salt and pepper, and gently place them in the skillet, skin side down. Spoon a bit of the broth over each piece. Cover and let simmer for 10-12 minutes, or until the fish flakes easily and reaches 140°F.
4. Move the hake to shallow bowls. Use a slotted spoon to divide the potatoes and chorizo between the bowls. Discard the bay leaf. Stir the lemon juice into the broth, season to taste, and ladle it over the fish. Sprinkle with parsley and drizzle a little olive oil over the top. Serve warm.

Provençal Braised Hake
Serves 4

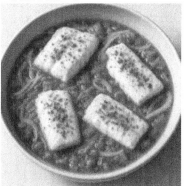

You'll Need:
- 2 tbsp extra-virgin olive oil, plus more for serving
- 1 onion, halved and thinly sliced
- 1 fennel bulb, stalks removed, halved, cored, and thinly sliced
- Salt and pepper
- 4 garlic cloves, minced

- 1 tsp fresh thyme (or ¼ tsp dried)
- 1 (14.5-oz) can diced tomatoes, drained
- ½ cup dry white wine
- 4 skinless hake fillets (4 to 6 oz each, 1 to 1½ inches thick)
- 2 tbsp chopped fresh parsley

How to Make it:
1. Heat 2 tablespoons of olive oil in a large skillet over medium. Add the onion, fennel, and ½ tsp salt. Cook for about 5 minutes, until softened. Stir in the garlic and thyme, cooking for about 30 seconds until fragrant.
2. Add the drained tomatoes and wine, and bring to a simmer.
3. Pat the fish dry, season with salt and pepper, and gently place them in the sauce, skin side down. Spoon some of the sauce over the top. Cover, reduce heat to medium-low, and cook for 10-12 minutes, or until the fish is cooked through and flakes easily.
4. Carefully transfer the fish to shallow bowls. Stir parsley into the sauce, season to taste, and spoon over the fish. Finish with a drizzle of olive oil and serve with warm bread.

Pan-Roasted Halibut with Chermoula
Serves 8 | Quick and Flavorful

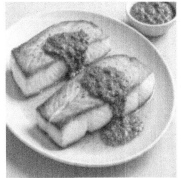

What You'll Need:
For the Chermoula:
- ¾ cup fresh cilantro leaves
- ¼ cup extra-virgin olive oil
- 2 tbsp lemon juice
- 4 garlic cloves, minced
- ½ tsp ground cumin
- ½ tsp paprika

- ¼ tsp salt
- ⅛ tsp cayenne pepper

For the Fish:
- 2 halibut steaks (about 1¼ lbs each, skin-on, 1 to 1½ inches thick, 10-12 inches long)
- Salt and pepper
- 2 tbsp extra-virgin olive oil

How to Make It:
1. Make the Chermoula:
   Toss all the chermoula ingredients into a food processor and blend until smooth, scraping down the sides as needed. Set aside.
2. Sear the Halibut:
   Move your oven rack to the middle and preheat the oven to 325°F. Pat the halibut dry and season with salt and pepper. Heat the oil in a 12-inch oven-safe nonstick skillet over medium-high until it's just starting to smoke. Add the halibut and cook for about 5 minutes until the bottom is nicely browned.
3. Finish in the Oven:
   Carefully flip the fish using two spatulas, then transfer the whole skillet to the oven. Roast for 6-9 minutes, or until the fish flakes easily and hits 140°F inside.
4. Serve:
   Let the halibut rest on a cutting board for 5 minutes under a loose foil tent. Remove the skin and separate the fish from the bones by sliding a knife or spatula between the sections. Serve with a generous spoonful of chermoula on top.

Braised Halibut with Leeks and Mustard
Serves 4

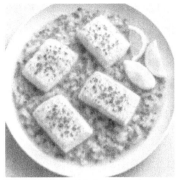

What You'll Need:
- 4 halibut fillets (4 to 6 oz each, skinless, ¾ to 1 inch thick)
- Salt and pepper
- ¼ cup extra-virgin olive oil, plus more for serving
- 1 lb leeks (white and light green parts only), halved lengthwise, thinly sliced, and cleaned
- 1 tsp Dijon mustard
- ¾ cup dry white wine
- 1 tbsp fresh parsley, minced
- Lemon wedges, for serving

How to Make It:
1. Pat the halibut dry and season with ½ tsp salt. Heat the oil in a large skillet over medium. Place the fish in the skillet, skinned side up, and cook for about 4 minutes—just until the bottom half starts to look opaque. It shouldn't brown. Gently transfer the fish, raw side down, to a plate.
2. Add the leeks, mustard, and ¼ tsp salt to the skillet. Cook over medium, stirring often, until the leeks are soft, about 10-12 minutes. Pour in the wine and bring it to a simmer.
3. Place the fish back in the pan, raw side down, on top of the leeks. Lower the heat to medium-low, cover, and let it cook gently for 6-10 minutes, or until the fish flakes easily and reaches 140°F.
4. Move the fish to a serving platter and loosely tent with foil. Turn the heat to high and simmer the leeks until the sauce thickens a bit, about 2-4 minutes. Taste and adjust seasoning.
5. Spoon the leek mixture around the fish, drizzle a little more olive oil on top, sprinkle with parsley, and serve with lemon wedges.

Baked Stuffed Mackerel with Red Pepper and Preserved Lemon
Serves 4

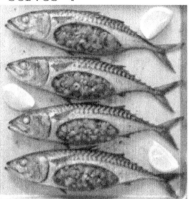

You'll Need:
- 3 tbsp extra-virgin olive oil
- 1 red bell pepper, chopped fine
- 1 red onion, chopped fine
- ½ preserved lemon (pulp and pith removed, rind rinsed and minced—about 2 tbsp)
- ⅓ cup pitted brine-cured green olives, chopped
- 1 tbsp fresh parsley, minced
- Salt and pepper
- 4 whole mackerel (8 to 10 oz each), gutted and fins trimmed
- Lemon wedges, for serving

How to Make It:
1. Preheat your oven to 500°F and set the rack to the middle. Heat 2 tablespoons of oil in a skillet over medium-high heat. Cook the bell pepper and onion for 8-10 minutes, until they're soft and well browned. Stir in the preserved lemon and cook for another 30 seconds. Take it off the heat, mix in the olives and parsley, and season with salt and pepper.
2. Grease a rimmed baking sheet with the remaining tablespoon of oil. Rinse the mackerel inside and out, then pat dry. Season the inside of each fish with salt and pepper. Stuff

each one with a quarter of the filling and place on the sheet, leaving at least 2 inches between each.

3. Roast the fish for 10-12 minutes, until the thickest part reaches 130-135°F. Let rest for 5 minutes. Serve with lemon wedges.

Quick Preserved Lemon Substitute (Makes about 1 tbsp):
 Combine 4 minced strips of lemon zest (about 2 inches each), 1 tsp lemon juice, ½ tsp water, ¼ tsp sugar, and ¼ tsp salt. Microwave at 50% power until the liquid's gone, about 1½ minutes, stirring and mashing every 30 seconds.

Want to Make the Real Thing?
 You'll need 12 lemons (Meyer if possible) and about ½ cup kosher salt. Cut 4 lemons nearly through into quarters, stuff each with 2 tbsp salt, and pack into a jar. Add juice from the rest of the lemons to cover, seal tightly, and shake. Refrigerate, shaking daily for 4 days. Let cure 6-8 weeks before using. They'll keep for at least 6 months.

Grilled Whole Mackerel with Lemon and Marjoram

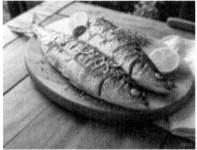

Serves 4 | Fast and Flavorful
What You'll Need:
- 2 tsp chopped fresh marjoram
- 1 tsp lemon zest, plus lemon wedges for serving
- Salt and pepper
- 4 whole mackerel (8 to 10 oz each), gutted, fins trimmed
- 2 tbsp mayonnaise
- ½ tsp honey
- 1 (13x9-inch) disposable aluminum roasting pan (for charcoal grill only)

How to Make It:
1. On a cutting board, combine marjoram, lemon zest, and 1 tsp salt. Chop until it's well mixed. Rinse the mackerel and pat dry inside and out. Season the inside with pepper and sprinkle the marjoram mixture evenly inside each fish. Let them rest for 10 minutes.
2. Mix the mayo and honey together, then brush it over the outside of each fish.

If Using a Charcoal Grill:
- Use kitchen shears to poke 12 holes in the bottom of the roasting pan.
- Open the bottom vent and set the pan in the middle of the grill.
- Fill a chimney starter with 4 quarts of charcoal and light it.
- Once the top coals are ashy, pour them evenly into the pan.
- Put the grate on, lid on, and let it heat up for 5 minutes.

If Using a Gas Grill:
- Turn all burners to high. Cover and heat for 15 minutes.

---

3.   Clean and oil the grill grate really well—do this 5 to 10 times until it's black and glossy.
4.   Place the mackerel directly over the heat. For gas grills, keep the lid closed. Cook for 2-4 minutes until the skin is browned and starting to blister.
5.   To flip: Gently lift the fish at the backbone with a thin spatula just enough to slide a second spatula underneath. Use both to carefully turn it over.
6.   Cook another 2-4 minutes on the other side, until the thickest part hits 130-135°F.
7.   Let the fish rest for 5 minutes, then serve with lemon wedges.

Pan-Roasted Halibut with Chermoula

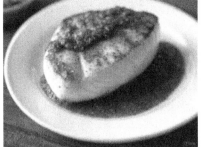

Serves 8 | Quick and Bold

You'll Need:

For the Chermoula:
- ¾ cup fresh cilantro leaves
- ¼ cup extra-virgin olive oil
- 2 tbsp lemon juice
- 4 garlic cloves, minced
- ½ tsp ground cumin
- ½ tsp paprika
- ¼ tsp salt
- ⅛ tsp cayenne pepper

For the Fish:
- 2 halibut steaks (about 1¼ lbs each, skin-on, 1 to 1½ inches thick, 10-12 inches long)
- Salt and pepper
- 2 tbsp extra-virgin olive oil

How to Make It:
1. Make the Chermoula:
   Blend all the chermoula ingredients in a food processor until smooth (about a minute), scraping down the sides as needed. Set aside.
2. Prep the Fish:
   Move your oven rack to the middle and preheat to 325°F. Pat the halibut dry and season with salt and pepper.
3. Sear:
   Heat the oil in a 12-inch oven-safe nonstick skillet over medium-high until it just starts to smoke. Add the halibut and sear for about 5 minutes, until the first side is nicely browned.
4. Roast:
   Flip the fish gently using two spatulas, then move the skillet to the oven. Roast for 6-9 minutes, until the fish flakes easily and reaches 140°F inside.
5. Finish & Serve:
   Let the halibut rest on a cutting board under loose foil for 5 minutes. Remove the skin, then use a knife or spatula to separate the meat from the bones into four neat sections per steak. Serve with generous spoonfuls of chermoula.

Pan-Roasted Halibut with Chermoula

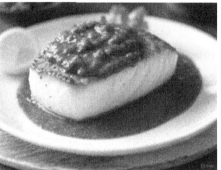

Serves 8 | Quick & Flavor-Packed

What You'll Need

For the Chermoula:
- ¾ cup fresh cilantro leaves
- ¼ cup extra-virgin olive oil
- 2 tablespoons lemon juice
- 4 garlic cloves, minced
- ½ teaspoon ground cumin
- ½ teaspoon paprika
- ¼ teaspoon salt
- ⅛ teaspoon cayenne pepper

For the Fish:
- 2 skin-on halibut steaks (about 1¼ lbs each, 1 to 1½ inches thick, 10-12 inches long)
- Salt and pepper
- 2 tablespoons extra-virgin olive oil

How to Make It
1. Make the Chermoula:
   Toss all the chermoula ingredients into a food processor and blend until smooth, about 1 minute. Scrape down the sides if needed. Set aside.
2. Prep the Fish:
   Preheat your oven to 325°F and move the oven rack to the middle. Pat the halibut dry and season both sides with salt and pepper.
3. Sear the Halibut:
   Heat the oil in a large oven-safe nonstick skillet over

medium-high heat until just starting to smoke. Add the halibut and sear for about 5 minutes, until the bottom is golden brown.

4. Finish in the Oven:
   Flip the fish gently using two spatulas, then transfer the skillet to the oven. Roast for 6 to 9 minutes, or until the fish flakes easily and hits 140°F inside.

5. Serve It Up:
   Let the fish rest on a cutting board under loose foil for 5 minutes. Remove the skin, then use a knife or spatula to separate the meat from the bones into clean sections. Spoon plenty of chermoula over the top and serve.

Braised Halibut with Leeks and Mustard

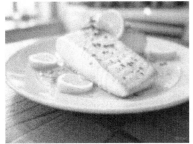

Serves 4 | One-Pan Comfort
You'll Need:
- 4 skinless halibut fillets (4 to 6 oz each, ¾ to 1 inch thick)
- Salt and pepper
- ¼ cup extra-virgin olive oil, plus more for drizzling
- 1 lb leeks (white and light green parts only), halved lengthwise, thinly sliced, thoroughly washed
- 1 tsp Dijon mustard
- ¾ cup dry white wine
- 1 tbsp minced fresh parsley
- Lemon wedges, for serving

How to Make It:
1. Sear the Halibut:
   Pat the fillets dry and sprinkle with ½ tsp salt. Heat the oil in a 12-inch skillet over medium until warm. Place the fish skinned side up in the skillet and cook for about 4 minutes, just until the bottom half turns opaque (you're not browning it). Carefully transfer fish, raw side down, to a plate.

2. Cook the Leeks:
   Add the leeks, mustard, and ¼ tsp salt to the same skillet. Cook over medium, stirring often, until softened, about 10-12 minutes. Stir in the wine and bring to a simmer.

3. Braise the Fish:
   Nestle the halibut (raw side down) into the leeks. Lower the heat to medium-low, cover, and cook gently for 6-10 minutes, or until the fish flakes easily and reads 140°F inside.

4. Finish the Sauce:
   Transfer the halibut to a serving platter and tent with foil. Turn the heat to high and simmer the leeks for 2-4 minutes until the sauce thickens slightly. Season with salt and pepper.

5. Serve It Up:
   Spoon the leeks around the halibut, drizzle with a bit more olive oil, sprinkle with parsley, and serve with lemon wedges.

Baked Stuffed Mackerel with Red Pepper and Preserved Lemon

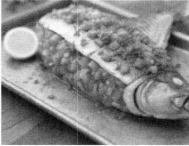

Serves 4 | Bold and Bright
You'll Need:
- 3 tbsp extra-virgin olive oil
- 1 red bell pepper, finely chopped
- 1 red onion, finely chopped
- ½ preserved lemon (remove pulp and white pith, rinse rind, mince to get 2 tbsp)

- ⅓ cup brine-cured green olives, chopped
- 1 tbsp fresh parsley, minced
- Salt and pepper
- 4 whole mackerel (8 to 10 oz each), gutted and fins trimmed
- Lemon wedges, for serving

How to Make It:
1. Prep the Filling:
   Preheat your oven to 500°F and set the rack to the middle. Heat 2 tablespoons of oil in a skillet over medium-high. Add the bell pepper and onion, and cook for 8-10 minutes until soft and browned. Stir in the preserved lemon and cook for 30 seconds. Remove from heat, mix in the olives and parsley, and season with salt and pepper.
2. Stuff the Fish:
   Grease a rimmed baking sheet with the remaining tablespoon of oil. Rinse the mackerel and pat them dry, inside and out. Season the inside of each with salt and pepper, then stuff with the filling—about a quarter per fish. Lay the fish on the sheet, spacing them at least 2 inches apart.
3. Bake:
   Roast the stuffed mackerel for 10-12 minutes, or until the thickest part hits 130-135°F. Transfer to a serving platter and let rest for 5 minutes. Serve with lemon wedges.

Grilled Whole Mackerel with Lemon and Marjoram

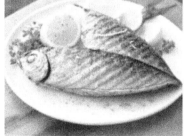

Serves 4 | Fast and Flavorful
You'll Need:
- 2 tsp chopped fresh marjoram
- 1 tsp grated lemon zest, plus lemon wedges for serving
- Salt and pepper

- 4 whole mackerel (8 to 10 oz each), gutted, fins trimmed
- 2 tbsp mayonnaise
- ½ tsp honey
- 1 (13x9-inch) disposable aluminum roasting pan (for charcoal grill only)

How to Make It:
1. On a cutting board, combine marjoram, lemon zest, and 1 tsp salt. Chop everything together until finely minced. Rinse and dry the fish inside and out. Open up each fish, season with pepper, and sprinkle the marjoram mix inside. Let sit for 10 minutes.
2. Mix the mayo and honey, then brush it all over the outside of each fish.

If Using a Charcoal Grill:
- Poke 12 holes in the bottom of the roasting pan using kitchen shears.
- Place it in the middle of the grill and open the bottom vent.
- Fill a chimney starter two-thirds full with charcoal (about 4 quarts). Light it.
- Once the coals are ashy on top, dump them into the pan in an even layer.
- Set the cooking grate on top (bars running parallel to the pan), cover the grill, and open the lid vent all the way. Heat for about 5 minutes.

If Using a Gas Grill:
- Turn all burners to high. Cover and heat for about 15 minutes until super hot.

3. Clean the grate well, then oil it with paper towels dipped in oil—do this several times until the grate looks black and glossy.
4. Place the fish directly over the heat. Cover the grill if using gas. Cook for 2 to 4 minutes on the first side, until the skin starts to blister and brown.
5. Flip gently: slide a spatula under the thick backbone edge, then use a second spatula to help flip it over. Cook for another 2 to 4

minutes, until the second side is browned and the thickest part of the fish hits 130-135°F.

6.   Let rest for 5 minutes, then serve with lemon wedges.

Pan-Roasted Monkfish with Oregano-Black Olive Relish

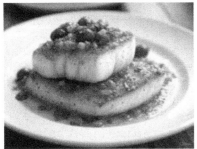

Serves 4 | Fast & Flavorful

You'll Need:

- ¼ cup extra-virgin olive oil
- 2 tbsp fresh oregano, minced
- 2 tbsp red wine vinegar
- 1 small shallot, minced
- 1 tsp Dijon mustard
- Salt and pepper
- ¼ cup kalamata olives, pitted and minced
- 4 monkfish fillets (4 to 6 oz each, 1 to 1½ inches thick, skinless and trimmed)
- ½ tsp sugar

How to Make It:

1. Make the Relish:
   In a medium bowl, combine 2 tablespoons of olive oil and the oregano. Microwave until it bubbles, about 30 seconds. Let it sit for 5 minutes to steep. Whisk in the vinegar, shallot, mustard, and ¼ tsp pepper. Stir in the chopped olives and set aside.

2. Prep the Fish:
   Preheat your oven to 425°F and move the rack to the middle. Pat the monkfish dry with paper towels, season both sides with salt and pepper, and sprinkle evenly with the sugar.

3. Sear and Roast:
   Heat the remaining 2 tablespoons of oil in a 12-inch oven-safe skillet over medium-high until just smoking. Add the monkfish and press lightly so it makes good contact with

the pan. Sear for 2 minutes until browned, then gently flip with two spatulas and sear the other side for 2 more minutes.

4. Finish in the Oven:
   Transfer the skillet to the oven and roast for 8 to 12 minutes, until the center of the fish reaches 160°F and turns opaque. Remove from the oven and let the fillets rest on a platter, loosely tented with foil, for 5 minutes.

5. Serve:
   Spoon the oregano-olive relish over the monkfish and serve warm.

Grilled Whole Sardines

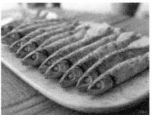

Serves 4 to 6 | Fast & Rustic

You'll Need:

- 12 whole sardines (2 to 3 oz each), scaled, gutted, fins trimmed
- Black pepper
- 2 tbsp mayonnaise
- ½ tsp honey
- Lemon wedges, for serving

How to Make It:

1. Rinse the sardines and pat dry, inside and out. Season the cavities with pepper. Mix the mayo and honey, then brush it all over the outside of the fish.

2A. For Charcoal Grill:
 Open the bottom vent and light a chimney starter full of charcoal (about 6 quarts). When ashy, spread the coals evenly. Place the grate on, cover, and open the lid vent. Let it heat for about 5 minutes.

2B. For Gas Grill:
 Turn all burners to high. Cover and heat for about 15 minutes.

3.   Clean and oil the grate well (5 to 10 times until glossy). Grill the sardines 2-4 minutes per side until the skin is blistered and browned,

and they lift easily from the grill.
Serve with lemon wedges.

Pan-Roasted Sea Bass

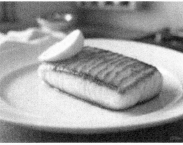

Serves 4 | Quick & Elegant
You'll Need:
- 4 sea bass fillets (4 to 6 oz each, 1 to 1½ inches thick, skinless)
- Salt and pepper
- ½ tsp sugar
- 1 tbsp extra-virgin olive oil
- Lemon wedges, for serving

How to Make It:
1. Move the oven rack to the middle and preheat to 425°F. Pat fish dry, season with salt and pepper, and sprinkle sugar on one side.
2. Heat oil in a 12-inch oven-safe skillet over medium-high until just smoking. Place the fish sugar-side down in the pan and press lightly for even contact. Sear for about 2 minutes until golden.
3. Carefully flip the fillets, transfer the skillet to the oven, and roast for 7-10 minutes, until the fish flakes easily and hits 140°F inside. Serve with lemon wedges.

Grilled Sea Bass with Citrus and Black Olive Salad

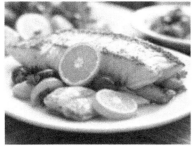

Serves 4 | Fast & Fresh
You'll Need:
- 2 oranges
- 1 red grapefruit

- ¼ cup kalamata olives, pitted and chopped
- 2 tbsp fresh parsley, minced
- ½ tsp ground cumin
- ½ tsp paprika
- Pinch of cayenne
- Salt and pepper
- 4 sea bass fillets (4 to 6 oz each, 1 to 1½ inches thick, skinless)
- 2 tbsp extra-virgin olive oil

How to Make It:
1. Make the Salad:
   Slice the peel and white pith off the oranges and grapefruit. Cut the oranges into quarters, then into ½-inch slices. Slice the grapefruit into 8 wedges, then into ½-inch chunks. Toss the citrus pieces (not the juice) with olives, parsley, cumin, paprika, cayenne, and a little salt. Cover and set aside.
2. Prep the Fish:
   Pat the fillets dry, rub them with olive oil, and season well with salt and pepper.

For a Charcoal Grill:
- Open the bottom vent. Light a chimney starter full of charcoal (about 6 quarts). When the coals are ashy, pour them over one side of the grill. Add the cooking grate, cover, open the lid vent, and heat for 5 minutes.

For a Gas Grill:
- Turn all burners to high. Cover and preheat for 15 minutes. Then leave one burner on high and set the others to medium-low.

3. Grill the Fish:
Scrub and oil the grate well—5 to 10 times until it's black and glossy. Place the fillets over the hot side and grill uncovered for about 10 minutes total, flipping gently halfway through with two spatulas.
4. Finish on the Cool Side:
Move the fish to the cooler part of the grill and cook uncovered for

another 3-6 minutes, until it flakes easily and hits 140°F inside.
5.   Serve:
 Plate the sea bass and spoon the citrus-olive salad over the top. Bright, smoky, and ready in no time.

Grilled Whole Sea Bass with Salmoriglio Sauce

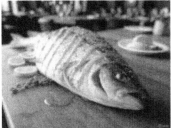

Serves 4 | Fast & Flavorful
You'll Need:
For the Salmoriglio Sauce:
- 1 small garlic clove, minced
- 1 tbsp lemon juice
- ⅛ tsp salt
- ⅛ tsp pepper
- 1½ tbsp fresh oregano, minced
- ¼ cup extra-virgin olive oil

For the Fish:
- 2 whole sea bass (1½ to 2 lbs each), scaled, gutted, fins trimmed
- 3 tbsp extra-virgin olive oil
- Salt and pepper

How to Make It:
1. Make the Sauce:
    Whisk the garlic, lemon juice, salt, pepper, oregano, and olive oil in a bowl. Cover and set aside.
2A. For a Charcoal Grill:
 Open the bottom vent. Light a full chimney of charcoal (about 6 quarts). When the coals are ashy on top, spread them out evenly. Put the grate on, cover, and open the lid vent. Heat for 5 minutes.
2B. For a Gas Grill:
 Turn all burners to high. Cover and heat for 15 minutes.
3.   Prep the Fish:
 Rinse and pat the sea bass dry. Use a sharp knife to make 3-4 shallow diagonal slashes on each side of the fish. Rub all over with olive oil, then season inside and out with salt and pepper.

4.   Grill the Fish:
 Clean the grate thoroughly, then oil it 5 to 10 times until glossy. Place the fish on the hot grill (cover if using gas) and cook for 6-8 minutes until the skin blisters and browns. Use two spatulas to gently flip. Grill the other side for 6-8 minutes until the fish hits 140°F.
5.   Serve:
 Let the fish rest for 5 minutes. To fillet, make a vertical cut behind the head and a horizontal cut down the top from head to tail. Slide a spatula between the flesh and bones to lift out the fillets. Repeat on the other side. Discard bones and serve with the salmoriglio sauce spooned over the top.

Poached Snapper with Crispy Artichokes and Sherry-Tomato Vinaigrette

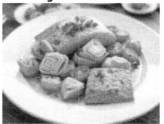

Serves 4 | Silky, Crispy, and Packed with Flavor
What You'll Need:
For the Fish & Garnish:
- 4 skinless red snapper fillets (4-6 oz each, about 1 inch thick)
- Salt
- 1 cup jarred whole baby artichokes (quartered, rinsed, patted dry)
- 1 tbsp cornstarch
- ¾ cup extra-virgin olive oil
- 3 garlic cloves, minced
- ½ onion, peeled

For the Vinaigrette:
- 6 oz cherry tomatoes (2 oz sliced into thin rounds for garnish)
- ½ small shallot, peeled
- 4 tsp sherry vinegar
- ½ tsp pepper
- ¼ tsp salt
- 1 tbsp fresh parsley, minced

How to Make It:
1. Prep the Fish:
   Preheat oven to 250°F with racks in the middle and lower positions. Pat the fish dry, season with salt, and let sit at room temp for 20 minutes.
2. Crisp the Artichokes:
   Toss artichokes with cornstarch. Heat ½ cup oil in a 10-inch oven-safe nonstick skillet over medium until shimmering. Shake off excess cornstarch and cook the artichokes until golden, 2-4 minutes. Add garlic and cook 30-60 seconds more. Strain oil through a fine mesh strainer into a bowl (don't wash the strainer). Transfer crispy bits to a paper towel-lined plate and season with salt.
3. Poach the Fish:
   Return the strained oil to the skillet and add remaining ¼ cup oil. Place the onion half in the center. Let the oil cool to about 180°F (takes 5-8 minutes). Nestle fish, skinned side up, around the onion, spooning oil over each fillet. Cover and transfer to the oven (upper rack). Cook for 15 minutes.
4. Finish Cooking:
   Carefully flip the fillets using 2 spatulas. Return skillet (covered) to the upper oven rack and place the plate with artichokes on the lower rack to rewarm. Cook another 9-14 minutes, until the fish hits 130-135°F. Transfer fillets to a platter, tent loosely with foil, and reserve ½ cup of the cooking oil.
5. Make the Vinaigrette:
   In a blender, combine the reserved oil, whole tomatoes, shallot, vinegar, pepper, and salt. Blend until smooth (about 2 minutes). Add any juices from resting fish and blend 10 seconds more. Strain through a mesh strainer into a bowl.

6. Serve It Up:
   Spoon the warm vinaigrette around the fish. Top each fillet with crisped artichokes, garlic, tomato slices, and a sprinkle of parsley.

Whole Roasted Snapper with Citrus Vinaigrette

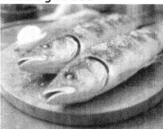

Serves 4 | Fast & Full of Flavor
You'll Need:
For the Vinaigrette:
- ¼ cup extra-virgin olive oil
- ¼ cup minced fresh cilantro
- 2 tbsp lime juice + 2 tsp lime zest
- 2 tbsp orange juice + 2 tsp orange zest
- 1 small shallot, minced
- ⅛ tsp red pepper flakes
- Salt and pepper to taste
For the Fish:
- 2 whole red snapper (1½ to 2 lbs each), scaled, gutted, and fins snipped
- 1½ tsp salt
- ½ tsp pepper
- 2 tbsp extra-virgin olive oil (for brushing)

How to Make It:
1. Preheat & Prep:
   Heat oven to 500°F and position the rack in the middle. Line a rimmed baking sheet with parchment and lightly grease it.
2. Make the Vinaigrette:
   In a bowl, whisk together ¼ cup oil, cilantro, citrus juices, shallot, and red pepper flakes. Season with salt and pepper to taste and set aside.
3. Season the Fish:
   Mix lime zest, orange zest, 1½ tsp salt, and ½ tsp pepper in a small bowl. Rinse and dry the snapper thoroughly. Make 3-4

shallow slashes on each side of the fish. Sprinkle 1 tsp of the citrus salt mixture inside the cavity of each fish. Brush 1 tbsp oil over the outside of each fish, then rub in the remaining citrus salt mixture. Let sit for 10 minutes.

4. Roast the Snapper:
   Roast for 15-20 minutes, until the flesh flakes easily and reads 140°F. Check for doneness by peeking into the slashes or looking through the bottom of the fish.

5. Serve:
   Let the fish rest for 5 minutes on a cutting board. To fillet, make a vertical cut just behind the head and a horizontal cut from head to tail along the top. Use a spatula to lift the fillets from the bones. Repeat for the other side. Discard the skeleton and head. Re-whisk the vinaigrette and spoon it over the fillets.

Sautéed Sole

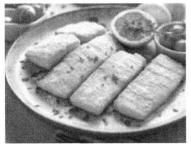

Serves 4 | Fast, Light & Classic
You'll Need:
- ½ cup all-purpose flour
- 8 skinless sole fillets (2 to 3 oz each, ¼ to ½ inch thick)
- Salt and pepper
- ¼ cup extra-virgin olive oil
- Lemon wedges, for serving

How to Make It:
1. Spread the flour out in a shallow dish. Pat the fish dry and season both sides with salt and pepper. Dredge the fillets in the flour, shaking off the extra.

2. Heat 2 tablespoons of oil in a nonstick skillet over medium-high until shimmering. Cook half the fillets, without crowding, for about 2-3 minutes on the first side, until golden. Flip gently and cook another 30-60 seconds until the fish flakes easily.

3. Transfer to a warm plate and tent loosely with foil. Wipe out the skillet, add the remaining oil, and cook the rest of the fillets the same way. Serve with lemon wedges.

Fresh Relish Ideas:
Tomato & Basil Relish
Bright, juicy, and perfect for summer
Mix together:
- 2 ripe tomatoes (cored, seeded, diced)
- 1 small shallot, minced
- 2 tbsp chopped fresh basil
- 1 tbsp extra-virgin olive oil
- 1 garlic clove, minced
- 1 tsp red wine vinegar

Let sit for 15 minutes. Season with salt and pepper. Spoon over the cooked fish.

Swordfish en Cocotte with Shallots, Cucumber, and Mint

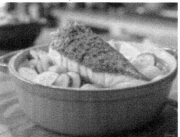

Serves 4 | Slow-Cooked & Packed with Bright, Herbal Flavor

What You'll Need:
- ¾ cup fresh mint leaves
- ¼ cup fresh parsley leaves
- 5 tbsp extra-virgin olive oil
- 2 tbsp lemon juice
- 4 garlic cloves, minced
- 1 tsp ground cumin
- ¼ tsp cayenne pepper
- Salt and pepper

- 3 shallots, thinly sliced
- 1 cucumber, peeled, seeded, and thinly sliced
- 4 swordfish steaks (4-6 oz each, skin-on, 1 to 1½ inches thick)

How to Make It:
1. Preheat the Oven:
   Set the rack to the lowest position and heat oven to 250°F.
2. Make the Herb Mixture:
   In a food processor, combine the mint, parsley, 3 tbsp olive oil, lemon juice, garlic, cumin, cayenne, and ¼ tsp salt. Blend until smooth, about 20 seconds, scraping the bowl as needed.
3. Cook the Shallots:
   Heat the remaining 2 tbsp oil in a Dutch oven over medium-low heat. Add shallots, cover, and cook, stirring now and then, until soft (about 5 minutes). Take off the heat and stir in the herb mixture and cucumber slices.
4. Add the Fish:
   Pat swordfish dry and season with salt and pepper. Lay the steaks on top of the cucumber mixture. Cover the pot tightly with foil, then the lid.
5. Bake Gently:
   Bake for 35 40 minutes, until the swordfish flakes easily with a paring knife and reaches 140°F inside.
6. Serve:
   Transfer the fish to a serving platter. Taste and season the cucumber mixture, then spoon it over the fish. Serve warm.

Grilled Swordfish with Italian Salsa Verde

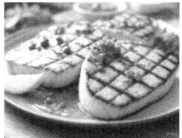

Serves 4 | Fast, Smoky & Zesty
What You'll Need:
- 4 swordfish steaks (4-6 oz each, skin-on, 1 to 1½ inches thick)
- 2 tbsp extra-virgin olive oil
- Salt and pepper
- ½ cup Italian Salsa Verde (homemade or store-bought)

How to Make It:
1. Prep the Fish:
   Pat the swordfish dry, rub with olive oil, and season well with salt and pepper.
2A. For a Charcoal Grill:
 Open bottom vent. Light a full chimney of charcoal (6 quarts). When coals are ashy, dump two-thirds on one side of the grill and the rest on the other. Set the grate in place, cover, open the lid vent, and heat for 5 minutes.
2B. For a Gas Grill:
 Turn all burners to high and heat, covered, for 15 minutes. Then leave one side on high, and lower the other to medium-high.
3.   Grill the Swordfish:
 Clean and oil the grate thoroughly (5-10 times until glossy). Place the steaks over the hot side. Grill uncovered for 6-9 minutes total, flipping gently halfway through, until the fish gets deep grill marks.
4.   Finish Cooking:
 Move the steaks to the cooler part of the grill and cook another 1-3 minutes per side, until the center is just cooked through (internal temp should hit 140°F).
5.   Serve:
 Plate the swordfish and top with a generous spoonful of Italian salsa verde.

Grilled Swordfish with Eggplant, Tomato, and Chickpea Salad

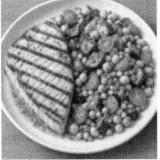

Serves 4 | Fast, Fresh & Mediterranean-Inspired

What You'll Need:

- 1 cup fresh cilantro leaves
- ½ red onion, chopped
- 6 tbsp extra-virgin olive oil
- 3 tbsp lemon juice
- 4 garlic cloves, chopped
- 1 tsp ground cumin
- 1 tsp paprika
- ¼ tsp cayenne pepper
- ⅛ tsp ground cinnamon
- Salt and pepper
- 4 swordfish steaks (4-6 oz each, skin-on, 1 to 1½ inches thick)
- 1 large eggplant, cut into ½-inch rounds
- 6 oz cherry tomatoes, halved
- 1 (15-oz) can chickpeas, rinsed

How to Make It:

1. Make the Cilantro Paste:
   In a food processor, blend cilantro, onion, 3 tbsp olive oil, lemon juice, garlic, cumin, paprika, cayenne, cinnamon, and ½ tsp salt until smooth (about 2 minutes). Set aside ½ cup for brushing the fish. Transfer the rest to a large bowl.
2. Prep the Fish & Eggplant:
   Brush swordfish with the reserved ½ cup cilantro mixture. Brush eggplant rounds with the remaining 3 tbsp olive oil, and season with salt and pepper.

3A. For a Charcoal Grill:
Light a chimney starter full of coals (6 quarts). Once ashy, pour two-thirds over one half of the grill and the rest over the other. Cover, heat the grate for 5 minutes, then scrub and oil it.

3B. For a Gas Grill:
Turn all burners to high, cover, and heat for 15 minutes. Leave one burner on high, lower the others to medium-high.

4. Grill the Swordfish & Eggplant:
Place both on the hot side of the grill. Grill the fish uncovered for 6-9 minutes total, flipping halfway through. Grill the eggplant until softened and nicely charred, flipping as needed (about 8 minutes). Transfer to a platter and loosely tent with foil.

5. Finish the Swordfish:
Move the fish to the cooler side of the grill and cook 1-3 more minutes per side, until the center hits 140°F. Tent loosely with foil and let it rest.

6. Make the Salad:
Coarsely chop the grilled eggplant. Add it to the bowl with the remaining cilantro mixture, along with the cherry tomatoes and chickpeas. Toss gently and season to taste.

7. Serve:
Plate the swordfish with a generous scoop of the eggplant-tomato-chickpea salad on the side.

Grilled Tuna Steaks with Romesco

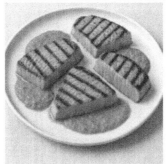

Serves 4 | Fast, Smoky & Bold

You'll Need:

For the Romesco Sauce:

- 1 slice hearty white bread (toasted, crusts removed, cut into ½-inch pieces - about ½ cup)
- 1½ tbsp slivered almonds, toasted

- 1 cup jarred roasted red peppers, rinsed, patted dry, chopped
- 1 plum tomato, cored, seeded, chopped
- ¼ cup extra-virgin olive oil
- 2¼ tsp sherry vinegar
- 1 garlic clove, minced
- ⅛ tsp cayenne pepper
- Salt and pepper, to taste

For the Tuna:
- 2 (8- to 12-oz) skinless tuna steaks, 1 inch thick, halved crosswise
- 2 tsp honey
- 1 tsp water
- 3 tbsp extra-virgin olive oil
- ½ tsp salt + a pinch of pepper

How to Make It:
1. Make the Romesco:
   In a food processor, pulse the bread and almonds until finely ground (about 10-15 seconds). Add the roasted peppers, tomato, 1 tbsp oil, vinegar, garlic, cayenne, and ½ tsp salt. Blend until smooth, 20-30 seconds, scraping the sides as needed. Season to taste and set aside.
2. Prep the Tuna:
   In a bowl, whisk together 3 tbsp oil, honey, water, ½ tsp salt, and a pinch of pepper. Pat tuna dry, then brush generously with the oil-honey mix.

3A. For a Charcoal Grill:
 Light a full chimney of coals (6 quarts), pour them over half the grill once ashed, and heat the grate for 5 minutes with the lid on and vent open.

3B. For a Gas Grill:
 Turn all burners to high and preheat for 15 minutes with the lid closed.

4.   Grill the Tuna:
 Scrub and oil the grate until glossy (5-10 times). Grill the tuna uncovered (or covered for gas) over high heat. For rare: grill 1-3 minutes on the first side, flip, and cook 1½ minutes more until the center is deep red and hits 110°F. For medium-rare: cook a bit longer until the center is reddish pink and registers 125°F.

5.   Serve:
 Plate the tuna and serve with generous spoonfuls of the romesco sauce.

Bouillabaisse

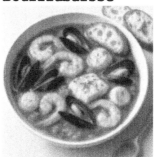

Serves 6 to 8 | Classic French Stew, Simplified

What You'll Need:
- ¼ cup extra-virgin olive oil
- 1 small fennel bulb, trimmed, cored, and finely chopped
- 1 onion, finely chopped
- 8 garlic cloves, minced
- 1 tsp fresh thyme (or ¼ tsp dried)
- ¼ tsp saffron threads, crumbled
- ⅛ tsp red pepper flakes
- ¾ cup dry white wine or dry vermouth
- 2 (8-oz) bottles clam juice
- 1 (14.5-oz) can whole peeled tomatoes, drained and chopped (save the juice)
- 2 bay leaves
- 1 lb halibut fillets (¾ to 1 inch thick), cut into 3-4 inch pieces
- 12 oz mussels, scrubbed and debearded
- 1 lb large sea scallops, tendons removed
- 8 oz medium-large shrimp (peeled and deveined)
- 2 tbsp fresh tarragon, minced
- Salt and pepper, to taste

How to Make It:
1. Build the Base:
   Heat olive oil in a Dutch oven over medium-high. Add fennel and onion and cook until

softened (about 5 minutes).
Stir in garlic, thyme, saffron,
and red pepper flakes. Cook 30
seconds until fragrant. Add
wine and let it reduce
slightly, about 30 seconds.

2. Simmer the Broth:
   Stir in clam juice, tomatoes
   with reserved juice, and bay
   leaves. Bring to a simmer and
   cook until the liquid reduces
   by half—about 7-9 minutes.

3. Cook the Fish:
   Pat halibut dry and season
   with salt and pepper. Nestle it
   into the pot, spoon broth over
   the top, and bring to a gentle
   simmer. Cover and cook over
   medium-low for 2 minutes.

4. Add the Shellfish:
   Add mussels and scallops to
   the pot, cover, and cook
   another 3 minutes. Add shrimp,
   cover again, and cook until all
   seafood is cooked through and
   mussels have opened (about 2
   more minutes). Discard any
   unopened mussels and bay
   leaves.

5. Finish and Serve:
   Off heat, stir in tarragon.
   Taste and season the broth with
   salt and pepper. Serve in
   shallow bowls with crusty bread
   or garlic toasts—and rouille if
   you want to go full Provençal.

Sicilian Fish Stew

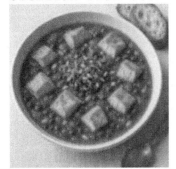

Serves 4 to 6 | Sweet, Savory &
Bold

You'll Need:
For the topping:
- ¼ cup pine nuts, toasted
- ¼ cup fresh mint, chopped
- 1 garlic clove (from the 4),
  minced
- 1 tsp grated orange zest

For the stew:
- 2 tbsp extra-virgin olive oil
- 2 onions, finely chopped
- 1 celery rib, minced
- Salt and pepper
- 1 tsp fresh thyme (or ¼ tsp
  dried)
- Pinch red pepper flakes
- 3 garlic cloves, minced
- ½ cup dry white wine
- 1 (28-oz) can whole peeled
  tomatoes, drained and chopped
  (reserve the juice)
- 2 (8-oz) bottles clam juice
- ¼ cup golden raisins
- 2 tbsp capers, rinsed
- 1½ lbs skinless swordfish
  steaks (1 to 1½ inches thick),
  cut into 1-inch chunks

How to Make It:
1. Mix the Topping:
   In a small bowl, combine
   toasted pine nuts, mint, 1
   minced garlic clove, and orange
   zest. Set aside.

2. Start the Stew Base:
   In a Dutch oven, heat the
   olive oil over medium heat. Add
   onions, celery, ½ tsp salt, and
   ¼ tsp pepper. Cook until soft,
   about 5 minutes. Stir in thyme,
   pepper flakes, and remaining
   garlic. Cook for 30 seconds
   until fragrant.

3. Build the Broth:
   Add wine and reserved tomato
   juice. Simmer until reduced by
   half, about 4 minutes. Add
   chopped tomatoes, clam juice,
   raisins, and capers. Bring to a
   simmer and let it cook for
   about 15 minutes to develop
   flavor.

4. Add the Fish:
   Pat swordfish dry, season with
   salt and pepper, and nestle
   into the pot. Spoon some broth

over the top, bring to a simmer, and cook uncovered for 4 minutes. Turn off the heat, cover the pot, and let it sit for about 3 minutes until the fish is just cooked through and flakes easily.

5. Serve:
    Taste and adjust seasoning. Ladle stew into bowls and top with the pine nut mixture. Serve with warm, crusty bread for dipping.

Monkfish Tagine

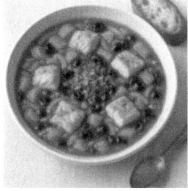

Serves 4 to 6 | Rich, Fragrant & Full of Moroccan Flavor

What You'll Need:
- 3 (2-inch) strips orange zest
- 5 garlic cloves, minced
- 2 tbsp extra-virgin olive oil
- 1 large onion, halved and sliced ¼ inch thick
- 3 carrots, peeled, halved lengthwise, and sliced ¼ inch thick
- Salt and pepper
- 1 tbsp tomato paste
- 1¼ tsp paprika
- 1 tsp ground cumin
- ½ tsp dried mint
- ¼ tsp saffron threads, crumbled
- 1 (8-oz) bottle clam juice
- 1½ lbs monkfish fillets (1 to 1½ inches thick), trimmed and cut into 3-inch pieces
- ¼ cup oil-cured black olives, pitted and quartered
- 2 tbsp fresh mint, minced
- 1 tsp sherry vinegar

How to Make It:

1. Make a Finishing Paste:
    Mince 1 strip of the orange zest and mix it with 1 tsp of garlic in a small bowl. Set aside.
2. Sauté Aromatics:
    In a Dutch oven, heat olive oil over medium. Add onion, carrots, ¼ tsp salt, and the remaining 2 orange zest strips. Cook until veggies soften and get a little color, about 10-12 minutes.
3. Add Spices & Broth:
    Stir in the remaining garlic, tomato paste, paprika, cumin, dried mint, and saffron. Cook for 30 seconds until fragrant. Pour in the clam juice and scrape up any browned bits.
4. Cook the Fish:
    Pat monkfish dry and season with salt and pepper. Nestle the pieces into the pot and spoon some broth over the top. Bring to a simmer, cover, and cook gently over medium-low until the fish is opaque and hits 160°F, about 8-12 minutes.
5. Finish the Tagine:
    Remove and discard the large orange zest strips. Stir in olives, fresh mint, sherry vinegar, and the reserved orange zest-garlic paste. Taste and adjust seasoning with salt and pepper.
6. Serve:
    Spoon into bowls with the broth and serve warm. Great with couscous, rice, or bread.

Greek-Style Shrimp with Tomatoes and Feta (Shrimp Saganaki)

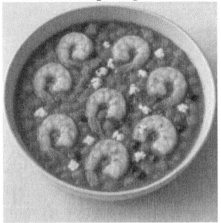

Serves 4 to 6 | Bright, Saucy & Packed with Flavor

What You'll Need:

- 1½ lbs extra-large shrimp (21-25 per lb), peeled and deveined
- ¼ cup extra-virgin olive oil
- 3 tbsp ouzo (or 3 tbsp Pernod OR 1 tbsp vodka + ⅛ tsp anise seeds)
- 5 garlic cloves, minced
- 1 tsp lemon zest
- Salt and pepper
- 1 small onion, chopped
- 1 red or green bell pepper, chopped
- ½ tsp red pepper flakes
- 1 (28-oz) can diced tomatoes, drained, with ⅓ cup juice reserved
- ¼ cup dry white wine
- 2 tbsp fresh parsley, chopped
- 6 oz feta, crumbled (about 1½ cups)
- 2 tbsp fresh dill, chopped

How to Make It:

1. Marinate the Shrimp:
   In a bowl, toss shrimp with 1 tbsp olive oil, 1 tbsp ouzo, 1 tsp garlic, lemon zest, ¼ tsp salt, and ⅛ tsp pepper. Let sit while you make the sauce.
2. Start the Sauce:
   In a 12-inch skillet, heat 2 tbsp olive oil over medium. Add onion, bell pepper, and ¼ tsp salt. Cover and cook, stirring occasionally, until softened and starting to release liquid (about 3-5 minutes). Uncover and cook another 5 minutes, stirring occasionally, until most of the liquid is gone.
3. Add Garlic & Tomatoes:
   Stir in remaining garlic and red pepper flakes. Cook 1 minute until fragrant. Stir in diced tomatoes, reserved juice, white wine, and remaining 2 tbsp ouzo. Bring to a simmer and cook for 5-8 minutes, until the sauce thickens slightly (it should still be a bit saucy). Stir in parsley and season with salt and pepper to taste.
4. Cook the Shrimp:
   Reduce heat to medium-low. Add shrimp and their marinade to the sauce and stir to coat. Cover and cook, stirring occasionally, for 6-9 minutes, until the shrimp are opaque and cooked through.
5. Finish and Serve:
   Take the skillet off the heat. Sprinkle feta and dill over the top and drizzle with the remaining 1 tbsp olive oil. Serve hot, with rice or crusty bread on the side.

Shrimp with White Beans

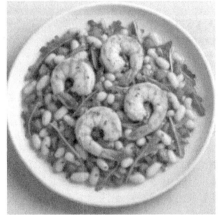

Serves 4 | Fast, Bright & Satisfying

What You'll Need:

- 1 lb extra-large shrimp (21-25 per pound), peeled and deveined
- Pinch of sugar
- Salt and pepper
- 5 tbsp extra-virgin olive oil
- 1 red bell pepper, finely chopped
- 1 small red onion, finely chopped
- 2 garlic cloves, minced
- ¼ tsp red pepper flakes
- 2 (15-oz) cans cannellini beans, rinsed
- 2 oz baby arugula (about 2 cups), roughly chopped
- 2 tbsp lemon juice

How to Make It:
1. Sear the Shrimp:
   Pat shrimp dry. Toss with a pinch of sugar, salt, and pepper. Heat 1 tbsp olive oil in a large nonstick skillet over high heat until just smoking. Add shrimp in a single layer and sear without stirring for about 1 minute, until spotty brown and the edges turn pink.
2. Finish the Shrimp:
   Take the skillet off the heat. Flip shrimp and let them finish cooking off-heat for about 30 seconds, until opaque. Transfer to a bowl and cover to keep warm.
3. Cook the Veggies:
   Return the skillet to medium heat and add the remaining ¼ cup olive oil. Once shimmering, add bell pepper, onion, and ½ tsp salt. Cook for about 5 minutes, until softened. Stir in garlic and red pepper flakes and cook for 30 seconds until fragrant.
4. Add Beans & Finish:
   Stir in the rinsed beans and heat through, about 5 minutes. Add shrimp (with any juices) and arugula, and toss gently until the arugula wilts—about 1 minute. Stir in lemon juice and season with salt and pepper to taste.

5. Serve:
   Dish it up warm, or chill for a light lunch or appetizer. Either way, it's delicious.

Garlicky Roasted Shrimp with Parsley and Anise

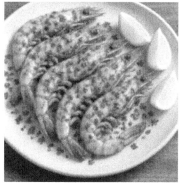

Serves 4 to 6 | Fast, Bold & Shell-On

What You'll Need:
- ¼ cup salt
- 2 lbs shell-on jumbo shrimp (16-20 per pound)
- ¼ cup extra-virgin olive oil
- 6 garlic cloves, minced
- 1 tsp anise seeds
- ½ tsp red pepper flakes
- ¼ tsp black pepper
- 2 tbsp fresh parsley, minced
- Lemon wedges, for serving

How to Make It:
1. Brine the Shrimp:
   In a large container, dissolve the salt in 4 cups cold water. Using kitchen shears or a sharp knife, cut through the shell and devein the shrimp, but don't remove the shell. Cut a little deeper—about ½ inch—without cutting the shrimp in half. Submerge in brine, cover, and chill for 15 minutes.
2. Prep for Broiling:
   Adjust your oven rack so it's 4 inches below the broiler, then heat the broiler. In a large bowl, mix olive oil, garlic, anise seeds, red pepper flakes, and black pepper. Drain and pat the shrimp dry, then toss with the oil mixture and parsley, making sure to get the seasoning into the cuts.

3. Broil:
   Arrange shrimp in a single layer on a wire rack set over a rimmed baking sheet. Broil for 2 to 4 minutes, rotating the pan halfway through, until the shells start to brown. Flip shrimp and broil the other side for another 2 to 4 minutes, again rotating halfway.
4. Serve:
   Serve immediately with lemon wedges for squeezing.

Grilled Marinated Shrimp Skewers

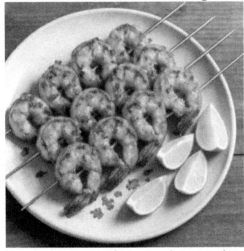

Serves 4 to 6 | Smoky, Juicy & Packed with Spice
What You'll Need:
Marinade:
- 3 tbsp extra-virgin olive oil
- 6 garlic cloves, minced
- 1 tsp grated lime zest
- ½ tsp smoked paprika
- ½ tsp ground ginger
- ½ tsp ground cumin
- ½ tsp salt
- ¼ tsp cayenne pepper

Shrimp:
- 1½ lbs extra-large shrimp (21–25 per pound), peeled and deveined
- ½ tsp sugar
- 1 tbsp chopped fresh cilantro
- Lime wedges, for serving

How to Make It:
1. Make the Marinade:
   In a medium bowl, whisk together olive oil, garlic, lime zest, paprika, ginger, cumin, salt, and cayenne.

2. Prep and Marinate the Shrimp:
   Pat shrimp dry. Use a sharp paring knife to butterfly each shrimp—make a shallow cut along the outside curve without slicing all the way through. Add to the marinade and toss well to coat. Cover and refrigerate for 30 to 60 minutes.
3. Prep the Grill:
   For Charcoal: Light a chimney starter with 6 quarts of charcoal. Once the top coals are ashed over, pour them over half the grill. Cover, open lid vent, and heat for 5 minutes.
   For Gas: Turn all burners to high, cover, and heat for 15 minutes.
4. Skewer & Season:
   Thread shrimp tightly onto four 12-inch metal skewers, alternating the direction of heads and tails. Sprinkle one side with sugar.
5. Grill the Shrimp:
   Place skewers sugar-side down on the hot side of the grill. Cook, covered if using gas, without moving for 3–4 minutes, until lightly charred. Flip and move to cooler side (or turn off burners on gas grill). Cover and cook 1–2 minutes more, until shrimp are just opaque.
6. Serve:
   Slide shrimp off skewers onto a platter. Season with salt and pepper, sprinkle with cilantro, and serve with lime wedges.

Seared Scallops with Orange-Lime Dressing

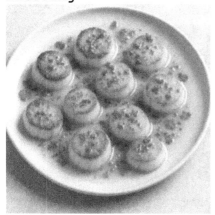

Serves 4 to 6 | Fast, Bright & Impressive
What You'll Need:
- 1½ lbs large sea scallops, tendons removed
- 6 tbsp extra-virgin olive oil·
- 2 tbsp orange juice
- 2 tbsp lime juice
- 1 small shallot, minced
- 1 tbsp fresh cilantro, minced
- ⅛ tsp red pepper flakes
- Salt and pepper

How to Make It:
1. Dry the Scallops:
   Lay scallops on a towel-lined baking sheet. Pat the tops dry with another towel and let them sit for 10 minutes, covered with the towel. This helps them sear instead of steam.
2. Make the Dressing:
   In a small bowl, whisk together ¼ cup olive oil, orange juice, lime juice, shallot, cilantro, red pepper flakes, and a pinch of salt. Set aside.
3. Sear the Scallops – First Batch:
   Heat 1 tbsp oil in a 12-inch nonstick skillet over medium-high until just smoking. Add half the scallops in a single layer. Don't move them—cook for about 1½ minutes until the bottoms are deeply browned. Flip and cook the other side for another 1½ minutes. Transfer to a platter and loosely cover with foil.

4. Second Batch:
   Repeat with remaining 1 tbsp oil and scallops.
5. Serve:
   Give the vinaigrette a quick whisk to recombine, then spoon it over the scallops. Serve right away.

Grilled Scallop and Zucchini Skewers with Basil Vinaigrette

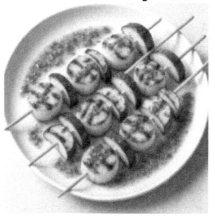

Serves 4 to 6 | Fast, Fresh & Smoky
What You'll Need:
- 1½ lbs large sea scallops, tendons removed
- ¾ cup fresh basil leaves
- 2 tbsp minced fresh chives
- 1 tbsp white wine vinegar
- 2 garlic cloves, minced
- 1¾ tsp sugar
- Salt and pepper
- ½ cup extra-virgin olive oil
- 2 zucchini, halved lengthwise, sliced into ¾-inch thick half moons
- 1 tbsp all-purpose flour
- 1 tsp cornstarch
- Eight 12-inch metal skewers (you'll use two per skewer)

How to Make It:
1. Prep the Scallops:
   Lay scallops on a towel-lined baking sheet. Cover with another towel and press gently to blot any moisture. Let sit for 10 minutes at room temp.
2. Make the Vinaigrette:
   In a food processor, pulse basil, chives, vinegar, garlic, ¾ tsp sugar, ¾ tsp salt, and ¼ tsp pepper until roughly chopped (about 5 pulses). With

the motor running, slowly
drizzle in 6 tbsp olive oil.
Blend until smooth, about 30
seconds.

Set aside all but 2 tbsp of
the vinaigrette. Toss those 2
tbsp with zucchini in a large
bowl and thread zucchini onto 2
skewers.
3. Skewer the Scallops:
Place scallops flat-side down
on a work surface. Thread them
onto doubled skewers (to keep
them from rotating), about 4 to
6 per pair of skewers. Return
to towel-lined sheet and chill
while prepping the grill.
4. Heat the Grill:
Charcoal: Punch holes in the
bottom of a disposable aluminum
roasting pan and place it in
the center of your grill. Fill
a chimney starter with 7 quarts
of coals. Once they're hot,
dump them in the pan.
Gas: Turn all burners to high
and preheat, lid closed, for
about 15 minutes.
5. Coat the Scallops:
In a small bowl, whisk
together 2 tbsp olive oil,
remaining 1 tsp sugar, flour,
and cornstarch. Brush both
sides of the scallops with the
mixture. Season with salt and
pepper.
6. Grill:
Clean and oil the grate
thoroughly—go over it 5-10
times until glossy. Grill
scallops and zucchini directly
over high heat. Don't move
them—let them sear for 2½ to 4
minutes. Flip and cook another
2 to 4 minutes, until the
scallops are just opaque and
the zucchini is tender with
grill marks.
7. Serve:
Slide scallops and zucchini
off the skewers onto a platter.
Spoon remaining vinaigrette
over everything and serve
immediately.

Mussels Steamed in White Wine

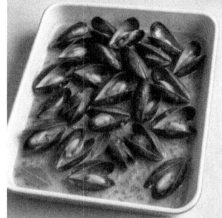

Serves 4 to 6 | Fast, Easy &
Flavor-Packed
You'll Need:
- 3 tbsp extra-virgin olive oil,
  divided
- 3 garlic cloves, minced
- Pinch of red pepper flakes
- 1 cup dry white wine
- 3 sprigs fresh thyme
- 2 bay leaves
- 4 lbs mussels, scrubbed and
  debearded
- ¼ tsp salt
- 2 tbsp minced fresh parsley

How to Make It:
1. Preheat the Oven:
Set the oven rack to the
lowest position and preheat to
500°F.
2. Build the Base:
In a large roasting pan over
medium heat, warm 1 tablespoon
olive oil. Add garlic and red
pepper flakes and cook,
stirring, for about 30 seconds
until fragrant. Pour in the
wine, toss in thyme and bay
leaves, and let it simmer for
about a minute to reduce
slightly.
3. Steam the Mussels:
Stir in the mussels and salt,
then cover the pan tightly with
foil. Transfer to the oven and
steam until most of the mussels
have opened, about 15 to 18
minutes.
4. Finish & Serve:
Remove from the oven. Discard
any unopened mussels, the thyme

sprigs, and bay leaves. Drizzle with the remaining 2 tablespoons olive oil, sprinkle with parsley, and give everything a good toss. Serve with crusty bread.

Clams Steamed in White Wine

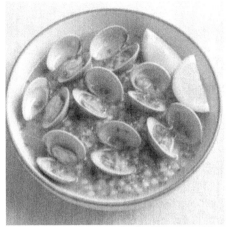

Serves 4 to 6 | Fast, Fresh, and Flavorful

You'll Need:
- 1½ cups dry white wine
- 3 shallots, minced
- 4 garlic cloves, minced
- 1 bay leaf
- 4 lbs littleneck clams, scrubbed
- 3 tbsp extra-virgin olive oil
- 2 tbsp minced fresh parsley
- Lemon wedges

How to Make It:
1. Build the Broth:
   In a Dutch oven over high heat, bring the wine, shallots, garlic, and bay leaf to a simmer. Let it go for about 3 minutes.
2. Steam the Clams:
   Add the clams, cover, and cook—give them a stir once or twice—until most have popped open, about 4 to 8 minutes. Scoop out the clams with a slotted spoon and discard any that stay closed.
3. Finish the Sauce:
   Off the heat, whisk in the olive oil to bring the broth together. Pour the sauce over the clams and sprinkle with

parsley. Serve with lemon wedges—and don't forget the bread to soak up that broth.

Clams with Pearl Couscous, Chorizo, and Leeks

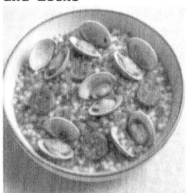

Serves 4 to 6 | Fast, Savory, and Satisfying
You'll Need:
- 2 cups pearl couscous
- Salt and pepper
- 2 tbsp extra-virgin olive oil
- 1½ lbs leeks (white/light green parts), halved, sliced thin, and cleaned
- 6 oz Spanish-style chorizo, halved and sliced thin
- 3 garlic cloves, minced
- 1 tbsp fresh thyme (or 1 tsp dried)
- 1 cup dry vermouth or dry white wine
- 3 tomatoes, cored, seeded, and chopped
- 4 lbs littleneck clams, scrubbed
- ½ cup fresh parsley, minced

How to Make It:
1. Cook the Couscous:
   Boil 2 quarts water in a medium saucepan. Add the couscous and 2 tsp salt. Cook until just tender, about 8 minutes. Drain and set aside.
2. Build the Base:
   Heat oil in a Dutch oven over medium. Add the leeks and

chorizo and cook until leeks soften, about 4 minutes. Stir in the garlic and thyme, and cook until fragrant, 30 seconds.

3. Steam the Clams:
   Add vermouth, let it reduce slightly (about a minute), then stir in the tomatoes and clams. Cover and cook until the clams open, 8 to 12 minutes.

4. Finish and Serve:
   Use a slotted spoon to remove clams (toss any that don't open). Stir couscous and parsley into the broth, season to taste. Spoon couscous mixture into bowls, top with clams, and serve warm.

Spanish Shellfish Stew (Zarzuela)

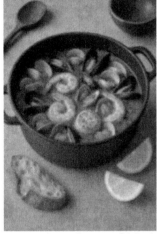

Serves 4 to 6 | Rich, Rustic, and Brimming with Flavor
What You'll Need:
Stew Base:
- ¼ cup extra-virgin olive oil
- 8 oz medium-large shrimp (31-40 per lb), peeled and deveined, shells reserved
- 1½ cups dry white wine or dry vermouth
- 1 onion, finely chopped
- 1 red bell pepper, finely chopped
- 3 garlic cloves, minced
- 1 tsp paprika
- ¼ tsp saffron threads, crumbled
- ⅛ tsp red pepper flakes
- 2 tbsp brandy
- 1 (28-oz) can whole peeled tomatoes, drained and chopped, juices reserved

- 2 bay leaves

Seafood:
- 1½ lbs littleneck clams, scrubbed
- 8 oz mussels, scrubbed and debearded
- 12 oz large sea scallops, tendons removed

To Finish:
- 1 batch Picada (see below)
- 1 tbsp chopped fresh parsley
- Salt and pepper
- Lemon wedges

How to Make It:
1. Make a Quick Shrimp Stock:
   Heat 1 tbsp oil in a medium saucepan over medium heat. Add shrimp shells and cook until spotty brown, about 2-4 minutes. Off heat, stir in wine, cover, and steep until needed.

2. Start the Sofrito:
   In a large Dutch oven, heat remaining 3 tbsp oil over medium-high. Add onion and bell pepper; cook until softened and starting to brown, about 5-7 minutes. Stir in garlic, paprika, saffron, and red pepper flakes. Cook until fragrant, about 30 seconds. Add brandy and scrape up any brown bits. Stir in tomatoes and juices, along with bay leaves, and simmer until slightly thickened, 5-7 minutes.

3. Strain the Stock & Combine:
   Strain shrimp wine mixture into the pot, pressing on shells to get all the liquid. Simmer for 3-5 minutes to meld the flavors.

4. Cook the Shellfish in Stages:
   o Nestle clams into the stew, cover, and cook for 4 minutes.
   o Add mussels and scallops, cover, and cook another 3 minutes.
   o Spread shrimp over the stew, cover again, and cook 1-2 more minutes, until shrimp are opaque

and all the shellfish
have opened.
5. Finish and Serve:
   Off heat, remove bay leaves
   and discard any clams/mussels
   that didn't open. Stir in the
   picada and parsley. Taste and
   season with salt and pepper.
   Serve with lemon wedges.

Grilled Squid with Lemon and Garlic

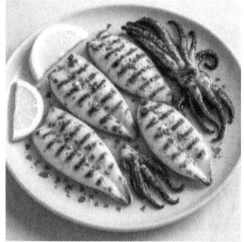

Serves 4 | Bright, Simple, and
Smoky
You'll Need:
- 5 tbsp extra-virgin olive oil
- 1 tbsp lemon juice, plus lemon
  wedges
- 2 tsp chopped fresh parsley
- 1 garlic clove, minced
- Salt and pepper
- 1 lb small squid (bodies 3-4
  inches)
- 2 tbsp baking soda

How to Make It:
1. In a bowl, mix 3 tbsp olive
   oil, lemon juice, parsley,
   garlic, and a bit of pepper.
   Set aside.
2. Slit the squid bodies
   lengthwise and flatten into
   planks. Mix baking soda and 2
   tbsp salt in 3 cups cold water.
   Add squid and refrigerate 15
   minutes.
3. Dry squid on paper towels,
   pressing with another towel on
   top. Let rest, covered, 10
   minutes.
4. Toss squid with remaining oil
   and pepper. Thread tentacles
   onto skewers.

5. Prep your grill: get it very
   hot. Brush grates until glossy.
6. Grill squid bodies and
   tentacles 5 minutes, flipping
   halfway, until lightly charred
   and just opaque. Tentacles
   might need 3 more minutes.
7. Slice bodies into strips, toss
   with vinaigrette and tentacles,
   and serve with lemon wedges.

Red Wine-Braised Octopus

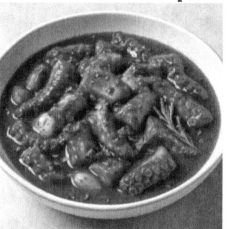

Serves 4 | Tender, Rich, and Rustic
You'll Need:
- 1 (4-lb) octopus, cleaned
- 1 tbsp olive oil
- 2 tbsp tomato paste
- 4 garlic cloves, smashed
- 1 rosemary sprig
- 2 bay leaves
- Pepper
- Pinch of cinnamon
- Pinch of nutmeg
- 1 cup dry red wine
- 2 tbsp red wine vinegar
- 2 tbsp unflavored gelatin
- 2 tsp chopped parsley

How to Make It:
1. Separate mantle and tentacles
   from the head. Simmer the
   octopus in a pot of water until
   tender, 45-75 minutes.
2. Reserve 3 cups cooking water
   and clean the octopus: remove
   skin, trim, and cut into
   chunks.
3. In the same pot, heat oil. Add
   tomato paste and cook a minute.
   Stir in garlic, herbs, spices,
   wine, vinegar, reserved liquid,
   and gelatin. Simmer 20 minutes.

4. Add octopus and juices, cook 20-25 minutes more until the sauce is thick and coats a spoon.
5. Finish with parsley and more pepper to taste. Serve with polenta or crusty bread.

Spanish Grilled Octopus Salad with Orange and Bell Pepper

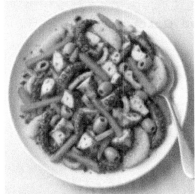

Serves 4 to 6 | Bright, Charred, and Mediterranean

You'll Need:
- 1 (4-lb) octopus, rinsed
- 2 cups dry white wine
- 6 garlic cloves (4 smashed, 2 minced)
- 2 bay leaves
- 1 tsp lemon zest + ⅓ cup lemon juice (from 2 lemons)
- 7 tbsp extra-virgin olive oil
- 3 tbsp sherry vinegar
- 2 tsp smoked paprika
- 1 tsp sugar
- Salt and pepper
- 1 large orange
- 2 celery ribs, thinly sliced on bias
- 1 red bell pepper, cut into 2-inch matchsticks
- ½ cup pitted green olives, halved
- 2 tbsp chopped fresh parsley

How to Make It:
1. Simmer the Octopus:
   Separate and discard the head. Place octopus in a large pot with wine, smashed garlic, bay leaves, and enough water to cover. Simmer gently until tender, 45-75 minutes.

2. Clean and Prep:
   Let cool slightly. Remove membrane from mantle and tentacles. Discard core, cut tentacles and mantle into chunks.
3. Make Marinade:
   Whisk together lemon juice/zest, 6 tbsp oil, vinegar, paprika, minced garlic, sugar, and some salt and pepper. Pour into a large zip-top bag.
4. Grill:
   Heat grill to high. Toss octopus with remaining 1 tbsp oil. Clean grates well and oil them thoroughly. Grill octopus until charred and streaked with grill marks, 8-10 minutes, flipping halfway.
5. Marinate:
   Slice grilled octopus ¼-inch thick. Add to bag with marinade and chill at least 2 hours, up to 24 hours, flipping occasionally.
6. Finish Salad:
   Let octopus come to room temp. Segment the orange over the bowl, add celery, bell pepper, olives, and parsley. Toss everything together gently. Season to taste and serve.

Poultry and Meat

Sautéed Chicken Cutlets with Romesco Sauce

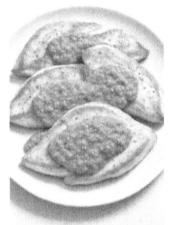

Serves 4 | Fast, Bold & Smoky
You'll Need:
For the Romesco Sauce
- ½ slice hearty white bread, cut into small cubes
- ¼ cup toasted, skinned hazelnuts
- 2 tbsp olive oil, divided
- 2 garlic cloves, thinly sliced
- 1 cup jarred roasted red peppers, rinsed and patted dry
- 1½ tbsp sherry vinegar
- 1 tsp honey
- ½ tsp smoked paprika
- ½ tsp salt
- Pinch of cayenne pepper

For the Chicken
- 4 boneless, skinless chicken breasts (4-6 oz each), trimmed
- Salt and pepper
- 4 tsp olive oil

How to Make It:
1. Make the Sauce:
   Heat 1 tbsp oil in a skillet over medium. Toast the bread cubes and hazelnuts, stirring, for about 3 minutes until golden. Add garlic, cook 30 seconds more, then transfer everything to a food processor. Pulse 5 times to break it down. Add the red peppers, vinegar, honey, paprika, salt, cayenne, and the last tbsp of oil. Pulse

again until the sauce is thick but spreadable—about 5-8 more pulses. Scoop into a bowl.
2. Prep the Chicken:
   Slice each breast horizontally into two thin cutlets. Place between plastic wrap and pound to about ¼ inch thick. Pat dry, then season with salt and pepper.
3. Cook the Chicken:
   Heat 2 tsp oil in a 12-inch skillet over medium-high until shimmering. Sauté 4 cutlets at a time for 2 minutes on one side without moving. Flip and cook 30 seconds more. Transfer to a platter, tent loosely with foil, and repeat with the remaining chicken and oil.
4. Serve:
   Spoon romesco over the chicken and dig in.

Sautéed Chicken Breasts with Cherry Tomatoes, Zucchini, and Yellow Squash

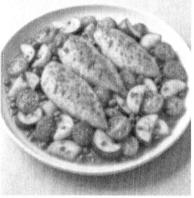

Serves 4 | Fast, Fresh, One-Pan
What You'll Need:
- ½ cup all-purpose flour
- 4 boneless, skinless chicken breasts (4-6 oz each), trimmed
- 1 tsp herbes de Provence
- Salt and pepper
- 3 tbsp + 2 tsp extra-virgin olive oil
- 2 zucchini, quartered lengthwise and sliced ½-inch thick
- 2 yellow squash, quartered lengthwise and sliced ½-inch thick
- 2 garlic cloves, minced
- 12 oz cherry tomatoes, halved

- 2 tbsp capers, rinsed
- ¼ cup shredded fresh basil or mint

How to Make It:
1. Prep the Chicken
    Pound the thick ends of the breasts so they're an even ½ inch thick. Pat dry. Season both sides with herbes de Provence, salt, and pepper. Dredge in flour and shake off any excess.
2. Cook the Chicken
    Heat 2 tbsp olive oil in a large nonstick skillet over medium-high until it's just starting to smoke. Add the chicken and cook, flipping as needed, until golden brown and cooked through (about 10 minutes total, or until it hits 160°F inside). Transfer to a plate and loosely tent with foil.
3. Sauté the Veggies
    In the same skillet, add 2 tsp oil and bring it back to medium-high. Toss in the zucchini and squash. Cook until nicely browned, about 10 minutes, stirring occasionally. Add garlic and cook another 30 seconds.
4. Finish It Off
    Stir in the cherry tomatoes and capers and cook just until the tomatoes soften a bit—about 2 minutes. Turn off the heat and stir in the fresh basil and last tablespoon of olive oil. Season to taste with salt and pepper.
5. Serve
    Plate the chicken and spoon the veggies over top. Dinner's ready.

Pan-Seared Chicken Breasts with Chickpea Salad

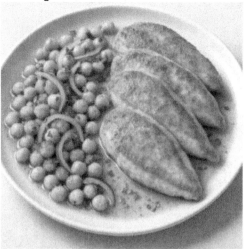

Serves 4 | Fast, Fresh, and Flavorful
What You'll Need:
- 6 tbsp extra-virgin olive oil
- ¼ cup lemon juice (from about 2 lemons)
- 1 tsp honey
- 1 tsp smoked paprika
- ½ tsp ground cumin
- Salt and pepper
- 2 (15-oz) cans chickpeas, rinsed
- ½ red onion, thinly sliced
- ¼ cup chopped fresh mint
- ½ cup all-purpose flour
- 4 boneless, skinless chicken breasts (4-6 oz each), trimmed

How to Make It:
1. Make the Dressing & Salad
    In a large bowl, whisk ¼ cup olive oil with the lemon juice, honey, paprika, cumin, ½ tsp salt, and ½ tsp pepper. Set aside 3 tbsp of this dressing. To the rest, add chickpeas, red onion, and mint. Toss well, season to taste, and set aside.
2. Prep and Cook the Chicken
    Pound the thickest part of each chicken breast so they're even—about ½ inch thick. Pat dry, season with salt and pepper, and dredge in flour, shaking off excess.
    Heat the remaining 2 tbsp olive oil in a 12-inch skillet over medium-high until it's just smoking. Add the chicken

and cook until golden and cooked through, flipping as needed—about 10 minutes total or until the internal temp hits 160°F. Let rest under foil for 5 minutes.
3. Serve It Up
   Drizzle the reserved dressing over the chicken. Serve alongside the chickpea salad.

Chicken in Turkish Walnut Sauce

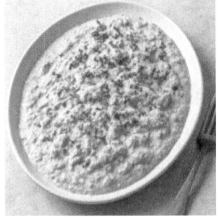

Serves 4 | Bold, Creamy & Comforting
What You'll Need:
- 4 boneless, skinless chicken breasts (4-6 oz each), trimmed
- Salt and pepper
- 3 tbsp extra-virgin olive oil, plus more for drizzling
- 3 cups chicken broth
- 1 onion, finely chopped
- 4 tsp paprika
- 3 garlic cloves, minced
- ½ tsp cayenne pepper
- 2 slices hearty white sandwich bread, crusts removed, torn into chunks
- 2 cups walnuts, toasted
- 2 tbsp chopped fresh parsley

How to Make It:
1. Cook the Chicken
   Pound chicken to ½ inch thick. Season with salt and pepper. Heat 1 tbsp oil in a large skillet over medium-high. Brown chicken on one side (about 4 minutes), flip, then add the broth. Cover, reduce heat, and simmer until the chicken hits 160°F—about 8 minutes. Remove

the chicken, let cool slightly, and shred it with two forks. Set aside. Strain and save the broth.
2. Start the Sauce
   Wipe out the skillet. Add 2 tbsp oil and the onion with ½ tsp salt. Cook until soft (about 5 minutes), then stir in paprika, garlic, and cayenne—cook just until fragrant, 30 seconds.
3. Make It Creamy
   In a food processor, blend the onion mix, bread, walnuts, and 2½ cups of the reserved broth until smooth. Add a bit more broth if it's too thick—you're aiming for a rich, pourable sauce. Toss with the shredded chicken and season to taste.
4. Finish and Serve
   Transfer to a platter, sprinkle with parsley, and drizzle with a little more olive oil. Great warm or at room temp with pita.

Spanish-Style Braised Chicken and Almonds

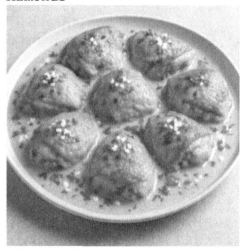

Serves 8 | Rich, Nutty & Aromatic
What You'll Need
- 8 bone-in chicken thighs (5-7 oz each), trimmed
- Salt and pepper
- 1 tbsp extra-virgin olive oil
- 1 onion, finely chopped
- 3 garlic cloves, minced
- 1 bay leaf
- ¼ tsp ground cinnamon

- ⅔ cup dry sherry (like fino or Manzanilla)
- 1 cup chicken broth
- 1 (14.5 oz) can whole peeled tomatoes, drained and finely chopped
- 2 hard-cooked large eggs, yolks and whites separated (whites chopped)
- ½ cup slivered almonds, toasted
- Pinch saffron threads, crumbled
- 2 tbsp chopped fresh parsley
- 1½ tsp lemon juice

How to Make It
1. Brown the Chicken
   Preheat oven to 300°F. Pat chicken dry, season with salt and pepper. In a 12-inch skillet, heat oil over medium-high. Brown the thighs, 5-6 minutes per side, then transfer to a plate. Pour off all but 2 tsp of fat.
2. Build the Base
   Add onion and ¼ tsp salt to the skillet. Cook until just soft, about 3 minutes. Stir in two-thirds of the garlic, bay leaf, and cinnamon—cook 1 minute. Add sherry and scrape up any browned bits. Cook until slightly thickened, about 2 minutes. Add broth and tomatoes, bring to a simmer.
3. Braise the Chicken
   Nestle the chicken back into the skillet. Cover and transfer to oven. Cook until thighs are super tender and reach 195°F, about 45-50 minutes.
4. Make the Sauce
   Remove skillet from oven. Transfer chicken to a platter, discard the skin, and tent loosely with foil. Discard bay leaf. In a blender, combine ¾ cup braising liquid with egg yolks, almonds, saffron, and remaining garlic. Blend until smooth, about 2 minutes.
5. Finish & Serve
   Pour almond sauce back into skillet, stir in 1 tbsp parsley and lemon juice. Simmer over medium heat until thickened, 3-

5 minutes. Season to taste. Spoon sauce over chicken, sprinkle with egg whites and remaining parsley, and serve.

Braised Chicken with Mushrooms and Tomatoes

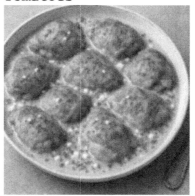

Serves 8 | Rustic, Earthy & Cozy
What You'll Need
- 8 bone-in chicken thighs (5-7 oz each), trimmed
- Salt and pepper
- 1 tbsp extra-virgin olive oil
- 1 onion, chopped
- 6 oz portobello mushroom caps, cut into ¾-inch pieces
- 4 garlic cloves, minced
- 2 tsp fresh thyme, minced
- 1½ tbsp all-purpose flour
- 1½ cups dry red wine
- ½ cup chicken broth
- 1 (14.5 oz) can diced tomatoes, drained
- 1 Parmesan rind (optional, but recommended)
- 2 tsp fresh sage, minced

How to Make It
1. Brown the Chicken
   Preheat oven to 300°F. Pat chicken dry, season with salt and pepper. In a Dutch oven, heat oil over medium-high. Brown thighs, 5-6 minutes per side. Transfer to a plate, discard the skin, and pour off all but 1 tbsp fat.
2. Build the Sauce
   Add onion, mushrooms, and ½ tsp salt to pot. Cook until softened and just browned, 6-8 minutes. Stir in garlic and thyme, cook 30 seconds. Stir in flour and cook 1 minute. Slowly

whisk in wine, scraping up any bits.
3. Braise the Chicken
   Add broth, tomatoes, and cheese rind if using. Bring to a simmer. Nestle chicken back in, cover, and transfer to oven. Cook until thighs reach 195°F, 35-40 minutes.
4. Finish & Serve
   Remove from oven. Transfer chicken to platter. Discard cheese rind. Stir sage into sauce, season to taste. Spoon sauce over chicken and serve.

Spanish-Style Braised Chicken and Almonds

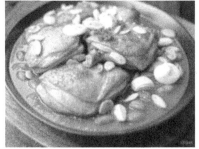

Serves 8 | Rich, Nutty & Aromatic
What You'll Need
8 bone-in chicken thighs (5-7 oz each), trimmed
Salt and pepper
1 tbsp extra-virgin olive oil
1 onion, finely chopped
3 garlic cloves, minced
1 bay leaf
¼ tsp ground cinnamon
⅔ cup dry sherry (like fino or Manzanilla)
1 cup chicken broth
1 (14.5 oz) can whole peeled tomatoes, drained and finely chopped
2 hard-cooked large eggs, yolks and whites separated (whites chopped)
½ cup slivered almonds, toasted
Pinch saffron threads, crumbled
2 tbsp chopped fresh parsley
1½ tsp lemon juice
How to Make It

1. Brown the Chicken
   Preheat oven to 300°F. Pat chicken dry, season with salt and pepper. In a 12-inch skillet, heat oil over medium-high. Brown the thighs, 5-6 minutes per side, then transfer to a plate. Pour off all but 2 tsp of fat.
2. Build the Base
   Add onion and ¼ tsp salt to the skillet. Cook until just soft, about 3 minutes. Stir in two-thirds of the garlic, bay leaf, and cinnamon—cook 1 minute. Add sherry and scrape up any browned bits. Cook until slightly thickened, about 2 minutes. Add broth and tomatoes, bring to a simmer.
3. Braise the Chicken
   Nestle the chicken back into the skillet. Cover and transfer to oven. Cook until thighs are super tender and reach 195°F, about 45-50 minutes.
4. Make the Sauce
   Remove skillet from oven. Transfer chicken to a platter, discard the skin, and tent loosely with foil. Discard bay leaf. In a blender, combine ¾ cup braising liquid with egg yolks, almonds, saffron, and remaining garlic. Blend until smooth, about 2 minutes.
5. Finish & Serve
   Pour almond sauce back into skillet, stir in 1 tbsp parsley and lemon juice. Simmer over medium heat until thickened, 3-5 minutes. Season to taste. Spoon sauce over chicken, sprinkle with egg whites and remaining parsley, and serve.

Braised Chicken with Mushrooms and Tomatoes

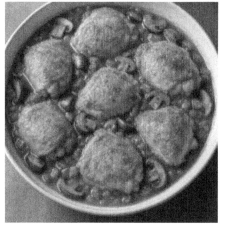

Serves 8 | Rustic, Earthy & Cozy
What You'll Need
- 8 bone-in chicken thighs (5-7 oz each), trimmed

- Salt and pepper
- 1 tbsp extra-virgin olive oil
- 1 onion, chopped
- 6 oz portobello mushroom caps, cut into ¾-inch pieces
- 4 garlic cloves, minced
- 2 tsp fresh thyme, minced
- 1½ tbsp all-purpose flour
- 1½ cups dry red wine
- ½ cup chicken broth
- 1 (14.5 oz) can diced tomatoes, drained
- 1 Parmesan rind (optional, but recommended)
- 2 tsp fresh sage, minced

How to Make It
1. Brown the Chicken
   Preheat oven to 300°F. Pat chicken dry, season with salt and pepper. In a Dutch oven, heat oil over medium-high. Brown thighs, 5-6 minutes per side. Transfer to a plate, discard the skin, and pour off all but 1 tbsp fat.

2. Build the Sauce
   Add onion, mushrooms, and ½ tsp salt to pot. Cook until softened and just browned, 6-8 minutes. Stir in garlic and thyme, cook 30 seconds. Stir in flour and cook 1 minute. Slowly whisk in wine, scraping up any bits.
3. Braise the Chicken
   Add broth, tomatoes, and cheese rind if using. Bring to a simmer. Nestle chicken back in, cover, and transfer to oven. Cook until thighs reach 195°F, 35-40 minutes.
4. Finish & Serve
   Remove from oven. Transfer chicken to platter. Discard cheese rind. Stir sage into sauce, season to taste. Spoon sauce over chicken and serve.

Za'atar-Rubbed Butterflied Chicken

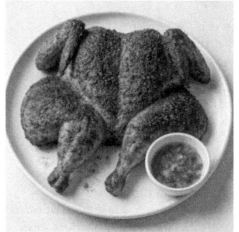

Serves 4 | Bold, Herby & Crispy
What You'll Need
- 2 tbsp za'atar
- 5 tbsp + 1 tsp extra-virgin olive oil
- 1 (3½-4 lb) whole chicken, butterflied
- Salt and pepper
- 1 tbsp minced fresh mint
- ¼ preserved lemon (rind only), minced (1 tbsp)
- 2 tsp white wine vinegar
- ½ tsp Dijon mustard

How to Make It
1. Prep Chicken
   Heat oven to 450°F. Mix za'atar with 2 tbsp oil. Butterfly chicken by removing the backbone and flattening it. Pound the breast to even it out. Season well with salt and pepper.
2. Sear Chicken
   In a large oven-safe skillet, heat 1 tsp oil over medium-high. Place chicken skin side down, reduce heat to medium, and place a heavy pot on top to press it flat. Cook until the skin is golden and crisp, about 25 minutes.
3. Roast Chicken
   Flip chicken carefully. Brush with za'atar paste. Transfer skillet to oven and roast, skin side up, until breast reaches 160°F and thighs 175°F, about 10-20 minutes.
4. Make Dressing & Serve
   Let chicken rest 10 minutes.

Meanwhile, whisk mint, preserved lemon, vinegar, mustard, ⅛ tsp salt, and pepper. Slowly whisk in remaining 3 tbsp oil. Carve chicken and serve with the dressing.

Grilled Chicken alla Diavola

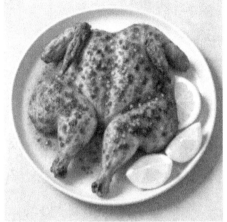

Serves 4 | Spicy, Garlicky & Juicy
What You'll Need
- 2 garlic heads + 4 cloves, minced
- 3 bay leaves
- Salt and pepper
- 1 (3½-4 lb) whole chicken, butterflied
- ¼ cup extra-virgin olive oil
- 2 tsp red pepper flakes
- Lemon wedges, for serving

How to Make It
1. Brine Chicken
   Smash garlic heads, bay leaves, and ½ cup salt in a bag. Add to 2 quarts water in a large container. Butterfly chicken and flatten. Submerge in brine for 1 hour in the fridge.
2. Make Garlic Oil
   In a small pan, heat oil, minced garlic, red pepper flakes, and 2 tsp black pepper until fragrant, about 3 minutes. Let cool. Reserve 2 tbsp for serving.
3. Season Chicken
   Remove chicken from brine, pat dry. Gently loosen skin over breast and thighs. Rub remaining garlic oil under the skin. Tuck wingtips behind the back.
4A. For Charcoal Grill:
   Set up a two-zone fire with a drip pan in the center. Light charcoal and distribute on both sides of the pan. Preheat grill, about 5 minutes.
4B. For Gas Grill:
   Heat all burners on high for 15 minutes. Then reduce to medium-low.
5.   Grill Chicken
   Clean and oil grate. Place chicken skin side down over indirect heat. Cover and grill until the skin is crisp and meat reaches 160°F (breast) and 175°F (thighs), about 30-45 minutes.
6.   Rest & Serve
   Let chicken rest 5-10 minutes, carve, and drizzle with reserved garlic oil. Serve with lemon wedges.

Grilled Chicken Kebabs with Tomato-Feta Salad

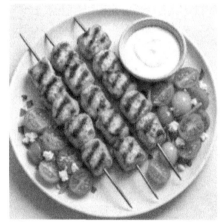

Serves 4 to 6 | Fresh, Juicy & Bright
What You'll Need
- ¼ cup extra-virgin olive oil
- 1 tsp lemon zest + 3 tbsp lemon juice
- 3 garlic cloves, minced
- 1 tbsp fresh oregano, minced
- Salt and pepper
- 1 lb cherry tomatoes, halved
- 4 oz feta cheese, crumbled (about 1 cup)
- ¼ cup red onion, thinly sliced
- ¼ cup plain yogurt
- 1½ lbs boneless, skinless chicken breasts, cut into 1-inch chunks

How to Make It

1. Mix the Marinade
   In a medium bowl, whisk together the oil, lemon zest and juice, garlic, oregano, ½ tsp salt, and ½ tsp pepper. Reserve half the mixture in another bowl. Toss tomatoes, feta, and onion with one half for the salad. Season and set aside.
2. Marinate the Chicken
   Whisk the yogurt into the reserved oil mixture. Set aside half for serving. Toss the chicken with the remaining yogurt mix and thread onto 4 skewers.
3. Grill the Kebabs
   Heat your grill (charcoal or gas) on high. Grill chicken skewers, turning occasionally, until browned and cooked through, about 10 minutes.
4. Serve
   Slide chicken off the skewers and serve with the tomato-feta salad and reserved yogurt sauce.

Grilled Chicken Souvlaki

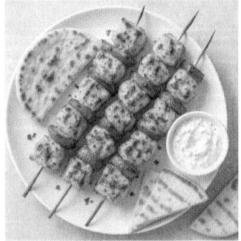

Serves 4 to 6 | Herby, Juicy & Classic
What You'll Need
- Salt and pepper
- 1½ lbs boneless, skinless chicken breasts, cut into 1-inch chunks
- ⅓ cup extra-virgin olive oil
- 2 tbsp fresh parsley, minced
- 1 tsp lemon zest + ¼ cup lemon juice
- 1 tsp honey
- 1 tsp dried oregano
- 1 green bell pepper, cut into chunks
- 1 small red onion, cut into chunks
- 4-6 (8-inch) pita breads
- 1 cup tzatziki

How to Make It
1. Brine the Chicken
   Mix 2 tbsp salt with 1 quart cold water. Add chicken and chill for 30 minutes. Meanwhile, combine oil, parsley, lemon zest and juice, honey, oregano, and ½ tsp pepper. Reserve ¼ cup in a large bowl.
2. Prep for the Grill
   Drain and dry the chicken, toss with the remaining oil mix. Thread chicken onto skewers, bookended with pepper and onion pieces.
3. Warm the Pitas
   Lightly dampen 2 pitas with water, sandwich remaining pitas between them, wrap in foil, and set aside for grilling.
4. Grill the Skewers
   Heat grill (charcoal or gas) to high. Grill skewers over hot side of grill, turning occasionally, until chicken is browned and reaches 160°F, about 10-12 minutes. Warm the pita over cooler side of grill.
5. Serve
   Toss grilled chicken in reserved oil mixture. Serve with warm pita and tzatziki.

Chicken Bouillabaisse

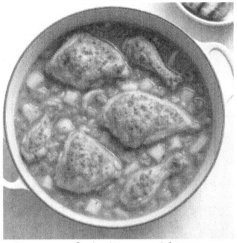

Serves 6 | Cozy, Citrusy & Bold

What You'll Need

- 3 lbs bone-in chicken (split breasts halved, thighs, and/or drumsticks), trimmed
- Salt and pepper
- 2 tbsp extra-virgin olive oil
- 1 large leek, halved and thinly sliced
- 1 small fennel bulb, halved and thinly sliced
- 4 garlic cloves, minced
- 1 tbsp tomato paste
- 1 tbsp all-purpose flour
- ¼ tsp saffron threads, crumbled
- ¼ tsp cayenne pepper
- 3 cups chicken broth
- 1 (14.5 oz) can diced tomatoes, drained
- 12 oz Yukon Gold potatoes, cut into ¾-inch chunks
- ½ cup dry white wine
- ¼ cup pastis or Pernod
- 1 (3-inch) strip orange zest
- 1 tbsp chopped fresh tarragon or parsley

How to Make It

1. Brown the Chicken
   Heat oven to 375°F, placing racks in the upper-middle and bottom positions. Pat chicken dry and season with salt and pepper. In a Dutch oven over medium-high, heat oil and brown the chicken well, about 5-8 minutes per side. Transfer to a plate.
2. Build the Broth
   In the same pot, sauté leek and fennel until soft, about 4 minutes. Stir in garlic, tomato paste, flour, saffron, and cayenne. Cook until fragrant, about 30 seconds. Whisk in broth, scraping up any browned bits. Add tomatoes, potatoes, wine, pastis, and orange zest. Simmer for 10 minutes.
3. Nestle in the Chicken
   Add thighs and drumsticks back to the pot with the skin above the broth. Cook uncovered for 5 minutes. Then add breast pieces, again keeping skin above the liquid.
4. Roast & Broil
   Transfer pot to upper oven rack and roast uncovered until breasts reach 145°F and thighs/drumsticks hit 160°F, about 10-20 minutes. Broil to crisp the skin and finish cooking (breasts to 160°F, thighs to 175°F), about 5-10 minutes more. Remove smaller pieces as they finish.
5. Finish & Serve
   Skim off any fat, stir in tarragon, and season to taste. Serve hot in shallow bowls with crusty bread or garlic toasts.

Pomegranate-Glazed Roasted Quail

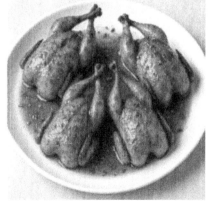

Serves 4 | Elegant, Sweet & Savory

What You'll Need

- 8 whole quail (5-7 oz each), giblets discarded
- Salt and pepper
- 2 tbsp extra-virgin olive oil
- 6 tbsp pomegranate molasses (store-bought or homemade, see below)

- 1 tbsp fresh thyme, minced
- 1 tsp ground cinnamon
- Vegetable oil spray

How to Make It
1. Brine the Quail
   Dissolve ½ cup salt in 2 quarts water in a large bowl. Submerge quail and refrigerate for 20 minutes. Meanwhile, set a wire rack inside a foil-lined baking sheet and coat with oil spray. Preheat oven to 500°F.
2. Prep the Birds
   Remove quail from brine, pat dry, and season with pepper. For tidy presentation, cut a small slit near the tip of one drumstick and tuck the opposite drumstick through it. Tuck wingtips behind backs.
3. Brown the Quail
   Heat 1 tbsp oil in a large skillet over medium-high until just smoking. Brown 4 quail on all sides, about 4 minutes. Transfer to the rack. Repeat with remaining oil and quail.
4. Glaze and Roast
   Mix pomegranate molasses, thyme, cinnamon, and a pinch of salt. Brush quail with half the glaze and roast for 5 minutes. Brush with remaining glaze and roast until browned and cooked through (160°F breast, 175°F thighs), 7-13 minutes more. Rest 5 minutes before serving.

Homemade Pomegranate Molasses

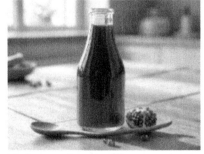

Makes about ⅔ cup | Fast & Easy
- 2 tbsp water
- 1 tbsp sugar
- 4 cups unsweetened pomegranate juice
- 2 tsp lemon juice

1. In a saucepan, mix water and sugar. Boil over medium-high

until golden, about 3 minutes, swirling gently. Once caramelized, remove from heat and let darken for 1 minute. Slowly add 2 tbsp pomegranate juice—it'll bubble. Then whisk in the rest with lemon juice.
2. Return to heat and simmer until thick and syrupy (⅔ cup), about 30-35 minutes. Cool and store.

Kibbeh

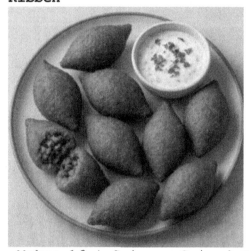

Makes 16 | Crispy, Spiced & Satisfying
What You'll Need
For the Dough
- 1 cup medium-grind bulgur, rinsed
- 1 cup water
- 8 oz ground lamb
- 1 small onion, chopped
- ½ tsp ground cinnamon
- ½ tsp salt
- ¼ tsp pepper

For the Filling
- 1 tsp olive oil
- 8 oz ground lamb
- Salt and pepper
- 1 small onion, finely chopped
- ½ cup pine nuts, toasted
- ½ tsp ground cinnamon
- ⅛ tsp ground allspice
- 1 tbsp pomegranate molasses

For Frying
- 2 cups vegetable oil

How to Make It
1. Make the Dough
   Soak bulgur in water for 30-40 minutes, then drain well. Add

to food processor with lamb, onion, cinnamon, salt, and pepper. Process until smooth, about 1 minute. Chill for 30 minutes.

2. Prepare the Filling
   Heat oil in a skillet. Brown lamb with ½ tsp salt and ¼ tsp pepper, about 3-5 minutes. Remove with slotted spoon. Cook onion in leftover fat until soft, about 5 minutes. Add pine nuts, cinnamon, and allspice, cook 30 seconds. Stir in lamb and pomegranate molasses. Season to taste.

3. Assemble Kibbeh
   Line a baking sheet with greased parchment. Roll dough into 16 balls (2 inches each). Working one at a time, flatten dough into a ¼-inch-thick cup, fill with 1 tbsp lamb mixture, and seal. Shape into torpedo form. Cover and chill for 30 minutes or up to 24 hours.

4. Cook the Kibbeh
   Heat oven to 200°F and prepare a paper towel-lined rack. Heat oil in skillet to 375°F. Fry kibbeh in batches until deep golden, 2-3 minutes per side. Drain on rack and keep warm in oven.

Grilled Beef Kebabs with Lemon and Rosemary Marinade

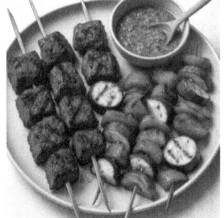

Serves 4 to 6 | Juicy, Herb-Infused & Flame-Kissed

What You'll Need
Marinade
- 1 onion, chopped
- ⅓ cup beef broth
- ⅓ cup extra-virgin olive oil
- 3 tbsp tomato paste
- 6 garlic cloves, chopped
- 2 tbsp chopped fresh rosemary
- 2 tsp lemon zest
- 2 tsp salt
- 1½ tsp sugar
- ¾ tsp pepper

Beef & Veggies
- 1½ lbs sirloin steak tips, cut into 2-inch chunks
- 2 zucchini or summer squash, halved and sliced 1 inch thick
- 2 red or green bell peppers, cut into 1½-inch pieces
- 2 red onions, cut into 1-inch thick pieces, layered

How to Make It
1. Blend the Marinade
   In a blender, blitz all marinade ingredients until smooth (about 45 seconds). Reserve ¾ cup in a large bowl for the veggies.

2. Marinate the Beef
   Toss the remaining marinade with the beef in a zip-top bag. Seal and chill for 1-2 hours, flipping the bag halfway through.

3. Prep the Veggies
   While beef marinates, toss zucchini, peppers, and onions with the reserved marinade. Let sit at room temp for 30 minutes.

4. Assemble the Skewers
   Pat beef dry. Thread it tightly onto 2 skewers. On 4 separate skewers, alternate zucchini, peppers, and onions.

5. Heat the Grill
   Charcoal: Build a hot center fire with a gap around the edges.
   Gas: Heat all burners on high, then reduce side burners to medium-low.

6. Grill
   Oil the grate. Grill beef skewers over high heat (covered if gas), turning every 3-4 minutes until medium-rare (120-

125°F), about 12-16 minutes. Rest under foil.

Grill veggie skewers until tender and charred, about 5 more minutes.
7. Serve
Slide everything off the skewers onto a platter and serve it up hot.

Spicy, smoky, and deeply aromatic!

Flank Steak Peperonata

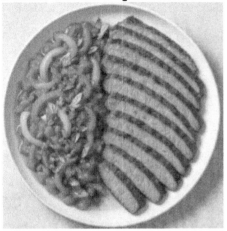

Serves 4 to 6 | Bright, Bold & Mediterranean
What You'll Need
- 2 tsp dried oregano
- Salt and pepper
- 1 (1½ lb) flank steak, trimmed
- ⅓ cup + 1 tbsp extra-virgin olive oil, plus more for drizzling
- 4 red or yellow bell peppers, sliced into ¼-inch strips
- 1 onion, sliced into ¼-inch strips
- 6 garlic cloves, lightly crushed and peeled
- 1 (14.5 oz) can diced tomatoes
- 2 tbsp capers + 4 tsp caper brine
- ⅛ tsp red pepper flakes
- ½ cup chopped fresh basil

How to Make It
1. Season the Steak
Mix oregano with 1 tsp salt. Cut the steak into 3 pieces (with the grain). Rub the oregano mix all over. Wrap in plastic and refrigerate for at least 30 minutes, or up to 24 hours.
2. Make the Peperonata
In a large skillet, heat ⅓ cup olive oil over medium-high until shimmering. Add peppers, onion, garlic, and ½ tsp salt. Cover and cook, stirring now and then, until softened, about 10 minutes.
3. Finish the Sauce
Stir in tomatoes, capers, caper brine, and red pepper flakes. Simmer uncovered until thickened slightly, about 5 minutes. Season with salt and pepper to taste. Transfer to a bowl and cover to keep warm.
4. Cook the Steak
Wipe out the skillet. Pat steak dry and season with pepper. Heat remaining 1 tbsp oil over medium-high. Sear steak pieces until well browned and 120-125°F for medium-rare, about 5-7 minutes per side. Let rest 10 minutes, loosely tented with foil.
5. Assemble & Serve
Stir basil into warm peperonata. Slice steak thinly against the grain on a bias. Season with salt, pepper, and drizzle with olive oil. Serve with peperonata on the side or over the top.

Grilled Flank Steak with Grilled Vegetables and Salsa Verde

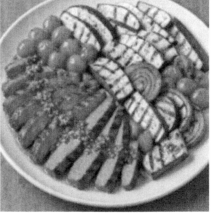

Serves 4 to 6 | Vibrant, Juicy & Perfect for a Party
What You'll Need

- 1 red onion, sliced into ½-inch-thick rounds
- 8 oz cherry tomatoes
- 2 zucchini, sliced lengthwise into ¾-inch-thick planks
- 1 lb eggplant, sliced lengthwise into ¾-inch-thick planks
- 2 tbsp extra-virgin olive oil
- 1½ lbs flank steak, trimmed
- Salt and pepper
- ½ cup Italian Salsa Verde (see below)

How to Make It

1. Prep the Veggies & Steak
   Thread onion slices onto two skewers and cherry tomatoes onto two more. Brush all vegetables with oil and season with salt and pepper. Pat steak dry and season well.
2. Grill Setup
   o Charcoal: Light a chimney full of coals and spread over the grill base. Heat grate 5 mins.
   o Gas: Preheat all burners to high for 15 minutes with the lid closed.
3. Grill Everything
   Place steak, veggie skewers, zucchini, and eggplant on the grill. Cook, flipping as needed, until steak hits 120-125°F for medium-rare and veggies are tender and slightly charred—about 7-12 minutes. Let steak rest 10 minutes.
4. Finish and Serve
   Slide onions and tomatoes off skewers. Cut all veggies into 2-3 inch pieces. Slice steak thinly against the grain. Serve steak and veggies on a platter, drizzled with ¼ cup salsa verde. Pass the rest at the table.

Italian Salsa Verde
Makes 1 cup
- 3 cups parsley leaves
- 1 cup mint leaves
- ½ cup olive oil
- 3 tbsp white wine vinegar
- 2 tbsp capers, rinsed
- 3 anchovy fillets, rinsed
- 1 garlic clove, minced
- ⅛ tsp salt

To Make: Pulse everything in a food processor until finely chopped but not smooth. (Refrigerate up to 2 days; bring to room temp before serving.)

Braised Oxtails with White Beans, Tomatoes, and Aleppo Pepper

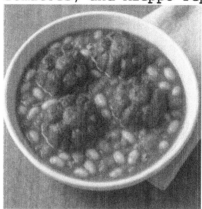

Serves 6 to 8 | Rich, Comforting & Hearty
What You'll Need
- 4 lbs oxtails, trimmed
- Salt and pepper
- 4 cups chicken broth
- 2 tbsp extra-virgin olive oil
- 1 onion, finely chopped
- 1 carrot, finely chopped
- 6 garlic cloves, minced
- 2 tbsp tomato paste
- 2 tbsp Aleppo pepper (or 1½ tsp paprika + 1½ tsp red pepper flakes)
- 1 tbsp fresh oregano, minced
- 1 (28 oz) can whole peeled tomatoes
- 1 (15 oz) can navy beans, rinsed
- 1 tbsp sherry vinegar

How to Make It
1. Roast the Oxtails
   Heat oven to 450°F. Season oxtails with salt and pepper and arrange in a single layer in a roasting pan. Roast 45 minutes. Discard fat and juices, then roast another 15-20 minutes until deeply

browned. Transfer oxtails to a bowl, tent with foil.
2. Deglaze & Sauté
   Deglaze roasting pan with broth, scraping up browned bits. Lower oven to 300°F. In a Dutch oven, heat oil over medium. Add onion and carrot, cook until softened. Stir in garlic, tomato paste, Aleppo pepper, and 1 tsp oregano; cook until fragrant.
3. Braise the Oxtails
   Add deglazing liquid and tomatoes (with juice). Bring to a simmer. Nestle oxtails in the pot, cover, and bake until fork-tender, about 3 hours.
4. Finish the Dish
   Remove oxtails. Strain liquid into a fat separator. Return solids to the pot. Once fat has separated, pour broth back into pot. Add beans, vinegar, and remaining oregano. Return oxtails and juices, simmer gently until heated through.
5. Serve
   Season with salt and pepper. Serve oxtails with 1 cup of sauce spooned over the top and extra sauce on the side.

Pomegranate-Braised Beef Short Ribs with Prunes and Sesame

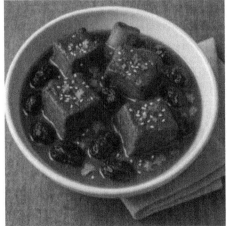

Serves 6 to 8 | Sweet, Tangy & Moroccan-Inspired
What You'll Need
- 4 lbs bone-in English-style short ribs, trimmed
- Salt and pepper
- 4 cups unsweetened pomegranate juice
- 1 cup water
- 2 tbsp extra-virgin olive oil
- 1 onion, finely chopped
- 1 carrot, finely chopped
- 2 tbsp ras el hanout
- 4 garlic cloves, minced
- ¾ cup prunes, halved
- 1 tbsp red wine vinegar
- 2 tbsp toasted sesame seeds
- 2 tbsp fresh cilantro, chopped

How to Make It
1. Roast the Ribs
   Heat oven to 450°F. Season ribs with salt and pepper and arrange bone side down in a single layer in a roasting pan. Roast for 45 minutes. Discard fat and juices, then roast another 15-20 minutes. Transfer ribs to a bowl, tent with foil.
2. Build the Base
   Deglaze roasting pan with pomegranate juice and water. Reduce oven to 300°F. In Dutch oven, heat oil, sauté onion and carrot with salt until soft. Stir in ras el hanout and garlic, cook until fragrant.
3. Braise the Ribs
   Stir in pomegranate mix and half the prunes. Bring to a simmer. Nestle ribs in, bone side up. Cover and cook in oven for about 2½ hours until tender.
4. Make the Sauce
   Remove ribs, discard loose bones. Strain braising liquid, transfer solids to a blender. Defat the liquid and blend with solids until smooth. Return sauce to pot, add vinegar and remaining prunes.
5. Finish & Serve
   Return ribs and juices to pot, simmer until warmed through. Season to taste. Serve ribs with sauce, sprinkled with sesame seeds and cilantro. Pass extra sauce at the table.

Grilled Spiced Pork Skewers with Onion and Caper Relish

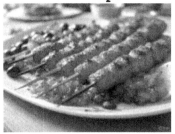

Serves 4 to 6 | Bold, Juicy & Smoky

What You'll Need
- 6 tbsp extra-virgin olive oil
- 5 garlic cloves, minced
- 1 tbsp lemon zest
- 1 tbsp ground coriander
- 2 tsp ground cumin
- ½ tsp ground nutmeg
- ½ tsp ground cinnamon
- Salt and pepper
- 1½ lbs boneless country-style pork ribs, cut into 1-inch pieces
- 2 tbsp honey
- 2 onions, sliced into ½-inch rounds
- ½ cup kalamata olives, chopped
- ¼ cup capers, rinsed
- 3 tbsp balsamic vinegar
- 2 tbsp fresh parsley, minced

How to Make It
1. Make the Marinade
   Whisk together ¼ cup oil, garlic, lemon zest, spices, 1½ tsp salt, and ½ tsp pepper. Set aside 2 tbsp. Toss remaining marinade with pork in a zip-top bag. Chill 1-2 hours, flipping halfway.
2. Prep the Skewers
   Whisk honey into reserved marinade and microwave until fragrant. Pat pork dry, thread onto 4 skewers. Thread onion rounds onto 2 skewers, brush with 1 tbsp oil, season with salt and pepper.
3. Grill
   Heat grill to medium-high. Grill pork and onion skewers, turning every 2 minutes and basting pork with honey marinade. Cook until pork hits 140°F and onions are charred and tender, 10-15 minutes.
4. Make the Relish
   Chop grilled onions and toss with olives, capers, vinegar, remaining oil, and parsley. Season to taste.

Serve
   Slide pork off skewers and serve with the onion-caper relish.

Greek-Style Braised Pork with Leeks

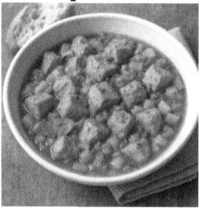

Serves 4 to 6 | Tender, Herby & Comforting

What You'll Need
- 2 lbs boneless pork butt, cut into 1-inch chunks
- Salt and pepper
- 3 tbsp extra-virgin olive oil
- 2 lbs leeks, sliced and rinsed
- 2 garlic cloves, minced
- 1 (14.5 oz) can diced tomatoes
- 1 cup dry white wine
- ½ cup chicken broth
- 1 bay leaf
- 2 tsp fresh oregano, chopped

How to Make It
1. Brown the Pork
   Preheat oven to 325°F. Season pork with salt and pepper. Brown in 2 batches in Dutch oven with 1 tbsp oil per batch, about 8 minutes per batch. Set pork aside.
2. Sauté the Veggies
   In same pot, add remaining 1 tbsp oil, leeks, and ½ tsp each salt and pepper. Cook until leeks are soft and lightly browned. Stir in garlic, cook 30 seconds. Add tomatoes, cook

until mostly evaporated, 10-12 minutes.
3. Braise
   Add wine, broth, bay leaf, and pork with juices. Simmer, cover, and transfer to oven. Cook until pork is very tender, 1 to 1½ hours. Remove bay leaf, stir in oregano, season to taste.
4. Serve
   Spoon into bowls with crusty bread or rice to catch the savory juices.

Spice-Rubbed Pork Tenderloin with Fennel, Tomatoes, Artichokes, and Olives

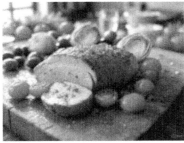

Serves 6 | Bright, Herby & Mediterranean
What You'll Need
- 2 large fennel bulbs, halved, cored, sliced ½-inch thick
- 2 cups jarred whole baby artichoke hearts (packed in water), quartered, rinsed, and patted dry
- ½ cup pitted kalamata olives, halved
- 3 tbsp extra-virgin olive oil
- 2 (12-16 oz) pork tenderloins, trimmed
- 2 tsp herbes de Provence
- Salt and pepper
- 1 lb cherry tomatoes, halved
- 1 tbsp lemon zest
- 2 tbsp chopped fresh parsley

How to Make It
1. Prep the Veggies
   Preheat oven to 450°F. Microwave fennel with 2 tbsp water in a covered bowl until softened, about 5 minutes. Drain well. Toss fennel with artichokes, olives, and olive oil.

2. Season the Pork
   Pat tenderloins dry. Rub all over with herbes de Provence, salt, and pepper. Spread veggie mix in a large roasting pan and place pork on top.
3. Roast
   Roast 25-30 minutes, flipping pork halfway, until internal temp hits 145°F. Transfer pork to cutting board and tent with foil to rest.
4. Finish the Veggies
   Stir tomatoes and lemon zest into veggies and return to oven. Roast 10 more minutes, until tomatoes soften and fennel is tender. Stir in parsley and season to taste.
5. Serve
   Slice pork into ½-inch rounds. Serve with roasted veggie mixture spooned over top.

Green Zhoug

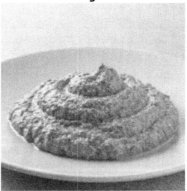

Makes ~½ cup | Bright, Spicy & Herby
Ingredients:
- 6 tbsp extra-virgin olive oil
- ½ tsp ground coriander
- ¼ tsp ground cumin
- ¼ tsp ground cardamom
- ¼ tsp salt
- Pinch ground cloves
- ¾ cup fresh cilantro leaves
- ½ cup fresh parsley leaves
- 2 green Thai chiles, chopped
- 2 garlic cloves, minced

Directions:
1. Microwave oil, spices, and salt in a covered bowl for about 30 seconds until fragrant. Let cool.

2. Add to food processor with
   herbs, chiles, and garlic.
   Pulse to a coarse paste.
Keeps in the fridge for 4 days.

Harissa

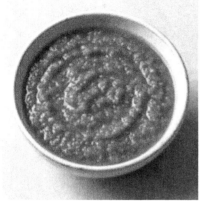

Makes ~½ cup | Bold, Smoky &
Versatile
Ingredients:
- 6 tbsp extra-virgin olive oil
- 6 garlic cloves, minced
- 2 tbsp paprika
- 1 tbsp ground coriander
- 1 tbsp ground Aleppo pepper (or
  ¾ tsp paprika + ¾ tsp crushed
  red pepper)
- 1 tsp ground cumin
- ¾ tsp caraway seeds
- ½ tsp salt

Directions:
Combine all ingredients in a bowl.
Microwave for 1 minute, stirring
halfway, until bubbling and
fragrant. Let cool.
Store in the fridge up to 4 days.

Rasel Hanout

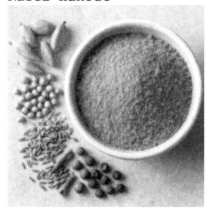

Makes ~½ cup | Warm, Fragrant &
Complex
Ingredients:

- 16 cardamom pods
- 4 tsp coriander seeds
- 4 tsp cumin seeds
- 2 tsp anise seeds
- ½ tsp allspice berries
- ¼ tsp black peppercorns
- 4 tsp ground ginger
- 2 tsp ground nutmeg
- 2 tsp ground Aleppo pepper (or
  ½ tsp paprika + ½ tsp red
  pepper flakes)
- 2 tsp ground cinnamon

Directions:
1. Toast whole spices in a dry
   skillet for 2 minutes until
   fragrant. Cool.
2. Grind with remaining
   ingredients into a fine powder.

Keeps in an airtight container for
up to a year.

Za'atar

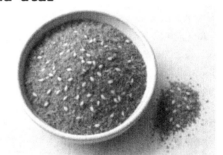

Makes ~½ cup | Tangy, Nutty &
Herbaceous
Ingredients:
- ½ cup dried thyme, ground
- 2 tbsp sesame seeds, toasted
- 1½ tbsp ground sumac

Directions:
Mix all ingredients together in a
bowl.
Store in an airtight container at
room temp for up to a year.

Dukkah

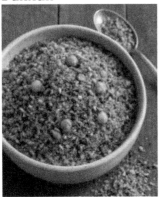

Makes 2 cups | Crunchy, Nutty & Warmly Spiced

Ingredients:
- 1 (15-oz) can chickpeas, rinsed
- 1 tsp extra-virgin olive oil
- ½ cup shelled pistachios, toasted
- ⅓ cup black sesame seeds, toasted
- 2½ tbsp coriander seeds, toasted
- 1 tbsp cumin seeds, toasted
- 2 tsp fennel seeds, toasted
- 1½ tsp black pepper
- 1¼ tsp salt

Directions:
1. Preheat oven to 400°F. Pat chickpeas dry and toss with olive oil. Roast on a rimmed baking sheet, stirring every 5-10 minutes, until crisp and browned, 40-45 minutes. Let cool.
2. Coarsely grind chickpeas in a food processor and transfer to a bowl.
3. Pulse pistachios and sesame seeds in processor until coarsely ground. Add to bowl.
4. Grind coriander, cumin, and fennel seeds finely. Add to chickpea mixture.
5. Stir in pepper and salt. Mix well.

Store in the fridge for up to 1 month.

Herbes de Provence

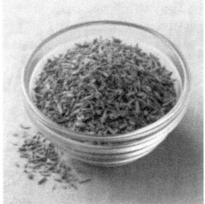

Makes ~½ cup | Floral, Savory & Classic

Ingredients:
- 2 tbsp dried thyme
- 2 tbsp dried marjoram
- 2 tbsp dried rosemary
- 2 tsp fennel seeds, toasted

Directions:
Mix all ingredients in a bowl. Store in an airtight container at room temp for up to 1 year.

Tips for Blends & Pastes:
- Storage: Keep blends away from light, heat, and moisture. Dry blends last ~1 year; whole spices can last 2 years.
- Freshness Test: Rub a pinch and smell—if the aroma is strong, it's still good.
- Pastes: Store in the fridge, especially if they contain garlic in oil (like harissa or zhoug). Use within 4 days.

Braised Greek Sausages with Peppers (Spetsofai)

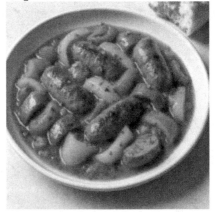

Serves 4 to 6 | Hearty, Bright & Bold

What You'll Need

- 1½ lbs loukaniko or Italian sausage
- 2 tbsp extra-virgin olive oil
- 4 bell peppers (any mix of red, yellow, green), cut into 1½-inch pieces
- 1 onion, chopped
- 2 jalapeño chiles, minced
- Salt and pepper
- 3 garlic cloves, minced
- 1 tbsp tomato paste
- 2 tsp grated orange zest
- 1 tsp ground fennel
- ½ cup dry white wine
- 1 (14.5 oz) can diced tomatoes
- ¾ cup chicken broth
- 1 tbsp fresh oregano, minced

How to Make It
1. Brown the Sausage
   Prick sausages a few times with a fork. In a large skillet, heat 1 tbsp oil over medium-high until just smoking. Sear sausages until nicely browned on all sides, about 8 minutes. Transfer to a board, let cool slightly, then cut into quarters.
2. Cook the Veggies
   In the same skillet, add remaining oil. Stir in bell peppers, onion, jalapeños, ½ tsp salt, and ½ tsp pepper. Cook until the peppers start to soften, about 5 minutes.
3. Build the Sauce
   Add garlic, tomato paste, orange zest, and fennel. Cook until fragrant, about 1 minute. Stir in white wine, scraping up the browned bits.
4. Simmer
   Add tomatoes (with juice), broth, and sausage pieces. Bring to a simmer, cover, and cook on low until sausage is fully cooked, about 5 minutes.
5. Finish & Serve
   Uncover, raise heat to medium, and cook until sauce thickens slightly, about 10 minutes. Stir in oregano and adjust seasoning. Serve with crusty bread or rice.

Sausage and White Beans with Mustard Greens

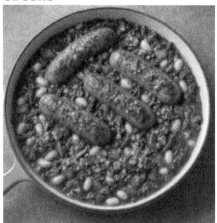

Serves 4 to 6 | Hearty, Rustic & Comforting
What You'll Need
- 1 lb hot or sweet Italian sausage
- 2 tbsp extra-virgin olive oil
- 1 onion, finely chopped
- Salt and pepper
- 2 tbsp fresh thyme (or 2 tsp dried)
- 6 garlic cloves, minced
- ½ cup dry white wine
- 1 (14.5 oz) can diced tomatoes, drained (juice reserved)
- 1½ cups chicken broth
- 1 (15 oz) can cannellini beans, rinsed
- 12 oz mustard greens, stemmed and chopped
- ½ cup Parmesan Bread Crumbs
- 2 tbsp chopped fresh parsley

How to Make It
1. Brown the Sausage
   Prick sausages a few times with a fork. Heat 1 tbsp oil in a Dutch oven over medium-high. Add sausages and brown well on all sides, about 8 minutes. Transfer to a plate.
2. Build the Base
   Add remaining oil to the pot. Cook onion with ¼ tsp salt until softened and just golden, 5-7 minutes. Stir in thyme and garlic and cook 30 seconds. Add wine and tomato juice, scraping

the pot. Simmer until nearly evaporated, about 5 minutes.

3. Simmer the Stew
   Stir in broth, tomatoes, and beans. Bring to a simmer, then stir in the mustard greens. Cook just until greens start to wilt, about 1 minute. Nestle sausages on top, cover, and reduce heat to low. Cook 10 minutes.

4. Finish & Serve
   Uncover and raise heat to medium-low. Cook another 15 minutes, stirring occasionally, until greens are tender and sausages are cooked through. Off heat, mash some of the beans against the side of the pot to thicken the stew. Serve topped with bread crumbs and parsley.

Lamb Meatballs with Leeks and Yogurt Sauce

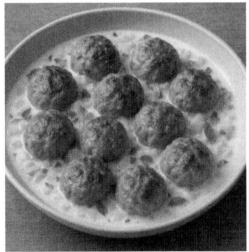

Serves 4 | Fragrant, Juicy & Bright

What You'll Need
- 1 cup whole Greek yogurt
- 3 tbsp panko bread crumbs
- 2 tbsp water
- 1 lb ground lamb
- 3 tbsp fresh mint, minced
- 1 large egg yolk
- 2 garlic cloves, minced
- 1 tsp ground cumin
- ¾ tsp ground cinnamon
- ⅛ tsp ground cloves
- Salt and pepper
- 2 tbsp extra-virgin olive oil
- 8 oz leeks, white/light green parts only, chopped and cleaned
- ½ tsp lemon zest + ½ tsp lemon juice
- 1 cup chicken broth

How to Make It

1. Mix the Meatballs
   In a large bowl, mash ⅓ cup yogurt, panko, and water into a paste. Add lamb, 2 tbsp mint, egg yolk, half the garlic, cumin, cinnamon, ¾ tsp salt, ⅛ tsp pepper, and cloves. Mix well with hands. Roll into 12 meatballs, about 1½ inches each.

2. Brown the Meatballs
   Heat oil in a 12-inch skillet over medium-high until just smoking. Brown meatballs on all sides, 6-8 minutes total. Transfer to a plate. Pour off all but 1 tbsp fat.

3. Make the Sauce Base
   Add leeks to skillet and cook over medium until soft and golden, about 5-7 minutes. Stir in lemon zest and remaining garlic and cook for 30 seconds. Pour in broth, scrape up any browned bits, and bring to a simmer.

4. Simmer the Meatballs
   Return meatballs to the skillet. Simmer, covered, over medium-low heat, turning occasionally, for 5 minutes. Uncover and cook 2 more minutes to reduce slightly.

5. Finish the Sauce
   Remove meatballs and keep warm. Slowly whisk about 1 cup of the hot broth into remaining ⅔ cup yogurt. Stir yogurt mixture and lemon juice into skillet until smooth. Season to taste with salt and pepper.

6. Serve
   Pour sauce over meatballs, sprinkle with remaining mint, and serve warm with orzo or couscous.

Grilled lamb koftas

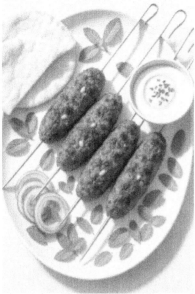

Serves: 4 to 6
Ingredients:
For the Koftas:
- ½ cup pine nuts
- 4 garlic cloves, peeled and smashed
- 1½ teaspoons hot smoked paprika
- 1 teaspoon salt
- 1 teaspoon ground cumin
- ½ teaspoon black pepper
- ¼ teaspoon ground coriander
- ¼ teaspoon ground cloves
- ⅛ teaspoon ground nutmeg
- ⅛ teaspoon ground cinnamon
- 1½ pounds ground lamb
- ½ cup grated onion, drained
- ⅓ cup minced fresh parsley
- ⅓ cup minced fresh mint
- 1½ teaspoons unflavored gelatin
- 8 (12-inch) metal skewers

For the Tahini-Yogurt Sauce:
- 1 cup plain Greek yogurt
- 2 tablespoons tahini
- 1 tablespoon fresh lemon juice
- 2 garlic cloves, minced
- ½ teaspoon salt

Instructions:
1. Prepare the Kofta Mixture:
    o In a food processor, combine pine nuts, garlic, paprika, salt, cumin, black pepper, coriander, cloves, nutmeg, and cinnamon. Process until a coarse paste forms, about 30 to 45 seconds.
    o Transfer the spice mixture to a large bowl. Add ground lamb, grated onion, parsley, mint, and gelatin. Using your hands, knead the mixture until thoroughly combined and slightly sticky, about 2 minutes.
2. Shape the Koftas:
    o Divide the lamb mixture into 8 equal portions. Shape each portion into a 5-inch-long cylinder about 1 inch in diameter.
    o Thread each cylinder onto a metal skewer, pressing gently to adhere.
    o Place the skewers on a lightly greased baking sheet, cover with plastic wrap, and refrigerate for at least 1 hour or up to 24 hours.
3. Prepare the Grill:
    o For a Charcoal Grill: Using kitchen shears, poke twelve ½-inch holes in the bottom of a disposable aluminum roasting pan. Open the bottom vent completely and place the pan in the center of the grill. Light a large chimney starter filled two-thirds with charcoal briquettes (about 4 quarts). When the top coals are partially covered with ash, pour them into the pan. Set the cooking grate in place, cover, and open the lid vent completely. Heat the grill until hot, about 5 minutes.
    o For a Gas Grill: Turn all burners to high, cover, and heat the grill until hot, about 15 minutes. Leave all burners on high.
4. Grill the Koftas:

- o Clean and oil the cooking grate. Place the skewers on the grill at a 45-degree angle to the grate.
- o Cook (covered if using gas) until browned and the meat easily releases from the grill, about 4 to 7 minutes.
- o Flip the skewers and continue to cook until browned on the second side and the meat registers 160°F, about 6 minutes longer.
- o Transfer the skewers to a serving platter.

5. Prepare the Tahini-Yogurt Sauce:
   - o In a bowl, whisk together Greek yogurt, tahini, lemon juice, minced garlic, and salt until smooth.
6. Serve:
   - o Serve the grilled koftas hot with the tahini-yogurt sauce on the side.
   - o Optionally, accompany with warm pita bread, sliced red onion, and chopped fresh mint.

Grilled Greek-Style Lamb Pita Sandwiches

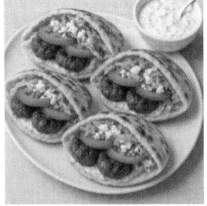

Serves 4 | Juicy, Flavorful, and Totally Satisfying

What You'll Need:
- 4 (8-inch) pita breads
- ½ onion, chopped
- 1 tbsp fresh oregano (or 1 tsp dried)
- 4 tsp lemon juice
- 2 garlic cloves, minced
- ½ tsp salt
- ¼ tsp black pepper
- 1 lb ground lamb
- 2 tsp extra-virgin olive oil
- 1 cup tzatziki
- 1 large tomato, thinly sliced
- 2 cups shredded iceberg lettuce
- 2 oz feta cheese, crumbled (½ cup)

How to Make It:
1. Prep the Pitas
   - o Slice the top quarter off each pita. Tear those tops into small 1-inch pieces—you'll use them in the lamb mixture.
   - o Lightly moisten 2 of the whole pitas with water. Sandwich the dry ones between them and wrap the stack in greased foil. Set aside.
2. Make the Patties
   - o In a food processor, blend the pita pieces, onion, oregano, lemon juice, garlic, salt, and pepper until smooth.
   - o Transfer to a large bowl, add the ground lamb, and knead until well combined.
   - o Divide the mixture into 12 equal parts, shape into balls, then flatten into ½-inch-thick disks.
3. Grill Setup
   - o Charcoal Grill: Light a chimney starter ¾ full with charcoal. When ready, pour over half the grill. Cover and preheat for 5 minutes.
   - o Gas Grill: Heat all burners on high, cover, and preheat for 15 minutes. Turn one burner to medium-high and the others off.
4. Grill the Patties
   - o Clean and oil the grates. Grill lamb patties over the hot side, covered if using gas, for 4-6

minutes per side until well browned and crusty.
  - Transfer to a plate and cover loosely with foil.
5. Warm the Pitas
  - Place the foil-wrapped pita stack on the cooler side of the grill. Flip occasionally until heated through, about 5 minutes.
6. Assemble & Serve
  - Spread about ¼ cup tzatziki inside each warm pita.
  - Stuff with 3 lamb patties, tomato slices, lettuce, and a sprinkle of feta.
  - Serve right away—these are best hot off the grill.

Grilled Lamb Shish Kebab

Serves 4 to 6 | Juicy, Bold & Flame-Kissed
What You'll Need
Marinade:
- 6 tbsp extra-virgin olive oil
- 7 fresh mint leaves
- 2 tsp chopped fresh rosemary
- 2 garlic cloves, peeled
- 1 tsp salt
- ½ tsp lemon zest + 2 tbsp lemon juice
- ¼ tsp black pepper

Lamb & Veggies:
- 2 lbs boneless leg of lamb, trimmed and cut into 2-inch pieces
- 2 zucchini (or yellow squash), halved and sliced 1 inch thick
- 2 red or green bell peppers, cut into 1½-inch chunks
- 2 red onions, cut into 1-inch, 3-layer-thick pieces

How to Make It
1. Make the Marinade
  - In a food processor, blend all marinade ingredients until smooth (about 1 minute). Set 3 tbsp aside in a large bowl for the vegetables.
2. Marinate the Lamb

- Place lamb and remaining marinade in a zip-top bag. Seal, shake to coat, and refrigerate 1-2 hours, flipping occasionally.
3. Marinate the Vegetables
  - Add zucchini, peppers, and onions to the reserved marinade. Toss well and let sit at room temp for 30 minutes.
4. Skewer Everything
  - Pat lamb dry. Thread tightly onto 2 metal skewers. Thread vegetables onto 4 skewers in alternating patterns.
5A. Charcoal Grill Setup
  - Light a full chimney of briquettes. Pour coals in center of grill, leaving a 2-inch gap from edges. Cover, vent open, and heat for 5 minutes.
5B. Gas Grill Setup
  - Turn all burners to high, cover, and preheat for 15 minutes. Leave one burner on high, others on medium-low.
6. Grill Time
  - Place lamb skewers over hot side of grill. Place veggie skewers over the cooler area. Cook, turning every 3-4 minutes:
    - Lamb: Until well-browned and 120-125°F (for medium-rare), 10-15 minutes. Let rest under foil.
    - Veggies: Until tender and lightly charred, 5-7 minutes.
7. Serve
  - Slide lamb and veggies off skewers onto a platter. Serve hot with warm pita, tzatziki, or a drizzle of lemon if you like.

Grilled Marinated Lamb Shoulder Chops with Asparagus

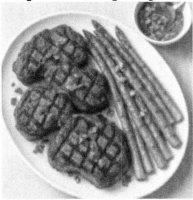

Serves 4 to 6 | Bold, Juicy & Herbaceous
What You'll Need
For the Vinaigrette:
- ¼ cup extra-virgin olive oil
- 3 tbsp red wine vinegar
- 2 tbsp chopped fresh mint
- 1 small shallot, minced
- 1 tsp Dijon mustard
- Salt and pepper

For the Marinade:
- ¼ cup extra-virgin olive oil
- 2 garlic cloves, minced
- 2 tsp minced fresh oregano
- 1 tsp baking soda
- ½ tsp salt
- ½ tsp pepper

Lamb & Asparagus:
- 4 lamb shoulder chops (8-12 oz each, ¾ to 1 inch thick)
- 1½ lbs thick asparagus, trimmed

How to Make It
1. Make the Vinaigrette
   o In a bowl, whisk together ¼ cup oil, vinegar, mint, shallot, mustard, ¼ tsp salt, and a pinch of pepper. Set aside.
2. Marinate the Chops
   o In another bowl, whisk together remaining ¼ cup oil, garlic, oregano, baking soda, salt, and pepper.
   o Add to a zip-top bag with lamb chops and toss to coat. Chill for 30 minutes to 1 hour, flipping halfway.
3. Prep the Grill

   o Charcoal: Light a chimney of coals, pour evenly over grill, cover, and heat 5 minutes.
   o Gas: Preheat all burners on high, covered, for 15 minutes.
4. Grill the Lamb
   o Clean and oil the grate. Grill chops 2-4 minutes per side, until browned and 120-125°F for medium-rare.
   o Transfer to platter, tent loosely with foil, and let rest.
5. Grill the Asparagus
   o Grill asparagus, turning now and then, until lightly charred and just tender, about 5 minutes.
6. Finish & Serve
   o Arrange lamb and asparagus on a platter. Drizzle everything with the vinaigrette and serve.

Braised Lamb Shoulder Chops with Tomatoes and Red Wine

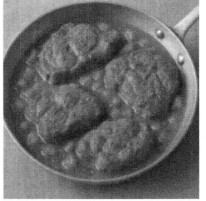

Serves 4 | Hearty, Tender & Flavorful
What You'll Need
- 4 lamb shoulder chops (8-12 oz each, ¾ inch thick), trimmed
- Salt and pepper
- 2 tbsp extra-virgin olive oil
- 1 small onion, finely chopped
- 2 garlic cloves, minced
- ⅓ cup dry red wine
- 1 cup canned whole peeled tomatoes, chopped
- 2 tbsp fresh parsley, minced

How to Make It
1. Brown the Chops
   Pat the lamb dry and season with salt and pepper. Heat 1 tbsp oil in a large skillet over medium-high. Brown the chops, 4-5 minutes per side. Do it in batches if needed. Transfer to a plate and pour off any fat.
2. Build the Sauce
   Add the rest of the oil to the skillet. Cook the onion over medium heat until soft, about 5 minutes. Stir in garlic and cook for 30 seconds. Add wine, scrape up browned bits, and simmer until reduced by half, 2-3 minutes. Stir in tomatoes.
3. Braise the Lamb
   Nestle chops back into the skillet with any juices. Bring to a simmer, cover, and cook on low until the meat is tender, 15-20 minutes. Move chops to a plate and tent with foil.
4. Finish the Sauce
   Stir parsley into the sauce and simmer 2-3 more minutes to thicken. Season to taste. Spoon sauce over chops and serve.

Braised Lamb Shanks with Bell Peppers and Harissa

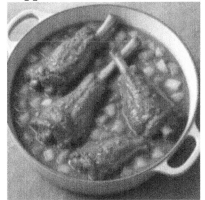

Serves 4 | Tender, Spiced & Rich

What You'll Need
- 4 lamb shanks (10-12 oz each), trimmed
- Salt and pepper
- 1 tbsp extra-virgin olive oil
- 1 onion, finely chopped
- 4 bell peppers (red, orange, and/or yellow), cut into 1-inch pieces
- ¼ cup harissa (plus more to taste)
- 2 tbsp tomato paste
- 4 garlic cloves, minced
- 2½ cups chicken broth
- 2 bay leaves
- 1 tbsp red wine vinegar
- 2 tbsp fresh mint, minced

How to Make It
1. Brown the Shanks
   Preheat oven to 350°F. Pat lamb shanks dry and season with salt and pepper. In a Dutch oven, heat oil over medium-high. Brown shanks on all sides, 8-10 minutes. Transfer to a bowl.
2. Build the Base
   Add onion, peppers, and ½ tsp salt to the pot. Cook over medium heat until soft, about 5 minutes. Stir in 3 tbsp harissa, tomato paste, and garlic. Cook until fragrant, about 30 seconds. Add broth and bay leaves, scraping up any browned bits. Bring to a simmer.
3. Braise the Lamb
   Nestle the shanks into the pot. Cover and transfer to the oven. Cook for 2 to 2½ hours, flipping shanks halfway through, until tender and peppers are soft. Remove shanks and tent with foil.
4. Blend the Sauce
   Strain the liquid into a fat separator. Discard bay leaves. Transfer solids to a blender. After 5 minutes, pour the defatted liquid into the blender and blend until smooth, about 1 minute.
5. Finish and Serve
   Return sauce to the pot and stir in vinegar and remaining 1 tbsp harissa. Add the lamb and any juices back in. Simmer gently, spooning sauce over shanks, until warmed through, about 5 minutes. Season to

taste, top with mint, and serve
with extra sauce on the side.

Eggs

Shakshuka

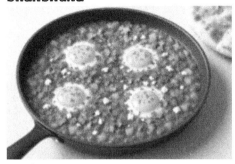

Serves 4 | Vegetarian
Ingredients
- 3 tbsp extra-virgin olive oil
- 2 onions, finely chopped
- 2 yellow bell peppers, stemmed, seeded, and diced into ¼-inch pieces
- 4 garlic cloves, minced
- 2 tsp tomato paste
- Salt and black pepper
- 1 tsp ground cumin
- 1 tsp ground turmeric
- ⅛ tsp cayenne pepper
- 1½ cups jarred piquillo peppers, coarsely chopped
- 1 (14.5 oz) can diced tomatoes
- ¼ cup water
- 2 bay leaves
- ⅓ cup chopped fresh cilantro
- 4 large eggs
- 2 oz feta cheese, crumbled (about ½ cup)

Instructions
1. Heat the olive oil in a 12-inch nonstick skillet over medium-high heat until hot. Add the onions and yellow bell peppers and cook, stirring occasionally, until they're soft and starting to brown—about 8 to 10 minutes. Toss in the garlic, tomato paste, 1½ teaspoons of salt, cumin, turmeric, a bit of pepper, and the cayenne. Cook for about 3 minutes, stirring often, until the tomato paste darkens slightly.
2. Stir in the chopped piquillo peppers, canned tomatoes with their juice, water, and bay leaves. Let it simmer, stirring now and then, until the sauce thickens a bit—about 10 to 15 minutes.
3. Take the pan off the heat, remove the bay leaves, and stir in ¼ cup of the cilantro. Scoop out 2 cups of the sauce and blend it until smooth—about a minute. Pour the blended sauce back into the skillet and bring everything back to a gentle simmer over medium-low heat.
4. Off the heat, use the back of a spoon to make four shallow wells (about 2 inches wide) in the sauce. Crack an egg into each one and season with a little salt and pepper. Cover the skillet and cook over medium-low until the egg whites are just set but the yolks are still soft—around 4 to 6 minutes.
5. Top with the crumbled feta and the rest of the cilantro, and serve right away.

Ratatouille with Poached Eggs

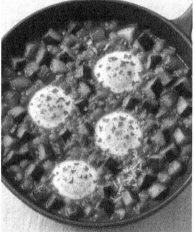

Serves 4 | Quick | Vegetarian
Ingredients
- ¼ cup extra-virgin olive oil
- 1 lb zucchini, cut into ¾-inch pieces
- 1 lb eggplant, cut into ¾-inch pieces
- Salt and pepper
- 1 onion, finely chopped
- 4 garlic cloves, minced
- 1 lb plum tomatoes, cored and chopped into ½-inch pieces

- ½ cup chicken or veggie broth
- 4 large eggs
- ¼ cup chopped fresh basil
- 1 oz Parmesan, grated (about ½ cup)

Instructions

1. Heat 1 tablespoon of olive oil in a 12-inch nonstick skillet over medium-high until it's almost smoking. Add the zucchini and cook until nicely browned, about 5 minutes. Transfer it to a bowl.
2. In the same skillet, add the eggplant, 2 tablespoons of oil, and ¼ teaspoon salt. Cook over medium-high heat until the eggplant is browned, about 5 to 7 minutes. Stir in the onion and the remaining tablespoon of oil. Cook until the onion softens, about 5 minutes. Add the garlic and cook for about 30 seconds, just until fragrant.
3. Stir in the tomatoes and broth. Let the mixture simmer until the veggies are tender, around 3 to 5 minutes. Add the zucchini back in along with any juices from the bowl. Season with salt and pepper to taste.
4. Turn off the heat. Use the back of a spoon to make four shallow wells (around 2 inches wide) in the ratatouille. Crack an egg into each one, sprinkle with a little salt and pepper, then cover the skillet. Cook over medium-low until the egg whites are just set and the yolks are still a little runny, 4 to 6 minutes.
5. Top with fresh basil and Parmesan. Serve right away.

Potato, Swiss Chard, and Lamb Hash with Poached Eggs

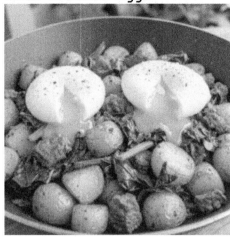

Serves 4

Ingredients

- 1½ lbs russet potatoes, peeled and cut into ½-inch pieces
- 2 tbsp extra-virgin olive oil
- Salt and pepper
- 1½ lbs Swiss chard, stems sliced ¼ inch thick, leaves sliced into ½-inch strips
- 8 oz ground lamb
- 1 onion, finely chopped
- 3 garlic cloves, minced
- 2 tsp paprika
- 1 tsp ground cumin
- 1 tsp ground coriander
- ¼ tsp cayenne pepper
- 4 large eggs
- 1 tbsp fresh chives, minced

Instructions

1. Toss potatoes with 1 tablespoon of oil, ½ teaspoon salt, and ¼ teaspoon pepper in a bowl. Cover and microwave until the potatoes are starting to look translucent on the edges, about 7 to 9 minutes, stirring once. Drain well.
2. In a 12-inch nonstick skillet, heat the remaining tablespoon of oil over medium-high. Add the chard stems with ¼ teaspoon salt and cook until softened and lightly browned, 5 to 7 minutes. Stir in the chard leaves by the handful, cooking until wilted, about 4 minutes. Transfer to the bowl with the potatoes.

3. In the empty skillet, cook the lamb over medium-high, breaking it up as it browns, about 5 minutes. Add the onion and cook until it softens and browns a bit, 5 to 7 minutes. Stir in garlic, paprika, cumin, coriander, and cayenne, and cook until fragrant, about 30 seconds.
4. Stir in the potato-chard mix. Press it all down gently with a spatula and cook without stirring for 2 minutes. Flip the hash in sections, pressing it back down after each flip. Keep flipping every few minutes until the potatoes are well browned, about 6 to 8 minutes total.
5. Off heat, make four shallow wells (about 2 inches wide) in the hash. Push the hash up around the edges and center to expose the skillet bottom in each divot. Crack an egg into each one, season with salt and pepper, cover, and cook over medium-low heat until the whites are just set and yolks are runny, about 4 to 6 minutes.
6. Sprinkle with chives and serve hot.

Fried Eggs with Potato and Parmesan Pancake

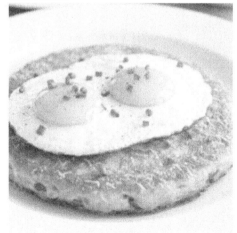

Serves 8 | Vegetarian
Ingredients
- 2½ lbs Yukon Gold potatoes, peeled and shredded
- 1½ tsp cornstarch
- Salt and pepper
- ¼ cup + 2 tsp extra-virgin olive oil
- 8 large eggs
- 1 oz Parmesan cheese, grated (½ cup)
- 1 tbsp fresh chives, minced

Instructions
1. Place shredded potatoes in a large bowl and fill with cold water. Swirl with your hands to release starch, then drain. Leave the potatoes in the colander.
2. Wipe the bowl dry. Working in three batches, squeeze the potatoes dry in a clean dish towel and return to the bowl.
3. Sprinkle in the cornstarch, 1 teaspoon salt, and a pinch of pepper. Mix until evenly combined.
4. Heat 2 tablespoons oil in a 12-inch nonstick skillet over medium heat. Add the potatoes and press into an even layer. Cover and cook for 6 minutes. Uncover, then press down gently with a spatula and continue cooking until the bottom is golden brown, 8 to 10 minutes.
5. Shake the skillet to loosen the pancake and slide it onto a plate. Add 2 more tablespoons oil to the skillet. Invert the pancake onto another plate, then slide it browned-side up back into the skillet. Cook the other side until deep golden brown, 8 to 10 minutes. Transfer to a cutting board and set aside while cooking the eggs.
6. Crack the eggs into 2 small bowls (4 eggs per bowl) and season with salt and pepper. Wipe the skillet clean and heat the remaining 2 teaspoons oil over medium. Quickly pour the eggs from both bowls into the skillet. Cover and cook for 2 minutes.
7. Take the skillet off the heat and let sit, covered, for 2 to 4 minutes depending on how set you want the yolks. Slide the

eggs onto plates. Sprinkle the pancake with Parmesan and chives, cut into wedges, and serve with the eggs.

Israeli Eggplant and Egg Sandwiches (Sabich-Style)

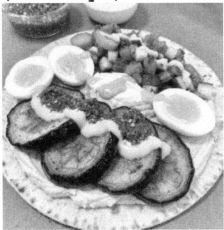

Serves 4 | Vegetarian
Ingredients
- 1 lb eggplant, cut into ½-inch rounds
- Salt and pepper
- ¼ cup extra-virgin olive oil
- 8 oz cherry tomatoes, quartered
- ½ cup finely chopped dill pickles
- ¼ cup finely chopped red onion
- ¼ cup fresh parsley leaves
- 1 tbsp lemon juice
- 1 garlic clove, minced
- 4 (8-inch) pita breads
- 1 cup hummus
- 6 large hard-cooked eggs, thinly sliced
- ½ cup Tahini-Yogurt Sauce
- ½ cup Green Zhoug
- 1 tsp ground Aleppo pepper (or paprika + red pepper flakes mix)

Instructions
1. Spread eggplant slices on a paper towel-lined baking sheet. Sprinkle both sides with 2 teaspoons salt and let them sit for 30 minutes.
2. Set oven rack 4 inches below broiler and heat broiler. Pat eggplant dry, arrange on a foil-lined baking sheet in a single layer, and brush both sides with 2 tablespoons of the oil. Broil until spotty brown

on both sides, about 5 minutes per side.
3. In a bowl, toss together the tomatoes, pickles, onion, parsley, lemon juice, garlic, and remaining 2 tablespoons olive oil. Season with salt and pepper to taste.
4. Lay out the pitas on plates. Spread each one with ¼ cup hummus, then top with broiled eggplant, tomato salad, and egg slices. Drizzle with Tahini-Yogurt Sauce and zhoug. Sprinkle with Aleppo pepper and serve right away.

Scrambled Eggs with Prosciutto and Asparagus

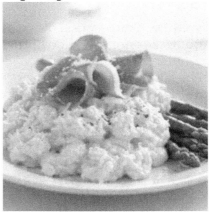

Serves 6 to 8 | Fast
Ingredients
- 3 tbsp extra-virgin olive oil
- 8 oz asparagus, trimmed and cut into ¼-inch diagonal pieces
- 12 large eggs
- 2 tbsp water
- ½ tsp salt
- ¼ tsp pepper
- 2 oz prosciutto, coarsely chopped
- 1 oz Parmesan, grated (about ½ cup)

Instructions
1. Heat 1 tablespoon olive oil in a 12-inch nonstick skillet over medium. Add asparagus and cook until just tender and lightly browned, 2 to 4 minutes. Transfer to a bowl and cover to keep warm.
2. In a bowl, beat eggs with water, salt, and pepper until

fully mixed and uniform in color—don't overdo it.
3. Wipe out the skillet and heat the remaining 2 tablespoons oil over medium. Pour in the eggs and use a rubber spatula to stir constantly, scraping the bottom and sides until eggs start to clump and trails form—about 1½ to 2 minutes.
4. Lower the heat and gently fold the eggs until they're soft and slightly glossy, about 30 to 60 seconds more. Take the skillet off the heat, fold in asparagus, prosciutto, and Parmesan, and serve right away.

Scrambled Eggs with Potatoes and Harissa

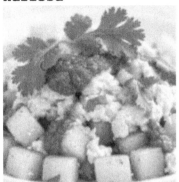

Serves 6 to 8 | Fast | Vegetarian
Ingredients
- 3 tbsp extra-virgin olive oil
- 8 oz red potatoes, unpeeled, cut into ½-inch pieces
- 8 oz cremini mushrooms, trimmed and halved or quartered
- ½ onion, finely chopped
- ½ cup + 2 tbsp water
- Salt and pepper
- 1 garlic clove, minced
- 12 large eggs
- 2 tbsp harissa, plus more for serving
- 2 tbsp chopped fresh cilantro

Instructions
1. In a 12-inch nonstick skillet, heat 1 tbsp oil over medium. Add potatoes, mushrooms, onion, ½ cup water, and ¼ tsp salt. Cover and cook, stirring now and then, for 8 to 10 minutes until tender. Uncover and keep cooking until the liquid's gone and the veggies start browning,

3 to 5 minutes. Stir in garlic and cook 30 seconds more. Transfer to a bowl and cover to keep warm.
2. In a bowl, whisk eggs with ¾ tsp salt, ¼ tsp pepper, and remaining 2 tbsp water until evenly yellow—don't overbeat.
3. Wipe out skillet and heat remaining 2 tbsp oil over medium. Pour in eggs and stir constantly with a rubber spatula until they start to clump and trails form on the skillet bottom, about 1½ to 2 minutes.
4. Turn heat to low and gently fold the eggs until just set but still glossy, about 30 to 60 seconds. Off heat, gently stir in the potato mixture. Drizzle with harissa and top with cilantro. Serve hot, with extra harissa on the side.

Scrambled Eggs with Piperade

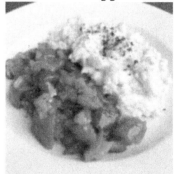

Serves 6 to 8 | Vegetarian
Ingredients
- 5 tbsp extra-virgin olive oil
- 1 large onion, chopped
- 1 bay leaf
- Salt and pepper
- 4 garlic cloves, minced
- 2 tsp paprika
- 1 tsp fresh thyme (or ¼ tsp dried)
- ¾ tsp red pepper flakes
- 3 red bell peppers, sliced into ½-inch strips
- 3 Cubanelle peppers, sliced into ½-inch strips (or green bell peppers)
- 1 (14 oz) can whole peeled tomatoes, drained (save ¼ cup juice), chopped

- 3 tbsp chopped fresh parsley
- 2 tsp sherry vinegar
- 12 large eggs
- 2 tbsp water

Instructions
1. Heat 3 tbsp oil in a 12-inch nonstick skillet over medium. Add onion, bay leaf, and ½ tsp salt. Cook until the onion's soft and lightly browned, 5 to 7 minutes. Stir in garlic, paprika, thyme, and red pepper flakes, and cook until fragrant—about 1 minute.
2. Add bell and Cubanelle peppers with 1 tsp salt. Cover and cook, stirring occasionally, until peppers soften, about 10 minutes. Lower heat to medium-low. Add tomatoes and reserved juice. Cook uncovered until mixture looks dry and peppers are tender, 10 to 12 minutes. Remove bay leaf. Stir in 2 tbsp parsley and vinegar, season to taste, and keep warm.
3. In a bowl, beat eggs with water, ½ tsp salt, and ¼ tsp pepper until fully mixed but not foamy.
4. Wipe out skillet, heat remaining 2 tbsp oil over medium. Pour in eggs and stir constantly with a spatula until they start to clump, about 1½ to 2 minutes.
5. Lower heat and fold eggs gently until just set, 30 to 60 seconds. Off heat, sprinkle with the last tablespoon of parsley and serve alongside the piperade.

Spanish Tortilla with Roasted Red Peppers and Peas

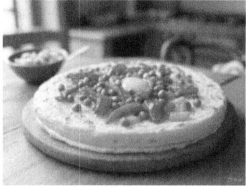

Serves 6 | Vegetarian

Ingredients
- 1½ lbs Yukon Gold potatoes, peeled, quartered, and thinly sliced (⅛ inch)
- 1 small onion, halved and thinly sliced
- 6 tbsp + 1 tsp extra-virgin olive oil
- Salt and black pepper
- 8 large eggs
- ½ cup jarred roasted red peppers, rinsed, dried, and cut into ½-inch pieces
- ½ cup frozen peas, thawed

Instructions
1. In a large bowl, toss the potatoes and onion with ¼ cup oil, ½ tsp salt, and ¼ tsp pepper. Heat 2 tbsp oil in a 10-inch nonstick skillet over medium-high until hot. Add the potato mixture, lower the heat to medium-low, cover, and cook for about 25 minutes, stirring every 5 minutes, until the potatoes are soft.
2. In the same (unwashed) bowl, beat the eggs with ½ tsp salt until fully combined and evenly yellow—don't overmix. Fold in the cooked potatoes, roasted red peppers, and peas, scraping all the cooked bits out of the skillet.
3. Wipe out the skillet if needed, then heat the remaining 1 tsp oil over medium-high. When it's just starting to smoke, pour in the egg mixture. Cook, shaking and gently folding with a spatula for about 15 seconds, then smooth the top. Reduce

heat to medium, cover, and cook for 2 minutes, shaking the pan every 30 seconds, until the bottom is browned and the top is just starting to set.

4. Take the pan off the heat. Use a spatula to loosen the tortilla around the edges and gently shake to make sure it's free. Slide it onto a large plate. Place another plate on top, flip, then slide it back into the skillet, browned side up. Tuck in the edges and cook for another 2 minutes over medium heat, shaking gently every 30 seconds.

5. Slide onto a cutting board and let it rest for a few minutes. Slice and serve warm, room temp, or chilled. Garlic aïoli on the side is a great touch.

Egyptian Eggah with Ground Beef and Spinach

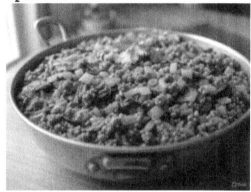

Serves 4 to 6 | Fast
Ingredients
- 8 oz (8 cups) baby spinach
- 6 tbsp water
- 4 tsp extra-virgin olive oil
- 1 lb leeks (white and light green parts only), halved lengthwise, thinly sliced, and well rinsed
- 8 oz 90% lean ground beef
- 1 garlic clove, minced
- 1 tsp ground cumin
- ¼ tsp ground cinnamon
- Salt and pepper
- 8 large eggs
- ¼ cup minced fresh cilantro
Instructions
1. Place spinach and ¼ cup water in a large bowl, cover, and

microwave until wilted—about 5 minutes. Let sit 1 minute, then transfer to a colander. Press out as much liquid as you can, then chop the spinach and press it again in the colander.

2. Heat 1 tsp oil in a 10-inch nonstick skillet over medium heat. Add leeks and cook until softened, about 5 minutes. Stir in beef and cook, breaking it up, until just browned, 5 to 7 minutes. Mix in garlic, cumin, cinnamon, ½ tsp salt, and ¼ tsp pepper. Cook 30 seconds. Add spinach and stir for 1 minute. Transfer to a bowl and let cool slightly.

3. In a clean bowl, beat eggs with remaining 2 tbsp water, ½ tsp salt, and ¼ tsp pepper until fully blended—don't overmix. Fold in the spinach mixture and cilantro.

4. Wipe out skillet and heat remaining 1 tbsp oil over medium-high. When oil is just smoking, pour in the egg mixture. Stir and fold for about 15 seconds while shaking the skillet. Smooth the top, reduce heat to medium, cover, and cook—shaking every 30 seconds—until the bottom is golden and the top is lightly set, about 3 minutes.

5. Off heat, loosen the edges with a spatula. Slide the eggah onto a plate. Cover with a second plate, flip, and slide it back into the skillet, browned side up. Tuck in edges, cook for another 2 minutes while shaking the pan, then slide onto a board. Let it rest a few minutes before slicing and serving.

Broccoli and Feta Frittata

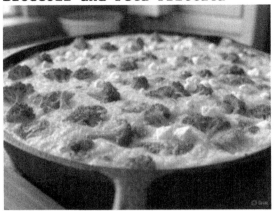

Serves 6 | Fast | Vegetarian

Ingredients

- 12 large eggs
- ⅓ cup whole milk
- Salt
- 1 tbsp extra-virgin olive oil
- 12 oz broccoli florets, cut into ½-inch pieces (about 3½ to 4 cups)
- Pinch red pepper flakes
- 3 tbsp water
- ½ tsp lemon zest + ½ tsp lemon juice
- 4 oz feta, crumbled into ½-inch pieces (1 cup

Instructions

1. Preheat oven to 350°F and set rack in the middle. Beat eggs, milk, and ½ tsp salt until well mixed and uniform in color.
2. Heat oil in a 12-inch nonstick skillet over medium-high. Add broccoli, red pepper flakes, and ¼ tsp salt. Cook, stirring often, until browned in spots and crisp-tender, 7 to 9 minutes. Add water, lemon zest, and juice, then cook another minute until broccoli is just tender and water is gone.
3. Add the feta and egg mixture. Stir constantly with a rubber spatula until large curds form and the bottom of the skillet shows trails—about 30 seconds. Smooth the surface, cook without stirring for 30 seconds, then move skillet to oven.
4. Bake until the frittata is slightly puffed and springs back when lightly pressed, 6 to

9 minutes. Let it rest 5 minutes, then loosen from the skillet, transfer to a cutting board, slice, and serve.

Baked Eggs with Tomatoes, Feta, and Croutons

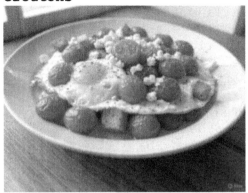

Serves 6 | Vegetarian

Ingredients

- 3 slices French or Italian bread, cut into ½-inch pieces (about 4 cups)
- ¼ cup extra-virgin olive oil, divided
- Salt and pepper
- 6 garlic cloves, thinly sliced
- 5 tsp minced fresh oregano
- 2 tsp tomato paste
- 1 tsp sugar
- 2 lbs cherry tomatoes
- 6 large eggs
- 2 oz feta cheese, crumbled (about ½ cup)

Instructions

1. Preheat oven to 450°F with racks in upper-middle and lower-middle positions. Toss bread with 1 tbsp oil, season with salt and pepper, and spread in a greased 9x13-inch baking dish.
2. In a bowl, mix garlic, 1 tbsp oil, 1 tbsp oregano, tomato paste, salt, sugar, and pepper. Add tomatoes and toss well. Transfer to a parchment-lined baking sheet, pushing tomatoes toward the center. Scrape any leftover mixture from the bowl into the tomatoes.
3. Roast the bread on the upper rack and tomatoes on the lower rack. Stir occasionally and roast bread until golden and

tomatoes start to soften—about 10 minutes. Remove croutons; roast tomatoes 10 more minutes until blistered.

4. Add roasted tomatoes and 1 tbsp oil to the croutons, fold gently, and spread into an even layer. Make 6 shallow wells with the back of a spoon. Crack 1 egg into each and season with salt and pepper.

5. Bake 10 to 12 minutes, until whites are just starting to set. Remove, tent loosely with foil, and let sit for 5 minutes. Top with feta, remaining oregano, and a final drizzle of oil. Serve immediately.

Greek-Style Zucchini and Egg Casserole (Sfougato-Inspired)

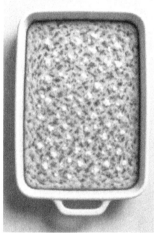

Serves 6 to 8 | Fast | Vegetarian
Ingredients
- 4 zucchini, shredded (use large holes of a box grater)
- Salt and pepper
- 1 tbsp extra-virgin olive oil
- 8 scallions, thinly sliced
- 2 garlic cloves, minced
- 6 large eggs
- ¼ cup whole milk
- 4 oz feta, crumbled (1 cup)
- ¼ cup minced fresh dill
- 1 tbsp chopped fresh oregano
Instructions
1. Preheat oven to 375°F. Toss shredded zucchini with 1 tsp salt and let drain in a strainer for 10 minutes. Wrap in a clean dish towel and squeeze out as much liquid as you can.

2. In a 12-inch nonstick skillet, heat oil over medium. Add scallions and garlic, cook until softened—about 2 minutes. Stir in zucchini, cover, and cook 4 to 6 minutes until it releases liquid. Uncover and cook 1 minute more until dry. Let cool a bit.

3. Beat eggs with milk and ½ tsp pepper until smooth but not foamy. Stir in zucchini mixture, feta, dill, and oregano. Pour into a greased 9x13-inch baking dish.

4. Bake 20 to 25 minutes until the eggs are just set and edges are golden. Let cool slightly before serving warm or at room temp.

Breads, Flatbreads

PizzasPita Bread

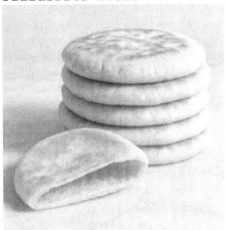

Makes eight 8-inch pitas |
Vegetarian
Ingredients
- 3⅔ cups (20⅛ oz) bread flour
- 2½ tsp instant or rapid-rise yeast
- 2 tsp salt
- 1⅓ cups water, room temp
- ¼ cup extra-virgin olive oil
- 2½ tsp sugar

Instructions
1. In a stand mixer bowl, whisk together the flour, yeast, and salt. In a separate container, whisk water, oil, and sugar until the sugar dissolves.
2. Using the dough hook on low, slowly add the liquid mixture to the flour mixture and mix for about 2 minutes until it comes together and no dry flour remains. Scrape down the sides as needed. Increase to medium-low and knead for 8 minutes until smooth and elastic.
3. Turn the dough out onto a lightly floured counter and knead into a smooth ball—about 30 seconds. Place seam side down in a lightly greased bowl, cover tightly, and let rise until doubled, 1 to 1½ hours.
4. Press the dough to deflate, then divide into 8 equal pieces. Cover loosely with greased plastic wrap.
5. Shape each piece into a ball by pulling the dough around your thumbs and pinching underneath so the top is smooth.
6. Flour each dough ball and roll out into an 8-inch round. Keep covered with greased plastic wrap. If the dough is tight, let it rest for 10-20 minutes and try again. Let the shaped rounds rest for 20 minutes.
7. One hour before baking, place a baking stone on the lower-middle rack and preheat the oven to 500°F. Gently place 2 dough rounds on a well-floured pizza peel.
8. Slide onto the hot stone and bake for 1 minute, until you see a puff starting. Quickly flip the pitas and bake for another 1 to 2 minutes until golden. Move to a plate and cover with a towel. Repeat in batches, letting the oven reheat for 5 minutes between each.

Let the pitas cool for 10 minutes before serving. Store extras in a zip-top bag at room temp for up to 5 days.

Socca

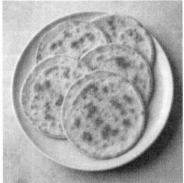

Makes five 6-inch flatbreads |
Serves 4 to 6 | Fast | Vegetarian
Ingredients
- 1½ cups (6¾ oz) chickpea flour (also called garbanzo bean or ceci flour)
- ½ tsp salt
- ½ tsp pepper
- ½ tsp ground turmeric
- 1½ cups water
- 6 tbsp + 1 tsp extra-virgin olive oil

Instructions

1. Adjust oven rack to middle position and heat to 200°F. Place a wire rack on a rimmed baking sheet and set in oven. In a bowl, whisk together chickpea flour, salt, pepper, and turmeric. Slowly whisk in water and 3 tbsp oil until smooth.
2. Heat 2 tsp oil in an 8-inch nonstick skillet over medium-high until shimmering. Pour in ½ cup batter and swirl to coat the bottom. Lower heat to medium and cook until the edges are crisp and the bottom is golden, 3 to 5 minutes.
3. Flip the socca and cook until the second side is browned, 2 to 3 minutes. Transfer to the wire rack in the warm oven. Repeat with the remaining oil and batter. Slice and serve as is or topped with one of the variations below.

Lavash with Tomatoes, Spinach, and Green Olives

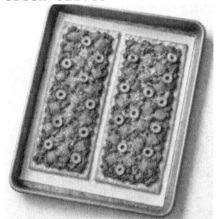

Makes two 12x9-inch flatbreads | Serves 4 to 6 | Fast | Vegetarian
Ingredients
- 10 oz frozen spinach, thawed and squeezed dry
- 4 oz fontina cheese, shredded (1 cup)
- 1 tomato, cored and diced
- ½ cup pitted brine-cured green olives, chopped
- 3 garlic cloves, minced
- ¼ tsp red pepper flakes
- ¼ tsp salt
- ¼ tsp black pepper
- 2 (12x9-inch) lavash breads

- 2 tbsp extra-virgin olive oil
- 1 oz Parmesan cheese, grated (½ cup)
Instructions
1. Preheat oven to 475°F with racks in the upper-middle and lower-middle positions. In a bowl, mix the spinach, fontina, tomato, olives, garlic, red pepper flakes, salt, and pepper.
2. Brush both sides of lavash with olive oil and place on 2 baking sheets. Toast in oven until golden and crisp, about 4 minutes total, flipping halfway through.
3. Spread the spinach mixture evenly over the toasted lavash and sprinkle with Parmesan. Return to oven and bake until cheese melts and browns slightly, 6 to 8 minutes, rotating and switching baking sheets halfway through. Slice and serve.

Pissaladière

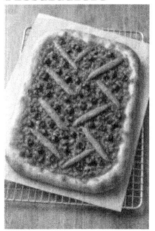

Makes two 14x8-inch tarts | Serves 4 to 6
Ingredients
- 3 cups (16½ oz) bread flour
- 2 tsp sugar
- ½ tsp instant or rapid-rise yeast
- 1⅓ cups ice water
- 1 tbsp extra-virgin olive oil
- 1½ tsp salt
Topping Ingredients
- ¼ cup extra-virgin olive oil, divided

- 2 lbs onions, halved and thinly sliced
- 1 tsp packed brown sugar
- ½ tsp salt
- 1 tbsp water
- ½ cup pitted niçoise olives, chopped
- 8 anchovy fillets, chopped (plus 12 more whole, optional)
- 2 tsp minced fresh thyme
- 1 tsp fennel seeds
- ½ tsp pepper
- 2 tbsp minced fresh parsley

Instructions
1. Make the Dough: In a food processor, pulse flour, sugar, and yeast. With the motor running, add ice water. Process 10 seconds, let rest 10 minutes. Add oil and salt, process 30-60 seconds until a sticky ball forms. Knead on a floured surface for 30 seconds. Transfer to greased bowl, cover, and refrigerate for 24 hours (or up to 3 days).
2. Prepare Toppings: Heat 2 tbsp oil in a skillet over medium. Add onions, sugar, and salt. Cover and cook 10 minutes, then uncover and continue cooking until golden, 10-15 more minutes. Stir in 1 tbsp water. Cool.
3. Shape Dough: One hour before baking, preheat oven to 500°F with a baking stone on the top rack. Divide dough in half and shape into tight balls. Cover and let rest for 1 hour.
4. Roll and Top: Heat broiler for 10 minutes. Roll one dough ball into a 14x8-inch oval. Transfer to a floured pizza peel. Poke all over with a fork. Brush with 1 tbsp oil and sprinkle with half the olives, chopped anchovies, thyme, fennel seeds, and pepper. Spread half the onions on top and arrange 6 whole anchovies if using.
5. Bake: Slide onto baking stone, turn oven back to 500°F, and bake until crust is crisp and browned, 13-15 minutes. Cool 5 minutes, sprinkle with 1 tbsp

parsley, slice, and serve. Repeat with remaining dough and toppings.

Mushroom Musakhan

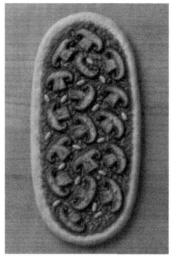

Makes two 15x8-inch flatbreads | Serves 4 to 6 | Vegetarian

DOUGH
- 1½ cups (8¼ oz) whole-wheat flour
- 1 cup (5½ oz) bread flour
- 2 tsp honey
- ¾ tsp instant or rapid-rise yeast
- 1¼ cups ice water
- 2 tbsp extra-virgin olive oil
- 1¾ tsp salt

TOPPINGS
- ½ cup extra-virgin olive oil, divided
- 2 tbsp minced fresh oregano (or 2 tsp dried)
- 4 garlic cloves, minced
- 1½ tbsp ground sumac
- ¼ tsp ground allspice
- ⅛ tsp ground cardamom
- 2 lbs onions, halved and thinly sliced
- 2 tsp packed light brown sugar
- Salt and pepper
- ¼ cup pine nuts
- 2 lbs portobello mushroom caps, gills removed, halved, and sliced ½ inch thick
- 2 tbsp minced fresh chives

Instructions
1. Make the Dough:
   In a food processor, pulse the whole-wheat flour, bread flour,

honey, and yeast. With the machine running, slowly pour in ice water and blend until just combined (about 10 seconds). Let it rest 10 minutes. Add oil and salt and process until a sticky, satiny dough ball forms, about 30-60 seconds. Knead briefly by hand on a lightly oiled surface to form a smooth ball. Place in a greased bowl, cover tightly, and refrigerate for at least 18 hours (or up to 2 days).

2. Make the Onion Jam:
 Mix 1 tbsp oil, oregano, garlic, sumac, allspice, and cardamom in a bowl. In a skillet, heat 2 tbsp oil over high. Add onions, sugar, and ½ tsp salt. Stir to coat and cook about 5 minutes, stirring occasionally. Reduce heat to medium and cook, stirring often, until deeply caramelized, 35-40 minutes. Push onions to the side of the skillet, add spice mix to the center, and mash it in until fragrant (about 30 seconds). Stir everything together. Transfer to a food processor and pulse to a jamlike texture, about 5 pulses. Stir in pine nuts and season to taste. Let cool.

3. Cook the Mushrooms:
 Wipe skillet clean. Heat 2 tbsp oil over medium-high. Cook half the mushrooms with ½ tsp salt until browned, 8-10 minutes. Repeat with remaining mushrooms, oil, and salt. Let cool.

4. Shape the Dough:
 One hour before baking, place a baking stone on the top rack and heat oven to 500°F. Deflate the dough and divide in half. Form each half into a taut ball, cover loosely, and let rest for 1 hour.

5. Shape the Flatbreads:
 After resting, flour one dough ball and roll it into a 12x8-inch oval. Transfer to a floured peel and stretch into a 15x8-inch oval. Poke the dough all over with a fork.

6. Bake the First Flatbread:
 Spread half the onion mixture across the dough, edge to edge. Top with half the mushrooms. Slide onto the stone and return oven to 500°F.

Bake until the crust is golden and crisp, about 10 minutes, rotating halfway. Let cool on a wire rack for 5 minutes. Drizzle with 1½ tsp olive oil and sprinkle with 1 tbsp chives. Slice and serve.

7. Repeat:
 Heat broiler for 10 minutes, then bake the second flatbread using the same method.

Lahmacun

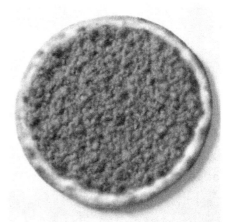

 Makes four 9-inch flatbreads | Serves 4 to 6

DOUGH
- 1¾ cups (9⅔ oz) bread flour
- 1 tsp sugar
- ¾ tsp instant or rapid-rise yeast
- ¾ cup ice water
- 2 tbsp extra-virgin olive oil
- 1 tsp salt

TOPPING
- 3 tbsp Turkish hot pepper paste*
- 1 tbsp tomato paste
- 1 garlic clove, minced
- ¾ tsp smoked hot paprika
- ¾ tsp ground allspice
- ½ tsp salt
- 1 cup chopped red bell pepper
- ⅔ cup chopped onion
- 4 oz ground lamb
- ¼ cup chopped fresh parsley

*No Turkish pepper paste? Use 3 tbsp tomato paste + 1 tsp smoked paprika + increase salt to ¾ tsp.

Instructions
1. Make the Dough:
 In a food processor, pulse flour, sugar, and yeast to combine. With

the machine running, slowly add the ice water and process about 10 seconds until a rough dough forms. Let it rest for 10 minutes.
Add olive oil and salt. Process 30-60 seconds until the dough becomes sticky, smooth, and clears the bowl. Turn it out onto a floured surface and knead into a ball. Place in a greased bowl, cover, and refrigerate at least 24 hours or up to 3 days.
2. Shape the Dough:
 Press dough down to deflate. Divide into 4 equal pieces. Shape each into a ball, cover loosely with greased plastic wrap, and let rest for 1 hour.
3. Make the Topping:
 In a food processor, blend pepper paste, tomato paste, garlic, paprika, allspice, and salt. Add bell pepper and onion; pulse until finely chopped. Add lamb and parsley; pulse until just combined.
4. Assemble:
 Heat oven to 350°F with racks in upper-middle and lower-middle positions. Grease two rimmed baking sheets.
Roll each dough ball into a 9-inch round on a floured surface. Place two rounds on each sheet, positioning them in opposite corners. Spread one-quarter of the lamb mixture over each round with the back of a spoon, leaving a ¼-inch border.
5. Bake and Broil:
 Bake for 10-12 minutes, switching and rotating sheets halfway through. The edges should be set but still pale. Remove from oven, turn on broiler.
Place one sheet on the upper rack and broil until the edges are crisp and lightly charred and the topping is set, 2-4 minutes. Transfer to a wire rack. Repeat with second batch. Let cool 5 minutes before serving. Serve warm with yogurt, pickled veggies, and herbs if desired.

Za'atar Bread

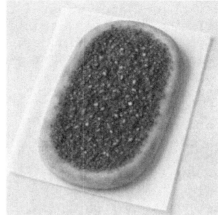

 Makes one flatbread | Serves 6 to 8 | Vegetarian
Ingredients
- 3½ cups (19¼ oz) bread flour
- 2½ tsp instant or rapid-rise yeast
- 2½ tsp sugar
- 1⅓ cups ice water
- ½ cup + 2 tbsp extra-virgin olive oil, divided
- 2 tsp salt
- ⅓ cup za'atar spice blend
- Coarse sea salt, for finishing

Instructions
1. In a food processor, pulse flour, yeast, and sugar to combine. With the machine running, slowly pour in the ice water and blend about 10 seconds until no dry flour remains. Let the dough rest for 10 minutes.
2. Add 2 tbsp olive oil and salt. Process until a sticky, satiny ball forms, 30 to 60 seconds. Turn dough onto a floured counter and knead briefly into a smooth ball. Place seam side down in a greased bowl, cover tightly, and refrigerate for at least 24 hours (up to 3 days).
3. Remove from fridge and let sit at room temp for 1 hour. Coat a rimmed baking sheet with 2 tbsp oil. Press the dough gently to release large air bubbles, then transfer it to the sheet. Use your fingertips to stretch it out evenly—don't worry if it doesn't reach the corners. Cover loosely with greased

plastic wrap and let rest for 1 hour.
4. Preheat oven to 375°F and position rack in the lower-middle. Use your fingertips to dimple the dough and gently press it into the corners of the pan.
5. Mix the remaining 6 tbsp olive oil with the za'atar. Spread the mixture evenly over the dough all the way to the edges.
6. Bake for 20 to 25 minutes, rotating halfway, until the bottom is deeply golden and the edges are crisp. Let cool in the pan for 10 minutes, then transfer to a board. Sprinkle with sea salt, slice, and serve warm.

Red Pepper Coques

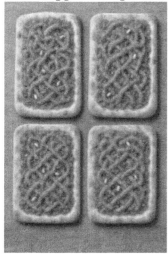

Makes 4 coques | Serves 6 to 8 | Vegetarian
DOUGH
- 3 cups (16½ oz) bread flour
- 2 tsp sugar
- ½ tsp instant or rapid-rise yeast
- 1⅓ cups ice water
- 3 tbsp extra-virgin olive oil
- 1½ tsp salt
TOPPING
- ½ cup extra-virgin olive oil
- 2 large onions, halved and thinly sliced
- 2 cups jarred roasted red peppers, patted dry and thinly sliced
- 3 tbsp sugar

- 3 garlic cloves, minced
- 1½ tsp salt
- ¼ tsp red pepper flakes
- 2 bay leaves
- 3 tbsp sherry vinegar
- ¼ cup pine nuts (optional)
- 1 tbsp minced fresh parsley

Instructions
1. Make the Dough:
  In a food processor, pulse together the flour, sugar, and yeast until combined. With the processor running, slowly add the ice water and process until the dough just comes together, about 10 seconds. Let it rest for 10 minutes.
Add olive oil and salt, then process until the dough forms a smooth, sticky ball that clears the sides of the bowl, about 30 to 60 seconds. Transfer the dough to a lightly floured surface and knead by hand for about 30 seconds to form a smooth round ball. Place the dough in a lightly greased large bowl, cover tightly with plastic wrap, and refrigerate for at least 24 hours or up to 3 days.
2. Prepare the Topping:
  Heat 3 tbsp olive oil in a 12-inch nonstick skillet over medium heat. Add onions, roasted red peppers, sugar, garlic, salt, red pepper flakes, and bay leaves. Cover and cook, stirring occasionally, until the onions are softened and have released their juices, about 10 minutes. Uncover and cook for another 10-15 minutes, stirring frequently, until the onions are golden brown.
Remove from heat, discard the bay leaves, and stir in the sherry vinegar. Let the topping cool completely before using.
3. Shape the Dough:
  Press down on the dough to deflate it. Transfer it to a lightly floured counter, divide into quarters, and cover loosely with greased plastic wrap. Working with one piece at a time (keep the remaining pieces covered), form a rough ball by stretching the dough around your

thumbs and pinching the edges together so the top is smooth. Place each ball seam-side down and, using cupped hands, drag it in small circles on the counter until it feels taut and round. Space the dough balls 3 inches apart, cover loosely, and let them rest for 1 hour.

4. Preheat Oven and Prepare Baking Sheets:
 Adjust oven racks to the upper-middle and lower-middle positions and preheat the oven to 500°F. Grease two rimmed baking sheets with 2 tbsp olive oil each.

5. Roll the Dough:
 Generously flour one dough ball and roll it out on a floured surface into a 14x5-inch oval. Place it on a prepared baking sheet, with one long edge fitting snugly against one side of the sheet. Reshape as needed. Repeat with the remaining dough, placing two ovals on each sheet, spaced ½ inch apart. Poke the surface of the dough 10 to 15 times with a fork.

6. Parbake the Dough:
 Brush the dough with the remaining 1 tbsp olive oil and bake for 6 to 8 minutes, rotating the sheets halfway through, until the dough is puffed and lightly golden.

7. Add Toppings and Bake Again:
 Spread the onion mixture evenly over the parbaked dough, from edge to edge. If using, sprinkle with pine nuts. Return to the oven and bake for another 12 to 15 minutes, rotating the sheets halfway through, until the edges of the flatbreads are golden brown and crisp, and the topping is heated through.

8. Finish and Serve:
 Remove from the oven, let cool for 10 minutes on the sheets, then transfer to a cutting board using a metal spatula. Sprinkle with minced parsley, slice, and serve warm.

Rosemary Focaccia

Makes two 9-inch round loaves | Serves 6 to 8 | Vegetarian
SPONGE

- ½ cup (2½ oz) all-purpose flour
- ⅓ cup room-temp water
- ¼ tsp instant or rapid-rise yeast

DOUGH
- 2½ cups (12½ oz) all-purpose flour
- 1¼ cups room-temp water
- 1 tsp instant or rapid-rise yeast
- 2 tsp kosher salt
- ¼ cup extra-virgin olive oil
- 2 tbsp chopped fresh rosemary

Instructions
1. Make the Sponge:
 In a large bowl, stir together sponge ingredients until well mixed. Cover with plastic wrap and let sit at room temperature until bubbly and starting to collapse, about 6 hours (up to 24 hours is fine).
2. Make the Dough:
 Add flour, water, and yeast to the sponge and mix with a wooden spoon until fully combined. Cover and rest for 15 minutes.
3. Add Salt:
 Stir in salt until thoroughly incorporated (about 1 minute). Cover again and let rest for 30 minutes.
4. Begin Folding:
 Using a greased spatula or bowl scraper, gently fold the dough over itself 8 times, turning the bowl 45 degrees between each fold. Cover and let rise for 30 minutes. Repeat this folding and resting process twice more. After the final fold, let the dough rise until almost doubled, about 30 to 60 minutes.
5. Prep for Baking:
 One hour before baking, place a baking stone on the upper-middle rack and heat oven to 500°F. Grease two 9-inch round cake pans with 2 tbsp olive oil each and sprinkle each with ½ tsp salt.
6. Shape the Dough:
 Transfer dough to a floured counter and dust the top. Divide in half and loosely cover with greased plastic. Shape each into a 5-inch round by gently tucking under the edges. Place seam-side up in prepared pans, coat with oil from the pan, then

flip seam-side down. Cover and let rest 5 minutes.

7. Stretch and Top:
Gently press dough to the edges of the pans with your fingertips (if it resists, wait 5-10 minutes). Poke the surface 25-30 times with a fork to pop bubbles. Sprinkle 1 tbsp rosemary on each, cover loosely, and let rest 10 minutes until slightly bubbly.

8. Bake:
Place pans on the baking stone and reduce oven temperature to 450°F. Bake until golden brown, 25 to 30 minutes, rotating pans halfway through. Cool in pans for 5 minutes, then transfer loaves to a wire rack. Brush tops with any remaining oil from the pans. Let cool 30 minutes before serving warm or at room temp.

Thin-Crust Pizza

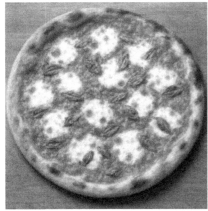

Makes two 13-inch pizzas | Serves 4 to 6 | Vegetarian

DOUGH
- 3 cups (16½ oz) bread flour
- 2 tsp sugar
- ½ tsp instant or rapid-rise yeast
- 1⅓ cups ice water
- 1 tbsp extra-virgin olive oil
- 1½ tsp salt

SAUCE AND TOPPINGS
- 1 (28 oz) can whole peeled tomatoes, drained (reserve juice)
- 1 tbsp extra-virgin olive oil
- 2 garlic cloves, minced
- 1 tsp red wine vinegar
- 1 tsp dried oregano
- ½ tsp salt
- ¼ tsp pepper
- 1 oz Parmesan, finely grated (½ cup)
- 8 oz whole-milk mozzarella, shredded (2 cups)

Instructions

1. Make the Dough:
In a food processor, pulse flour, sugar, and yeast to combine. With machine running, slowly add ice water and process for 10 seconds until fully combined. Let rest 10 minutes.
Add oil and salt and process 30-60 seconds until dough forms a sticky, smooth ball. Knead briefly on an oiled surface, then shape into a ball. Place in a greased bowl, cover tightly, and refrigerate at least 24 hours or up to 3 days.

2. Make the Sauce:
In a clean processor bowl, blend tomatoes, oil, garlic, vinegar, oregano, salt, and pepper until smooth, about 30 seconds. Measure out 2 cups using reserved tomato juice as needed. Set aside 1 cup for the pizzas and refrigerate or freeze the rest.

3. Shape the Dough:
One hour before baking, set a baking stone on a rack 4 inches below the broiler and heat oven to 500°F. Deflate dough, divide in half, and loosely cover both pieces with greased plastic wrap. Shape one piece into a ball by folding the edges toward the center and dragging it seam-side down on the counter until taut. Repeat with the second piece. Let rest for 1 hour.

4. Stretch and Top:
Turn on broiler for 10 minutes. Generously flour one dough ball and the counter. Flatten into an 8-inch circle, keeping the edge slightly thicker. Stretch to a 12-inch round by rotating and gently pulling at the edges.
Transfer to a floured pizza peel and stretch to a 13-inch circle. Spread ½ cup tomato sauce over the top, leaving a ¼-inch border. Sprinkle with ¼ cup Parmesan and 1 cup mozzarella.

5. Bake:
Slide onto the hot stone and return

oven to 500°F. Bake 8-10 minutes until crust is deeply browned and cheese is bubbling and browned in spots. Rotate halfway through for even cooking. Transfer to wire rack and cool 5 minutes before slicing.

6. Repeat:
 Heat broiler again for 10 minutes. Shape and top the second dough ball and repeat the baking process. Serve immediately.

Whole-Wheat Pizza with Feta, Figs, and Honey

Makes two 13-inch pizzas | Serves 4 to 6 | Vegetarian

DOUGH
- 1½ cups (8¼ oz) whole-wheat flour
- 1 cup (5½ oz) bread flour
- 2 tsp honey
- ¾ tsp instant or rapid-rise yeast
- 1¼ cups ice water
- 2 tbsp extra-virgin olive oil
- 1¾ tsp salt

GARLIC OIL AND TOPPINGS
- 2 tbsp extra-virgin olive oil
- 2 garlic cloves, minced
- ½ tsp black pepper
- ½ tsp dried thyme
- ⅛ tsp salt
- 1 cup fresh basil leaves
- 4 oz feta cheese, crumbled (1 cup)
- 8 oz fresh figs, stemmed and quartered (1½ cups)
- 2 tbsp honey

Instructions

1. Make the Dough:
 In a food processor, pulse both flours, honey, and yeast. With machine running, slowly add ice water. Process 10 seconds until fully combined. Rest for 10 minutes. Add olive oil and salt, then process 45-60 seconds until a sticky, satiny dough forms. Knead briefly on an oiled counter to form a ball. Place in a greased bowl, cover, and refrigerate for 18 to 48 hours.

2. Prepare the Garlic Oil:
 In a small skillet, heat oil over medium-low. Add garlic, pepper, thyme, and salt. Stir constantly for 30 seconds until fragrant. Transfer to a bowl and cool completely.

3. Shape the Dough:
 One hour before baking, preheat oven to 500°F with baking stone placed 4 inches below the broiler. Deflate dough, divide in half, and cover loosely. Shape one piece into a ball by folding edges in and turning seam-side down. Let rest for 1 hour.

4. Stretch and Top:
 Turn on broiler for 10 minutes. Flour one dough ball and the counter. Flatten dough to an 8-inch round, keeping the edge slightly thicker. Gently stretch to a 12-inch round, then transfer to a floured pizza peel and stretch to 13 inches. Brush with half the garlic oil, leaving a ¼-inch border. Layer with ½ cup basil, ½ cup feta, and ¾ cup figs.

5. Bake and Finish:
 Slide onto hot stone and return oven to 500°F. Bake 8-10 minutes until the crust is browned and cheese is lightly golden. Transfer to wire rack and drizzle with 1 tbsp honey. Cool for 5 minutes before slicing.

6. Repeat:
 Broil again for 10 minutes, then shape, top, and bake the second pizza the same way. Serve warm.

Turkish Pide with Eggplant and Tomatoes

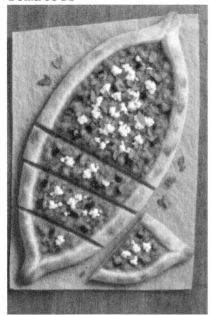

Makes 6 pide | Serves 6 to 8 | Vegetarian

DOUGH

- 3 cups (16½ oz) bread flour
- 2 tsp sugar
- ½ tsp instant or rapid-rise yeast
- 1⅓ cups ice water
- 1 tbsp extra-virgin olive oil
- 1½ tsp salt

TOPPINGS

- 1 (28 oz) can whole peeled tomatoes
- 5 tbsp extra-virgin olive oil, divided
- 1 lb eggplant, cut into ½-inch pieces
- ½ red bell pepper, chopped
- Salt and pepper
- 3 garlic cloves, minced
- ¼ tsp red pepper flakes
- ½ tsp smoked paprika
- 6 tbsp chopped fresh mint, divided
- 6 oz feta cheese, crumbled (1½ cups)

Instructions

1. Make the Dough:
  In a food processor, pulse flour, sugar, and yeast. With the motor running, slowly add ice water. Blend about 10 seconds until combined. Rest dough 10 minutes.
Add olive oil and salt; process 30–60 seconds until a sticky, satiny ball forms. Knead briefly by hand to make a smooth ball. Place in a greased bowl, cover, and refrigerate at least 24 hours or up to 3 days.

2. Make the Topping:
  Pulse tomatoes and juice until coarsely chopped (about 12 pulses). Heat 2 tbsp oil in a skillet over medium-high. Add eggplant, bell pepper, and ½ tsp salt. Cook 5-7 minutes until soft and browned. Stir in garlic, pepper flakes, and paprika; cook 30 seconds until fragrant.
Add pulsed tomatoes and simmer until thick and reduced to 3½ cups, about 10 minutes. Off heat, stir in ¼ cup mint. Season with salt and pepper and let cool completely.

3. Prepare for Baking:
  One hour before baking, preheat oven to 500°F with baking stone on upper-middle rack (4 inches from broiler). Deflate dough and divide into 6 equal pieces (about 4¾ oz each). Shape each into a ball, cover, and let rest 1 hour.

4. Shape the Pide:
  Cut six 16x6-inch pieces of parchment. Roll each dough ball into a 14x5½-inch oval and place on a piece of parchment. Repeat for three dough balls.

5. Top and Bake:
  Brush dough with oil. Add ½ cup eggplant mixture and ¼ cup feta to each, leaving a ¾-inch border. Fold long edges over the filling and pinch ends to seal into a canoe shape. Brush edges with more oil. Transfer to a pizza peel and slide each pide with parchment onto the hot stone. Bake 10-15 minutes until golden and crisp. Cool 5 minutes, sprinkle with 1 tbsp mint, slice, and serve.

6. Repeat:
  Shape and bake the remaining three pide as above. Serve warm.

Fennel, Olive, and Goat Cheese Hand Pies

Makes 15 triangles | Serves 6 to 8 |
Vegetarian
FILLING

- 1 tbsp extra-virgin olive oil
- 1 large fennel bulb, stalks removed, halved, cored, and thinly sliced
- 3 garlic cloves, minced
- ½ cup dry white wine
- 6 oz goat cheese, crumbled (1½ cups)
- ¼ cup pitted kalamata olives, finely chopped
- 2 tbsp chopped fresh oregano
- 2 tsp lemon zest + 1 tbsp lemon juice
- Salt and pepper

PIES

- 10 sheets phyllo dough (14x9-inch), thawed
- ¼ cup extra-virgin olive oil

Instructions
1. Make the Filling:
 Heat 1 tbsp olive oil in a 12-inch skillet over medium heat. Add fennel and cook until soft and lightly browned, 8-10 minutes. Stir in garlic and cook 30 seconds. Add wine, cover, and cook for 5 minutes. Uncover and simmer until the liquid evaporates and fennel is very tender, 3-5 more minutes.
Transfer fennel mixture to a bowl and let cool to room temperature, about 15 minutes. Stir in goat cheese, olives, oregano, lemon zest, and lemon juice. Season with salt and pepper to taste.
2. Prepare the Pies:
 Preheat oven to 375°F and set rack in lower-middle position. Line a rimmed baking sheet with parchment paper.
Place 1 phyllo sheet on the counter (long side facing you), brush lightly with olive oil, and top with a second sheet. Cut the stacked phyllo lengthwise into three strips, each about 9x4⅔ inches.

Place a heaping tablespoon of filling in the bottom left corner of each strip. Fold the corner over the filling to form a triangle, then continue folding like a flag until you reach the end. Brush the outside with oil and place seam-side down on the baking sheet.
Repeat with the remaining phyllo sheets and filling to make 15 triangles total.
3. Bake and Serve:
 Bake for 10 to 15 minutes, rotating the sheet halfway through, until golden brown. Cool for 5 minutes on the baking sheet. Serve warm.

Mushroom Tart

Makes one 9-inch tart | Serves 4 to 6 | Vegetarian
CRUST

- 1¾ cups (8¾ oz) all-purpose flour
- 1 tbsp sugar
- ¾ tsp salt
- ⅔ cup extra-virgin olive oil
- ⅓ cup water

FILLING

- 2 tbsp extra-virgin olive oil, divided
- 1 lb white mushrooms, thinly sliced
- ½ tsp salt
- 2 tsp fresh thyme, minced
- 1 garlic clove, minced
- 1 oz Parmesan cheese, grated (½ cup)
- 4 oz part-skim ricotta cheese (½ cup)
- 1 oz mozzarella cheese, shredded (¼ cup)
- Salt and pepper to taste

Instructions
1. Make the Crust:
 Preheat oven to 350°F. Whisk flour, sugar, and salt in a bowl. Add oil and water and stir until clumps form and no dry flour remains.
Sprinkle walnut-size clumps of dough evenly in a 9-inch tart pan. Press into an even layer and up the sides.

Level off the top edge. Use any
leftover dough to patch holes.
Place the tart pan on a baking sheet
and bake on the lower oven rack
until golden and set, about 50
minutes, rotating halfway through.
Let cool completely.
2. Cook the Mushrooms:
 Heat 1 tbsp oil in a large skillet
over medium-high heat. Add mushrooms
and salt, and cook about 15 minutes,
stirring occasionally, until browned
and dry. Add thyme and garlic; cook
1 more minute. Set aside to cool
slightly.
3. Assemble and Bake:
 Mix Parmesan, ricotta, mozzarella,
and remaining 1 tbsp oil in a bowl.
Season with salt and pepper. Spread
cheese mixture in cooled tart shell.
Top with mushrooms.
Bake tart (still on sheet) until
filling is hot and bubbling at the
edges, 20-25 minutes. Let cool 10
minutes before slicing and serving.

Spanakopita (Greek Spinach Pie)

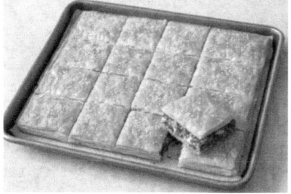

Serves 10 to 12 | Vegetarian
FILLING
- 20 oz curly-leaf spinach,
  stemmed
- ¼ cup water
- 8 oz feta cheese, crumbled (2
  cups)
- ¾ cup whole-milk Greek yogurt
- 4 scallions, thinly sliced
- 2 large eggs, lightly beaten
- ¼ cup chopped fresh mint
- 2 tbsp chopped fresh dill
- 3 garlic cloves, minced
- 1 tsp lemon zest + 1 tbsp lemon
  juice
- 1 tsp ground nutmeg
- ½ tsp pepper
- ¼ tsp salt
- ⅛ tsp cayenne pepper

PHYLLO LAYERS
- 7 tbsp extra-virgin olive oil
- 8 oz phyllo (14 by 9-inch
  sheets), thawed
- 1½ oz Pecorino Romano cheese,
  grated (¾ cup)
- 2 tsp sesame seeds (optional)

Instructions
1. Prep the Spinach Filling:
 In a large bowl, combine spinach
and water. Microwave until wilted
(about 5 minutes), then let sit
covered for 1 minute. Press out
moisture in a colander, chop the
spinach, and press again to remove
excess water. Mix spinach with
remaining filling ingredients.
2. Assemble the Base Layers:
 Preheat oven to 425°F with rack in
lower-middle position. Line a rimmed
baking sheet with parchment. Brush a
14x9-inch rectangle of oil on the
parchment. Lay down 1 phyllo sheet,
brush with oil, and repeat with 9
more sheets (10 total).
3. Add Filling and Top Layers:
 Spread spinach mixture evenly over
phyllo, leaving a ¼-inch border. Add
6 more phyllo sheets on top,
brushing each with oil and
sprinkling each with ~2 tbsp
Pecorino. Add 2 final sheets,
brushing each with oil (no cheese on
these top layers).
4. Score and Bake:
 Press gently to remove air pockets.
Use a sharp knife to score the top 3
layers into 24 pieces. Sprinkle with
sesame seeds (optional). Bake for
20-25 minutes until golden and
crisp.
5. Cool and Serve:
 Let cool on the baking sheet for at
least 10 minutes. Slide spanakopita
with parchment onto a cutting board,
slice along scored lines, and serve
warm or at room temp.

Pumpkin Borek

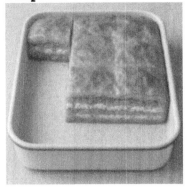

Serves 10 to 12 | Vegetarian

FILLING
- 1 tbsp extra-virgin olive oil
- 1 large onion, chopped
- 1½ tsp salt
- 3 garlic cloves, minced
- 1 tsp grated fresh ginger
- ½ tsp pepper
- 1½ cups dry white wine
- 3 (15 oz) cans unsweetened pumpkin puree
- 5 large eggs
- 12 oz halloumi cheese, grated (3 cups)
- 8 oz (1 cup) cottage cheese
- ½ cup chopped fresh mint

LAYERS
- ⅓ cup whole milk
- 1 large egg
- 2 lbs phyllo dough (14x9-inch sheets), thawed

Instructions

1. Make the Pumpkin Filling:
 Heat oil in a skillet over medium-high. Sauté onion and salt for 5 minutes until soft. Stir in garlic, ginger, and pepper; cook 30 seconds. Add wine, simmer, and cook until slightly reduced and onion is tender, 15-20 minutes (should yield 1¼ cups).
Transfer mixture to food processor and let cool slightly. Add pumpkin and eggs and blend until smooth, about 3 minutes.

2. Make the Cheese Filling:
 In a separate bowl, mix grated halloumi, cottage cheese, and mint. Set aside.

3. Prep the Dough and Oven:
 Preheat oven to 400°F. Whisk milk and egg together in a bowl. Trim 50 phyllo sheets to 12½x8½ inches. Grease a 13x9-inch baking dish.

4. Assemble the Borek:
- Spread 1 cup pumpkin filling on bottom of dish.
- Layer 5 phyllo sheets, brush with egg wash, top with 5 more sheets.
- Brush again, spread 2⅓ cups pumpkin filling.
- Repeat phyllo layering (5 sheets, egg wash, 5 more sheets).
- Spread half of cheese filling.
- Repeat phyllo layering.
- Press gently to compress layers.
- Repeat pumpkin and cheese layers once more, each time separated by 10 phyllo sheets (5+5 with egg wash in between).
- Top with remaining pumpkin filling.

5. Finish with Full-Size Phyllo:
 Trim 10 sheets to 13x9 inches. Lay 5 sheets, brush with egg wash, then 5 more sheets. Press down to flatten and clean up any spillover. Brush top with remaining egg wash.

6. Bake:
 Bake for 40-45 minutes, until top is puffed and golden brown and center hits 165°F. Let rest 30 minutes before slicing and serving.

Chicken B'stilla (Moroccan Savory-Sweet Pie)

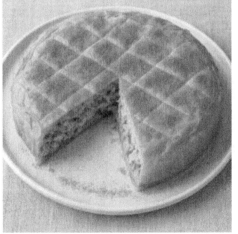

Serves 10 to 12

Ingredients

- ½ cup extra-virgin olive oil
- 1 onion, finely chopped
- ¾ tsp salt
- 1 tbsp grated fresh ginger
- ½ tsp black pepper
- ½ tsp ground turmeric
- ½ tsp paprika
- 1½ cups water
- 2 lbs boneless, skinless chicken thighs, trimmed
- 6 large eggs
- ½ cup minced fresh cilantro
- 1 lb phyllo dough (14x9-inch sheets), thawed
- 1½ cups slivered almonds, toasted and chopped
- ¼ cup confectioners' sugar
- 1 tbsp ground cinnamon

Instructions

1. Cook Chicken and Broth:
 In a 12-inch nonstick skillet, heat 1 tbsp oil over medium. Add onion and salt; cook until soft, 5 minutes. Stir in ginger, pepper, turmeric, and paprika; cook 30 seconds. Add water and chicken; bring to a simmer. Cover, reduce heat to low, and cook until chicken hits 175°F, 15-20 minutes. Transfer chicken to a cutting board, let cool, then shred with two forks. Transfer to a large bowl.

2. Make Custard:
 Whisk eggs in a small bowl. Bring remaining cooking liquid to a boil over high and reduce to 1 cup, about 10 minutes. Reduce heat to low. Whisking constantly, slowly add eggs to the broth and cook until mixture is like loose scrambled eggs, 6-8 minutes. Add to bowl with chicken and stir in cilantro. Wipe skillet clean and let it cool.

3. Build the Phyllo Base:
 Preheat oven to 375°F. Brush 1 phyllo sheet with oil and place it in the cooled skillet, letting the edges hang over. Turn skillet 30° and repeat with a second oiled sheet. Continue layering 10 more oiled sheets in a pinwheel pattern (12 total).

4. Add Almond Layer:
 Mix almonds with 3 tbsp sugar and 2 tsp cinnamon. Sprinkle over the phyllo base. Lay 2 more phyllo sheets over the almonds, brush with oil, rotate the skillet 90°, and add 2 more sheets (don't oil these).

5. Add Chicken Filling:
 Spoon the chicken mixture on top in an even layer.

6. Top and Seal:
 Stack 5 phyllo sheets, brush the top with oil, fold in half crosswise, brush again, and place over the filling. Fold the overhanging bottom layers over the top, pleating as you go. Press gently to seal and brush the top with oil.

7. Bake and Finish:
 Bake until crisp and golden, 35-40 minutes. Let cool for 15 minutes in the skillet. Mix remaining 1 tbsp sugar and 1 tsp cinnamon. Carefully slide b'stilla onto a cutting board, dust with cinnamon sugar, slice, and serve.

Fruit and Sweets

Apricot Spoon Sweets

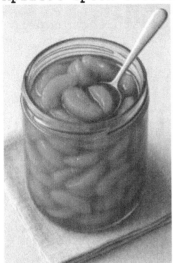

Makes 4 cups

Ingredients

- 1½ cups sugar
- 1 cup honey
- ¾ cup water
- 1½ lbs ripe but firm apricots, pitted and cut into ½-inch wedges
- 2 tbsp lemon juice

Instructions

1. In a Dutch oven, bring sugar, honey, and water to a boil over high heat. Cook, stirring occasionally, until syrup is reduced to about 2 cups, 10 minutes.
2. Add apricots and lemon juice. Return to a boil, then reduce heat to medium-low. Simmer until apricots soften and release some juices, about 5 minutes.
3. Remove from heat and let cool completely.
4. Transfer to an airtight container and refrigerate for 24 hours before serving. Keeps up to 1 week.

Dried Fruit Compote

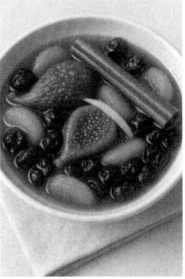

Serves 6

Ingredients

- 4 cups water
- 3 tbsp honey
- 2 (2-inch) strips lemon zest + 1 tbsp lemon juice
- 2 cinnamon sticks
- 1¼ tsp ground coriander
- 2 cups (12 oz) dried Turkish or Calimyrna figs, stemmed
- ¾ cup dried apricots
- ½ cup dried cherries

Instructions

1. In a large saucepan, bring water, honey, lemon zest and juice, cinnamon, and coriander to a boil over medium-high heat. Stir until honey dissolves, about 2 minutes.
2. Stir in figs and apricots. Return to a boil, then reduce heat to medium-low. Simmer until plump and tender, about 30 minutes.
3. Add cherries and cook until everything is tender and the liquid is syrupy, 15 to 20 minutes.
4. Remove from heat. Discard zest and cinnamon sticks. Let cool slightly and serve warm, at room temp, or chilled.

Turkish Stuffed Apricots with Rose Water and Pistachios

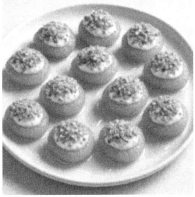

Serves 6
Ingredients
- ½ cup plain Greek yogurt
- ¼ cup sugar
- ½ tsp rose water
- ½ tsp lemon zest + 1 tbsp lemon juice
- Pinch of salt
- 2 cups water
- 4 green cardamom pods, cracked
- 2 bay leaves
- 24 dried apricots (about 1½ inches in diameter)
- ¼ cup shelled pistachios, toasted and finely chopped

Instructions
1. Make the filling:
   In a small bowl, mix yogurt, 1 tsp sugar, rose water, lemon zest, and a pinch of salt. Chill until ready to use.
2. Candy the apricots:
   In a small saucepan, combine water, cardamom pods, bay leaves, lemon juice, and remaining sugar. Bring to a simmer over medium-low heat and stir until sugar dissolves, about 2 minutes.
   Add apricots and simmer gently, stirring occasionally, until they're plump and tender, about 25-30 minutes. Transfer apricots to a plate with a slotted spoon and let cool.
3. Thicken the syrup:
   Discard the cardamom pods and bay leaves. Increase heat and boil the syrup until it thickens and reduces to about 3 tablespoons, 4-6 minutes. Let cool.
4. Stuff the apricots:
   Spoon the filling into a small zip-top bag and snip a ½-inch opening at one corner. Pipe yogurt into the cavity of each apricot. Press the filled side into the pistachios to coat.

Serve:
Arrange stuffed apricots on a platter and drizzle with the cooled syrup. Serve at room temp or slightly chilled.

Honey-Glazed Peaches with Hazelnuts

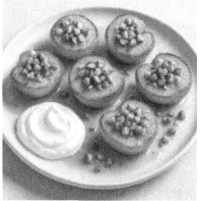

Serves 6 | Fast
Ingredients
- 2 tbsp lemon juice
- 1 tbsp sugar
- ¼ tsp salt
- 6 ripe but firm peaches, peeled, halved, and pitted
- ⅓ cup water
- ¼ cup honey
- 1 tbsp extra-virgin olive oil
- ¼ cup hazelnuts, toasted, skinned, and chopped

Instructions
1. Prep peaches:
   Adjust oven rack 6 inches from the broiler and heat the broiler. In a large bowl, mix lemon juice, sugar, and salt. Toss peaches in the mixture to coat evenly.
2. Broil the first time:
   Arrange peaches cut side up in a 12-inch broiler-safe skillet. Spoon any leftover lemon mixture into the centers. Pour water around the peaches. Broil

until they start to brown, 11–15 minutes.

3. Glaze and broil again:
   Mix honey and oil in a small bowl and microwave until warm, about 20 seconds. Stir to combine. Carefully remove skillet from oven. Brush half the honey mixture onto the peaches, then return to broiler until nicely glazed, 5–7 minutes.

4. Finish and serve:
   Take peaches out of the skillet and place on a platter. Simmer the leftover juices in the skillet over medium heat until syrupy, about 1 minute. Drizzle over peaches and sprinkle with hazelnuts. Serve warm.

Warm Figs with Goat Cheese and Honey

Serves 4 to 6 | Fast
Ingredients
- 1½ oz goat cheese
- 8 fresh figs, halved lengthwise
- 16 walnut halves, toasted
- 3 tbsp honey

Instructions
1. Heat oven to 500°F and adjust rack to the middle position.
2. Line a rimmed baking sheet with parchment. Top each fig half with about ½ tsp goat cheese and place on the sheet.
3. Bake until warmed through, about 4 minutes. Transfer to a serving platter.
4. Place a walnut half on each fig and drizzle with honey. Serve warm.

Peaches and Cherries Poached in Spiced Red Wine

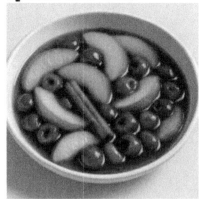

Serves 6 | Fast
Ingredients
- 1 lb fresh sweet cherries, pitted and halved
- 1 lb ripe but firm peaches, peeled, halved, pitted, and sliced ¼ inch thick
- ½ cinnamon stick
- 2 whole cloves
- 2 cups dry red wine
- 1 cup sugar

Instructions
1. Combine cherries, peaches, cinnamon stick, and cloves in a large bowl.
2. In a small saucepan, bring wine and sugar to a boil over high heat, stirring until the sugar dissolves—about 5 minutes.
3. Pour the hot syrup over the fruit mixture. Cover and let cool to room temperature.
4. Discard the cinnamon and cloves. Serve the fruit with some of the syrup, on its own or with Greek yogurt or crème fraîche.
5. serve.

Roasted Pears with Dried Apricots and Pistachios

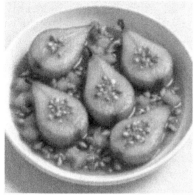

Serves 4 to 6
Ingredients
- 2 tbsp extra-virgin olive oil
- 4 ripe but firm Bosc or Bartlett pears (6-7 oz each), peeled, halved, and cored
- 1¼ cups dry white wine (like Sauvignon Blanc or Chardonnay)
- ½ cup dried apricots, quartered
- ⅓ cup sugar
- ¼ tsp ground cardamom
- ⅛ tsp salt
- 1 tsp lemon juice
- ⅓ cup shelled pistachios, toasted and chopped

Instructions
1. Prep and Sear the Pears
   Heat oven to 450°F and adjust rack to the middle position. Heat olive oil in a 12-inch oven-safe skillet over medium-high heat. Add pears cut side down and cook without moving until just beginning to brown, 3-5 minutes.
2. Roast in Oven
   Transfer skillet to oven and roast pears for 15 minutes. Carefully flip the pears and roast until a toothpick slips in and out easily, another 10-15 minutes.
3. Make the Sauce
   Using oven mitts, remove skillet from oven and transfer pears to a serving dish. Add wine, apricots, sugar, cardamom, and salt to the hot skillet. Bring to a simmer over medium-high heat, scraping up the browned bits, and cook until the sauce reduces to a

syrupy consistency, 7-10 minutes. Off heat, stir in lemon juice.
4. Finish and Serve
   Spoon the sauce and apricots over the pears. Sprinkle with pistachios and serve warm, optionally with Greek yogurt.

White Wine-Poached Pears with Lemon and Herbs

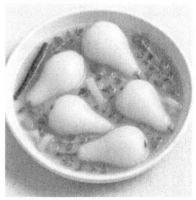

Serves 6 to 8
Ingredients
- 1 vanilla bean
- 1 (750-ml) bottle dry white wine (like Sauvignon Blanc or Chardonnay)
- ¾ cup sugar
- 6 (2-inch) strips lemon zest
- 5 sprigs fresh mint
- 3 sprigs fresh thyme
- ½ cinnamon stick
- ⅛ teaspoon salt
- 6 ripe but firm Bosc or Bartlett pears (about 8 oz each), peeled, halved, and cored

Instructions
1. Make the Poaching Liquid
   Split the vanilla bean lengthwise and scrape out the seeds. Add seeds and pod to a large saucepan along with the wine, sugar, lemon zest, mint, thyme, cinnamon stick, and salt. Bring to a boil over high heat, stirring occasionally, until sugar dissolves, about 5 minutes.
2. Poach the Pears
   Add the halved pears to the pot. Return to a boil, then reduce heat to medium-low. Cover and simmer until the

pears are tender and a toothpick slips in easily, 10-20 minutes, turning the pears gently every 5 minutes to ensure even cooking.
3. Finish the Syrup
Use a slotted spoon to transfer the pears to a shallow dish. Bring the poaching liquid back to a simmer and reduce until slightly thickened and measuring about 1¼ to 1½ cups, 15 minutes. Strain the syrup through a fine-mesh sieve over the pears, discarding the solids.
4. Chill and Serve
Let pears cool to room temperature in the syrup, then cover and chill in the fridge for at least 2 hours or up to 3 days. Serve chilled, spooning syrup over the pears. They're great on their own or with a spoonful of crème fraîche.

Melon, Plums, and Cherries with Mint and Vanilla

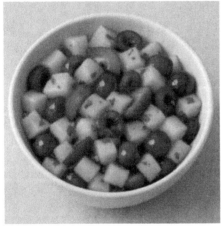

Serves 4 to 6 | Fast
Ingredients
- 4 tsp sugar
- 1 tbsp minced fresh mint
- 3 cups cantaloupe, cut into ½-inch pieces
- 2 plums, halved, pitted, and cut into ½-inch pieces
- 8 oz fresh sweet cherries, pitted and halved
- ¼ tsp vanilla extract
- 1 tbsp lime juice, plus more to taste
Instructions

1. In a large bowl, mash the sugar and mint together with a spatula until the sugar looks damp, about 30 seconds.
2. Add the cantaloupe, plums, cherries, and vanilla. Gently toss to combine.
3. Let the fruit sit at room temperature for 15 to 30 minutes, stirring now and then, until it releases its juices.
4. Stir in lime juice and adjust with more to taste. Serve.

Variation: **Peaches, Blackberries, and Strawberries with Basil and Pepper**

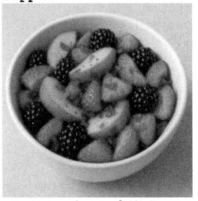

Serves 4 to 6 | Fast
Ingredients
- 4 tsp sugar
- 2 tbsp chopped fresh basil
- ½ tsp pepper
- 3 peaches, halved, pitted, and cut into ½-inch pieces
- 10 oz (2 cups) blackberries
- 10 oz strawberries, hulled and quartered (2 cups)
- 1 tbsp lime juice, plus more to taste
Instructions
1. Mash sugar, basil, and pepper in a large bowl until the sugar looks damp.
2. Add the peaches, blackberries, and strawberries and toss gently.
3. Let sit 15 to 30 minutes, stirring occasionally. Stir in lime juice and adjust to taste. Serve.

Strawberries with Balsamic Vinegar

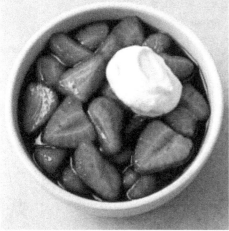

Serves 6 | Fast

Ingredients

- ⅓ cup balsamic vinegar
- 2 tsp granulated sugar
- ½ tsp lemon juice
- 2 lb strawberries, hulled and sliced ¼ inch thick (5 cups)
- ¼ cup packed light brown sugar
- Pinch of pepper

Instructions

1. Simmer vinegar, granulated sugar, and lemon juice in a small saucepan over medium heat until thickened and reduced to about 3 tbsp, around 3 minutes. Let cool.
2. Toss strawberries with brown sugar and pepper in a large bowl. Let sit at room temp for 10 to 15 minutes until juicy.
3. Drizzle with the balsamic syrup and toss gently to coat. Serve as is or with a dollop of sweetened mascarpone.

Nectarines and Berries in Prosecco

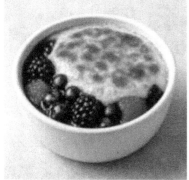

Serves 6 to 8 | Fast

Ingredients

- 10 oz (2 cups) blackberries or raspberries
- 10 oz strawberries, hulled and quartered (2 cups)
- 1 lb nectarines, pitted and sliced into ¼-inch wedges
- ¼ cup sugar, plus more to taste
- 1 tbsp orange liqueur (like Grand Marnier or triple sec)
- 1 tbsp chopped fresh mint
- ¼ tsp grated lemon zest
- 1 cup chilled prosecco

Instructions

1. In a large bowl, gently toss the berries, nectarines, sugar, orange liqueur, mint, and lemon zest together.
2. Let the mixture sit at room temperature for 10 to 15 minutes, stirring occasionally, until the fruit starts to release its juices.
3. Right before serving, pour prosecco over the fruit and stir gently. Taste and add more sugar if needed. Serve immediately.

Individual Fresh Berry Gratins

(Serves 4)

Ingredients

Berry Mixture

- 11 oz (2¼ cups) blackberries, blueberries, and/or raspberries
- 4 oz strawberries, hulled and halved or quartered (¾ cup)
- 2 tsp granulated sugar
- Pinch of salt

Zabaglione

- 3 large egg yolks
- 3 tbsp granulated sugar (divided)
- 3 tbsp dry white wine
- 2 tsp packed light brown sugar
- 3 tbsp heavy cream, chilled

Instructions

1. Prep the Berries
   Line a baking sheet with foil. In a bowl, toss all the berries with sugar and a pinch of salt. Divide evenly among four 6-

ounce gratin dishes on the baking sheet. Set aside.

2. Make the Zabaglione
   Whisk the egg yolks, 2 tbsp + 1 tsp of the sugar, and the wine in a medium glass bowl until sugar dissolves (about a minute). Set the bowl over a pot of barely simmering water and whisk constantly until it's frothy, then keep going until it thickens a bit—creamy and glossy, about 5-10 minutes. It should fall in soft mounds from the whisk. Remove from heat and whisk for another 30 seconds. Chill in the fridge for about 10 minutes until completely cool

3. Preheat the Broiler
   Position oven rack 6 inches from the broiler and turn it on. Mix the brown sugar with the remaining 2 tsp granulated sugar in a small bowl.

4. Finish the Zabaglione
   Whip the cream until it forms soft peaks (30-90 seconds). Gently fold it into the cooled egg mixture with a spatula. Spoon this over the berries in the ramekins and sprinkle the sugar mixture evenly on top. Let sit for 10 minutes at room temp so the sugar starts to dissolve.

5. Broil and Serve
   Broil until the tops are bubbly and caramelized—should take 1 to 4 minutes. Serve right away.

Greek Sesame-Honey Bars (Makes 32 bars)

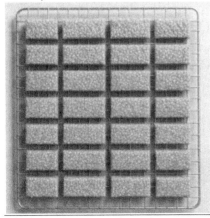

Ingredients
- 1¾ cups sesame seeds
- ¾ cup honey
- ¼ teaspoon salt

Instructions
1. Prep the Pan
   Adjust your oven rack to the middle and heat the oven to 350°F. Line an 8-inch square baking pan with two pieces of foil, crisscrossed with overhang on all sides. Press the foil into the corners and grease it lightly.

2. Toast the Seeds
   Spread the sesame seeds in a single layer on a rimmed baking sheet. Toast in the oven, stirring often, until golden—about 10 to 12 minutes. Move them to a bowl right away to stop the cooking.

3. Cook the Honey
   In a large saucepan, heat the honey over medium-high until it starts to bubble. Lower the heat to medium-low and cook, swirling the pan gently every so often, until the honey turns a deep amber and reaches 300-310°F on a thermometer (should take 4 to 5 minutes). Take it off the heat and stir in the toasted sesame seeds and salt until well mixed.

4. Shape the Bars
   Working quickly, pour the hot mixture into the prepared pan and use a greased spatula to spread it to the edges. Let it cool for about 5 minutes—just until it's cool enough to touch but still flexible. Use greased fingers to press it into an even layer.

5. Cool and Cut
   Let it cool until firm, about 20 minutes. Don't wait much longer or it'll be hard to cut. Use the foil to lift the block out of the pan and place it on a cutting board. Remove the foil and slice into thirty-two 2-by-1-inch bars. Place on a

wire rack to cool completely—
about 1 hour.
6. Let Them Crisp Up
   Transfer the bars to an
   airtight container and let them
   sit at room temp until fully
   crisp, about 8 hours. They'll
   keep for up to a month.

Lemon-Anise Biscotti (Makes about 48
cookies)

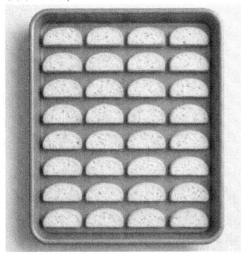

Ingredients
* 2 cups (10 oz) all-purpose
  flour
* 1 tsp baking powder
* ¼ tsp salt
* 1 cup (7 oz) sugar
* 2 large eggs
* 1 tbsp grated lemon zest
* 1 tbsp anise seeds
* ¼ tsp vanilla extract

Instructions
1. Set Up the Pan
   Preheat oven to 350°F. On a
   piece of parchment, draw two
   13x2-inch rectangles about 3
   inches apart. Place the
   parchment, marked side down, on
   a greased baking sheet.
2. Make the Dough
   In a small bowl, whisk
   together flour, baking powder,
   and salt. In a large bowl,
   whisk the sugar and eggs until
   the mixture is pale. Stir in
   lemon zest, anise seeds, and
   vanilla. Add the flour mixture
   and stir just until it comes
   together.

3. Shape and Bake
   Split the dough in half. With
   floured hands, shape each half
   into a 13x2-inch log on the
   parchment, using the lines as a
   guide. Smooth the tops and
   sides with a spatula lightly
   sprayed with oil. Bake until
   the loaves are golden and start
   to crack on top, about 35
   minutes, rotating the sheet
   halfway through.
4. Slice and Bake Again
   Let the loaves cool on the
   sheet for 10 minutes. Lower the
   oven temp to 325°F. Move loaves
   to a cutting board and slice on
   a slight angle into ½-inch-
   thick cookies using a serrated
   knife.
5. Final Bake
   Lay slices cut side down on
   the baking sheet, spacing them
   about ½ inch apart. Bake until
   golden and crisp on both sides,
   about 15 minutes, flipping
   halfway through. Let them cool
   on a wire rack. Store in an
   airtight container for up to a
   month.

Pignoli (Makes about 18 cookies)

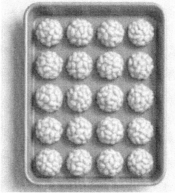

Ingredients
* 1⅔ cups slivered almonds
* 1⅓ cups (9⅓ oz) sugar
* 2 large egg whites
* 1 cup pine nuts

Instructions
1. Prep the Oven and Pans
   Set oven racks to the upper-
   middle and lower-middle
   positions. Preheat to 375°F.

Line two baking sheets with parchment paper.

2. Make the Dough
   In a food processor, blend the almonds and sugar until finely ground, about 30 seconds. Scrape down the sides, add the egg whites, and blend again until the mixture is smooth and sticky, about 30 seconds. Transfer to a bowl. Pour the pine nuts into a shallow dish.

3. Shape the Cookies
   Scoop about 1 tablespoon of dough and roll into a ball. Roll the ball in pine nuts to coat and place on the prepared baking sheet. Repeat with the rest of the dough, spacing cookies about 2 inches apart.

4. Bake
   Bake until the cookies are light golden brown, about 13 to 15 minutes, rotating and switching the sheets halfway through. Let cool on the baking sheet for 5 minutes, then transfer to a wire rack to cool completely.

Fig Phyllo Cookies
(Makes about 24 cookies)

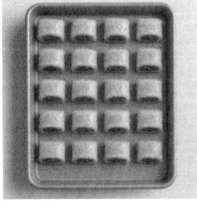

Ingredients
Sugar Syrup
- ¼ cup granulated sugar
- 2 tbsp water
- 2 tbsp honey
- 2 (2-inch) strips orange zest + 2 tbsp orange juice

Fig Filling
- 1½ cups (9 oz) dried figs, stemmed and halved
- ¾ cup water
- ½ cup sugar
- 1 tsp orange zest
- ½ tsp anise seeds
- ½ cup walnuts, toasted and chopped
- 1 tbsp dry sherry

Pastry
- 6 phyllo sheets (14x9-inch), thawed
- ¼ cup extra-virgin olive oil
- 2 tbsp confectioners' sugar

Instructions

1. Make the Syrup
   In a small saucepan, combine sugar, water, honey, and orange zest and juice. Bring to a boil over medium-high heat, stirring occasionally until sugar dissolves (about 2 minutes). Reduce heat and simmer until slightly thickened, about 3 minutes. Remove zest and set syrup aside.

2. Prepare the Filling
   In the same saucepan, combine figs, water, sugar, orange zest, and anise seeds. Simmer over medium heat until thick and syrupy, about 5 minutes. Let cool to room temp, about 1 hour.

3. Process the Filling
   Blend the fig mixture in a food processor until a thick paste forms (about 15 seconds). Add walnuts and sherry, then pulse until walnuts are finely chopped. Scoop mixture into a zip-top bag and snip a 1-inch opening in one corner.

4. Assemble the Cookies
   Preheat oven to 375°F and line a baking sheet with parchment. Lay out one phyllo sheet (long side facing you), brush lightly with olive oil, and dust with 1 tsp powdered sugar. Repeat twice more to make a 3-layer stack.

5. Fill and Roll
   Pipe half the fig filling in a line along the bottom edge, leaving a 1½-inch border. Fold the edge over the filling, then roll up tightly into a log. Place seam-side down and slice

into 12 pieces with a serrated knife. Place on baking sheet, spacing them about 1½ inches apart. Repeat with the rest of the phyllo and filling.
6. Bake and Finish
Bake for 15–20 minutes, rotating halfway, until cookies are golden. Drizzle the warm cookies with the syrup, let sit for 5 minutes, then transfer to a wire rack to cool completely.

Baklava
(Makes 32 to 40 pieces)

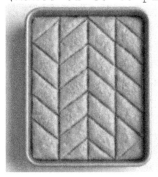

Ingredients
Sugar Syrup
- 1¼ cups (8¾ oz) sugar
- ¾ cup water
- ⅓ cup honey
- 3 (2-inch) strips lemon zest + 1 tbsp lemon juice
- 1 cinnamon stick
- 5 whole cloves
- ⅛ tsp salt

Nut Filling
- 1¾ cups slivered almonds
- 1 cup walnuts
- 2 tbsp sugar
- 1¼ tsp ground cinnamon
- ¼ tsp ground cloves
- ⅛ tsp salt

Pastry
- 5 tbsp extra-virgin olive oil
- 1 lb phyllo dough (14x9-inch sheets), thawed

Instructions
1. Make the Syrup
In a small saucepan, combine all syrup ingredients and bring to a boil over medium-high heat, stirring occasionally. Simmer until sugar dissolves, about 5 minutes. Pour into a measuring cup and let cool. Discard the zest, cinnamon stick, and cloves.
2. Make the Filling
Pulse almonds in a food processor until finely chopped (about 20 pulses), then do the same with walnuts (about 15 pulses). Mix together in a bowl and set aside 1 tablespoon for garnish. Stir in sugar, cinnamon, cloves, and salt.
3. Assemble the Layers
Preheat oven to 300°F and adjust rack to the lower-middle position. Grease a 13x9-inch pan. Lay 1 sheet of phyllo in the bottom, brush with oil, and repeat with 7 more sheets (8 total).
4. Add Nuts and Build
Sprinkle 1 cup nut filling evenly over phyllo. Add 6 more phyllo sheets, brushing each with oil, then another cup of nuts. Repeat again with 6 sheets and the final cup of nuts.
5. Finish the Top Layers
Add 8 more sheets on top, brushing each with oil except the final one. Gently press the layers with your palms to flatten and get rid of air bubbles. Use the remaining oil (about 2 tbsp) to brush the top.
6. Cut and Bake
Cut the baklava into diamonds using a serrated knife. Bake for 1½ hours, rotating the pan halfway through, until golden and crisp.
7. Add Syrup
Right after baking, pour all but 2 tablespoons of the syrup into the cut lines (it'll sizzle). Drizzle the rest over the top and sprinkle each piece with a pinch of the reserved ground nuts.
8. Let It Rest
Let it cool in the pan for about 3 hours, then cover with foil and let sit at room temperature for 8 hours before

serving.

Almond Cake
(Serves 12)

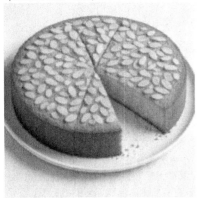

Ingredients
- 1½ cups + ⅓ cup blanched sliced almonds, toasted
- ¾ cup (3¾ oz) all-purpose flour
- ¾ tsp salt
- ¼ tsp baking powder
- ⅛ tsp baking soda
- 4 large eggs
- 1¼ cups (8¾ oz) + 2 tbsp sugar
- 1 tbsp + ½ tsp grated lemon zest (from 2 lemons)
- ¾ tsp almond extract
- ½ cup extra-virgin olive oil

Instructions
1. Prep the Pan
   Adjust oven rack to the middle position and preheat to 300°F. Grease a 9-inch round cake pan and line the bottom with parchment paper.
2. Make the Almond Mixture
   In a food processor, combine 1½ cups of the almonds with the flour, salt, baking powder, and baking soda. Pulse 10 to 15 times until the almonds are finely ground. Transfer to a bowl.
3. Mix the Wet Ingredients
   In the now-empty food processor, blend the eggs, 1¼ cups sugar, 1 tbsp lemon zest, and almond extract for about 30 seconds until pale and frothy. While the processor is running, slowly drizzle in the olive oil. This should take about 10 seconds.

4. Finish the Batter
   Add the almond-flour mixture and pulse 4 to 5 times until just combined. Pour the batter into your prepared pan and smooth the top.
5. Top the Cake
   In a small bowl, rub together the remaining 2 tbsp sugar and ½ tsp lemon zest with your fingers until it smells fragrant. Sprinkle the remaining ⅓ cup sliced almonds over the cake, then top evenly with the lemon-sugar mix.
6. Bake
   Bake until the center is set and springs back when lightly pressed, and a toothpick comes out clean—about 55 to 65 minutes. Rotate the pan halfway through baking.
7. Cool and Serve
   Let the cake cool in the pan for 15 minutes, then run a paring knife around the edge to loosen it. Remove the cake, discard the parchment, and cool completely on a wire rack (about 2 hours). Serve and enjoy!

Orange Polenta Cake
(Serves 12)

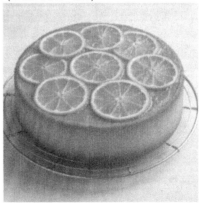

Why This Works:
Ingredients
- 1½ cups (8¼ oz) instant polenta
- 1½ cups whole milk
- 2 oranges + 2 tsp grated orange zest
- ⅓ cup (2⅓ oz) packed brown sugar
- 2 tsp cornstarch
- Salt

- 1 cup (5 oz) all-purpose flour
- 1 tsp baking powder
- ½ tsp baking soda
- 3 large eggs
- 1 cup (7 oz) granulated sugar
- 6 tbsp extra-virgin olive oil
- 2 tsp vanilla extract

Instructions
1. Toast and Soak the Polenta
   Preheat oven to 350°F. Spread polenta on a baking sheet and toast until fragrant, about 10 minutes. Transfer to a large bowl, stir in milk and orange zest, and let it sit for 10 minutes to absorb. Break up any clumps with your hands into fine crumbs. Set aside.
2. Prepare the Pan and Oranges
   Grease a 9-inch round cake pan, line with parchment, and grease the parchment. In a small bowl, mix brown sugar, cornstarch, and ⅛ tsp salt. Sprinkle the mixture evenly in the pan. Peel the oranges, removing the pith, then slice them into thin ⅛-inch rounds. Arrange the slices in a single layer over the sugar mixture (a little overlap is fine).
3. Make the Batter
   In a medium bowl, whisk flour, baking powder, baking soda, and ½ tsp salt. In a stand mixer fitted with the paddle, beat eggs and granulated sugar on medium until pale and tripled in volume—about 6-8 minutes. Reduce speed to low and mix in oil and vanilla. Add the polenta crumbs and mix until combined. Add the flour mixture in 3 additions, scraping down the bowl as needed. Give the batter one final stir by hand.
4. Bake the Cake
   Pour the batter over the orange slices and smooth the top. Bake for 50 to 60 minutes, rotating halfway, until golden and a toothpick in the center comes out clean.
5. Cool and Unmold
   Let the cake cool in the pan for 15 minutes. Run a paring knife around the edges. Set a wire rack over the pan and invert the cake onto the rack. Let it sit for a minute so the cake releases, then lift off the pan. If any orange slices stick, carefully remove and place them back on top. Let the cake cool completely—about 2 hours.

Serve as is or with lightly sweetened whipped cream.

Olive Oil-Yogurt Cake
(Serves 12)

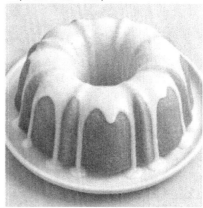

Ingredients
Cake:
- 3 cups (15 oz) all-purpose flour
- 1 tbsp baking powder
- 1 tsp salt
- 1¼ cups (8¾ oz) granulated sugar
- 4 large eggs
- 1¼ cups extra-virgin olive oil
- 1 cup plain whole-milk yogurt

Lemon Glaze:
- 2-3 tbsp lemon juice
- 1 tbsp plain whole-milk yogurt
- 2 cups (8 oz) confectioners' sugar

Instructions
1. Preheat & Prep
   Set oven rack to lower-middle position and heat to 350°F. Grease a 12-cup nonstick Bundt pan.
2. Make the Batter
   In a bowl, whisk flour, baking powder, and salt. In a large separate bowl, whisk sugar and

eggs until pale and frothy—about 1 minute. Whisk in olive oil and yogurt until smooth. Add dry ingredients and stir with a rubber spatula until no dry flour remains.

3. Bake
   Pour the batter into the pan, smooth the top, and tap it gently on the counter to settle. Bake for 40 to 45 minutes, rotating halfway through, until a skewer comes out clean.

4. Make the Glaze
   Whisk together 2 tbsp lemon juice, yogurt, and powdered sugar. Add more juice a little at a time until it's thick but pourable (it should leave a faint trail when drizzled).

5. Glaze & Cool
   Let the cake cool in the pan for 10 minutes, then turn it out onto a wire rack. Drizzle with half the glaze while still warm. Let cool for an hour, then drizzle with the rest. Let cool completely before serving.

Lemon Yogurt Mousse with Blueberry Sauce (Serves 6)

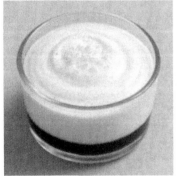

Ingredients
Blueberry Sauce:
- 4 oz (¾ cup) blueberries
- 2 tbsp sugar
- 2 tbsp water
- Pinch of salt

Mousse:
- ¾ tsp unflavored gelatin
- 3 tbsp water
- ½ cup whole Greek yogurt
- ¼ cup heavy cream
- 1½ tsp grated lemon zest + 3 tbsp lemon juice
- 1 tsp vanilla extract
- ⅛ tsp salt
- 3 large egg whites
- ¼ tsp cream of tartar
- 6 tbsp (2⅔ oz) sugar

Instructions
1. Make the Sauce
   Simmer blueberries, sugar, water, and salt over medium heat until sugar dissolves and berries are warmed, about 2-4 minutes. Blend until smooth, then strain. Spoon into six 4-oz ramekins and chill for 20 minutes.

2. Start the Mousse
   Sprinkle gelatin over 3 tbsp water and let it sit for 5 minutes. In a bowl, whisk together yogurt, cream, lemon zest and juice, vanilla, and salt.

3. Cook Egg Whites
   In a stand mixer bowl, whisk egg whites, cream of tartar, and sugar. Set the bowl over barely simmering water and whisk constantly until tripled in volume and about 160°F, 5-10 minutes.

4. Finish the Mousse
   Off heat, quickly whisk in the softened gelatin until dissolved. Transfer to the stand mixer with whisk attachment and beat on medium-high until stiff, shiny peaks form—about 4-6 minutes. Add yogurt mixture and mix just until combined.

5. Chill and Set
   Divide mousse over the chilled sauce in ramekins. Cover with plastic wrap and refrigerate until set, 6-8 hours. Serve chilled.

Semolina Pudding with Almonds and Dates
(Serves 6 to 8)

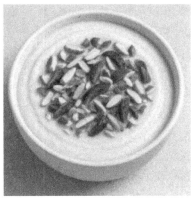

Ingredients

- 1 tbsp extra-virgin olive oil
- ¾ cup fine semolina flour
- 4½ cups whole milk, plus more if needed
- ½ cup sugar
- ½ tsp ground cardamom
- ⅛ tsp saffron threads, crumbled
- ⅛ tsp salt
- ½ cup slivered almonds, toasted and chopped
- 3 oz pitted dates, thinly sliced (about ½ cup)

Instructions

1. Toast the Semolina
   Heat olive oil in a 12-inch skillet over medium until shimmering. Add semolina and cook, stirring occasionally, until golden and fragrant—about 3 to 5 minutes. Transfer to a bowl.
2. Make the Pudding Base
   In a large saucepan, bring milk, sugar, cardamom, saffron, and salt to a simmer over medium heat. Slowly whisk in the semolina, one tablespoon at a time, stirring constantly. Cook until it thickens slightly and just starts to bubble—about 3 minutes. Take it off the heat, cover, and let it rest for 30 minutes.
3. Finish and Serve
   Stir to loosen the pudding and add a splash of warm milk if it seems too thick. Spoon into bowls and top with almonds and sliced dates. Serve warm for the creamiest texture.

Greek Lemon Rice Pudding

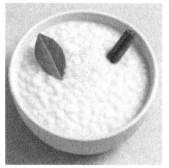

Serves: 8

Ingredients:
- 2 cups water
- 1 cup Arborio rice
- ½ teaspoon salt
- 1 vanilla bean, seeds scraped
- 4½ cups whole milk, plus extra if needed
- ½ cup sugar
- ½ cinnamon stick
- 2 bay leaves
- 2 teaspoons grated lemon zest

Directions:
1. Bring water to a boil in a saucepan. Add rice and salt. Cover and simmer gently on low until water is nearly absorbed (15-20 minutes).
2. Stir in vanilla bean with seeds, milk, sugar, cinnamon stick, and bay leaves. Simmer uncovered, stirring frequently, until rice is tender and pudding thickens to yogurt consistency (35-45 minutes).
3. Remove from heat; discard vanilla bean, cinnamon, and bay leaves. Mix in lemon zest. Cool completely (about 2 hours), stir gently, adjust consistency with extra milk, and serve chilled or at room temperature.

Raspberry Sorbet

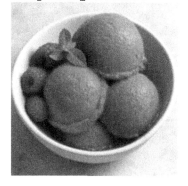

Makes: 1 quart (serves 8)
Ingredients:
- 1 cup water
- 1 teaspoon low/no-sugar fruit pectin
- ⅛ teaspoon salt
- 1¼ pounds (4 cups) fresh/frozen raspberries, thawed if frozen
- ½ cup plus 2 tablespoons sugar
- ¼ cup light corn syrup

Directions:
1. In a saucepan, heat water, pectin, and salt, stirring occasionally, until pectin dissolves (~5 min). Let cool slightly (10 min).
2. Blend raspberries, sugar, corn syrup, and cooled water-pectin mixture until smooth. Strain to remove seeds, pressing to extract liquid. Place 1 cup puree into a small bowl and freeze; refrigerate remaining puree (at least 4 hrs or overnight).
3. Combine frozen puree with chilled puree, mixing until completely smooth. Transfer to ice cream maker and churn until thick and lighter in color (15–25 min).
4. Pack sorbet tightly into a container to remove air pockets. Freeze until firm (at least 2 hrs, up to 5 days). Let

stand at room temperature for 5 min before serving.

Lemon Ice

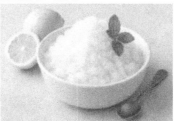

Makes: 1 quart (serves 8)
Ingredients:
- 2¼ cups spring water (preferred)
- 1 cup fresh lemon juice (from about 6 lemons)
- 1 cup sugar
- 2 tablespoons vodka (optional)
- ⅛ teaspoon salt

Directions:
1. In a bowl, whisk all ingredients until sugar dissolves. Pour mixture into 2 ice cube trays; freeze until solid, at least 3 hours (up to 5 days).
2. Chill a medium bowl in freezer. Pulse half of the frozen cubes in a food processor until creamy (about 18 pulses); transfer to chilled bowl. Repeat with remaining cubes. Serve immediately.

CHAPTER 10 - The Metaboost Diet for Life

Maintaining Your Progress on the Metaboost Diet

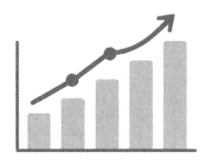

At some point on your health journey, you'll reach the stage where your goal is no longer weight loss, but maintaining the progress you've made—keeping the weight off and preserving your new, healthier habits. Most diet plans don't clearly address this phase, but the **Metaboost Diet** does. Its maintenance approach isn't just about staying at your current weight—it's about fully embracing and sustaining the **lifestyle** that got you there. The most successful individuals are those who consistently maintain the positive dietary and lifestyle patterns that helped them reach their goals.

After a month of following the Metaboost Diet, you've likely adapted to **intermittent fasting** and begun to naturally include **anti-inflammatory foods**, proper **macronutrient balance**, and optimal **micronutrient intake** into your routine. These behaviors, once habitual, become the foundation for long-term success.

Think of your new habits like trails in a forest. The more you walk them, the more well-worn they become—making them the easiest and most enjoyable routes to follow. That's how it should feel when you return to these new lifestyle habits—natural, rewarding, and sustainable.

The Metaboost Diet is about **restoring health and wellness**, especially during midlife—a period that can span 40% or more of your life. You've not only reached a healthy weight but also improved your overall health, and now you want to **stay on track**.

Transitioning to Maintenance Mode

To sustain your progress, enter what we call **"maintenance mode."** This means reinforcing your positive habits while allowing for more flexibility. The key is to **build stability**, not abandon your routine. Here's how:

Keep Up With Intermittent Fasting

By now, fasting should feel like second nature. What might have started as a temporary experiment has likely become a **long-term wellness tool**—supporting weight management, reducing inflammation, and boosting how you feel day to day.

Though intermittent fasting may not cause dramatic weight loss on its own, its real strength lies in helping you **keep the weight off**. It's now a core part of weight maintenance advice given to countless women.

There's science behind this: Traditional calorie-counting has proven ineffective for long-term results, with 95% of dieters regaining weight within a year—often adding more. Worse, they often lose valuable **muscle mass** in the process.

A 2021 study by researchers at the University of Kansas Medical Center confirmed that **intermittent fasting** can be more effective than calorie counting for long-term weight maintenance.
Bottom line: Intermittent fasting is a reliable, lifelong strategy for managing weight and inflammation.

Stick with Anti-Inflammatory Eating
You've seen firsthand how your diet impacts inflammation, metabolism, weight, and overall health. Unlike quick-fix programs, the Metaboost Diet is a **sustainable eating pattern** with anti-inflammatory nutrition at its core.
The goal now is to **expand your food choices** while still prioritizing high-antioxidant, fiber-rich, nutrient-dense foods like fruits, vegetables, healthy fats, and lean protein.
You can now reintroduce additional **anti-inflammatory foods**, such as:
- Extra servings of fruit like grapes, melons, papaya, peaches, or pineapple
- More starchy carbs like sweet potatoes, squash, root vegetables, and whole grains

These foods are powerful inflammation fighters—just be sure to continue **tracking your macros** to align with your maintenance goals.

Adjust Your Macronutrient Ratios Gradually

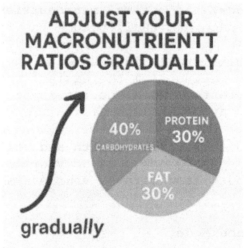

As your health improves, you can begin to shift your **macro ratios** to support maintenance rather than fat-burning. This means slightly **increasing carbs**, decreasing fats, and keeping protein moderate.
Here's a suggested progression:
- **Start with**: 60% fat, 20% protein, 20% carbohydrates
- **Transition to**: 50% fat, 20% protein, 30% carbohydrates
- **Maintain at**: 40% fat, 20% protein, 40% carbohydrates

Take your time—each shift may take several weeks to become habit. Be mindful of how your body responds to each change, and **track progress**, both in weight and non-scale victories like energy, waist-to-hip ratio, or inflammation symptoms.
A **5-pound weight fluctuation** is usually nothing to worry about. But if weight gain exceeds that or your health markers regress, consider temporarily

reverting to the original fat-burning macro ratios (70% fat, 20% protein, 10% carbs).

Tips for adjusting macros in maintenance:

- Use recipes in the book, tweaking them to suit new macro needs
- Add in whole grains, legumes, starchy veggies, and fruits in place of lower-carb foods
- Slightly cut back on fat—try using half an avocado instead of a whole one
- Focus on **whole, unprocessed foods**. If it grows from the ground and doesn't need a label, it's usually a yes. If it comes in a box and looks man-made, it's likely a no.

Don't forget to **read labels** on sauces and condiments—look out for added sugars and inflammatory ingredients.

Embrace the Joy of Lasting Change

The transformation you've made is profound—and it's just the beginning.

Valerie, for example, experienced significant changes after a hysterectomy at 43. By 50, she had gained weight, particularly around her midsection. After following the Metaboost Diet, she dropped to her goal weight of 120 pounds, eliminated bloating, and got rid of her sugar cravings—all without restrictive gimmicks.

Laurie, navigating menopause, lost 12 pounds in six weeks and experienced major relief from chronic hip pain. A busy midwife, she now feels vibrant and healthy, with no need for drastic interventions.

Mayra saw her blood markers normalize—no longer prediabetic or borderline high cholesterol—and her menopause symptoms disappeared entirely.

Debbie, a long-term intermittent faster, lost 77 pounds and has maintained her weight—ending her years of yo-yo dieting. "I wish I had discovered fasting earlier in life," she said.

Maintenance Meal Plans

To support your maintenance journey, sample menus are provided—both traditional and vegetarian—featuring modified recipes that align with your adjusted macro needs. These are designed to help you stay on track while enjoying greater food flexibility.

Conventional Menu

Day 1

- **Breakfast:** Meredith Shirk's Parfait
- **Midday Snack:** Nutty Banana Toast
- **Lunch/Dinner:** Meatloaf served with Mashed Cauliflower and a Baked Sweet Potato
- **Evening Snack:** Date Night

Macros:

- Fat: 43%
- Protein: 21%
- Net Carbohydrates: 36%
- Fiber: 29g

Day 2

- **Breakfast:** Mini Avocado "For Life" Toast
- **Midday Snack:** Chickpea and Tomato Salad

- **Lunch/Dinner**: Lemon-Caper Chicken with Farro
- **Evening Snack**: Summer Fruit Salad

Macros:
- Fat: 40%
- Protein: 24%
- Net Carbohydrates: 36%
- Fiber: 34g

Vegetarian Menu
Day 1
- **Breakfast**: Tofu with Peanut Sauce and Brown Rice
- **Midday Snack**: Two hard-boiled eggs
- **Lunch/Dinner**: Vegan Protein Lower-Fat Salad
- **Evening Snack**: Baked Cinnamon Apple with Raisins

Macros:
- Fat: 47%
- Protein: 16%
- Net Carbohydrates: 37%
- Fiber: 27g

Day 2
- **Breakfast**: Oat Cakes topped with Almond Butter and Blueberries
- **Midday Snack**: Green Almond Butter Smoothie
- **Lunch/Dinner**: Slow Cooker Mushroom Stroganoff with Creamy Brown Rice
- **Evening Snack**: Lemon-Ricotta Dip served with Pear Slices

Macros:
- Fat: 48%
- Protein: 16%
- Net Carbohydrates: 36%
- Fiber: 31g

Dining Out While Following the Metaboost Diet

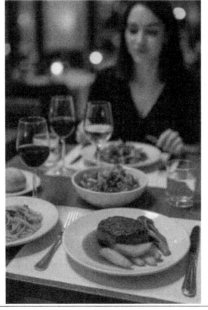

One of the best parts of the Metaboost Diet is its flexibility—it's not just designed for home-cooked meals. Eating out is absolutely doable, as long as you make smart choices aligned with your goals.

Restaurants today are increasingly offering healthier, fresher options. Many menus now feature grilled meats, fresh fish, a wide variety of vegetables, and other wholesome ingredients, making it easier than ever to stay on track while dining out.

A good rule of thumb is to build your plate around a **lean protein**, some **non-starchy vegetables** (like a side salad or steamed veggies), and a **nutrient-dense starch** such as a small portion of sweet potato or brown rice.

For your main course, opt for items like grilled steak, roasted chicken or turkey, or fish prepared by baking, broiling, or grilling. Pair your protein with vegetables or a fresh salad with vinaigrette dressing.

Don't hesitate to request substitutions—most restaurants are happy to accommodate. For example, ask to swap out fries for extra veggies. This way, tempting foods don't even land on your plate.

Watch out for restaurant-sized portions, which are often much larger than you'd prepare at home. Eat until satisfied, and take leftovers home for another meal.

Dining Out Tips by Cuisine

Sandwich and Burger Joints:
Many places now offer lettuce wraps as a bun alternative. Request your sandwich or burger on a lettuce leaf to avoid processed carbs.

Bowls and Entrée Salads:
Look for customizable bowls—often found at Mexican or Southwestern spots—that can include protein, greens, legumes, a bit of cheese, salsa, and guacamole. Entree salads with grilled meats, beans, avocado, and vinaigrette are also great options. Some Mexican restaurants even offer fiber-rich tortillas.

Asian Cuisine:
Stir-fry dishes with meat or seafood and vegetables are common. Ask for a light sauce and a small serving of brown rice. Dishes like moo shu chicken or moo goo gai pan are typically full of vegetables. Start your meal with a light, broth-based soup to help fill you up.

Steakhouses:
It's easy to find diet-friendly meals at steakhouses—think grilled steak, fish, or chicken with veggie sides or salads. Just avoid sugary glazes and opt for simple toppings like sautéed mushrooms.

Mediterranean and Greek:
Grilled meats and Greek salads are ideal picks. If you're vegetarian, order hummus with cucumber slices instead of pita bread.

Italian Restaurants:
Focus on the *secondi* (main dish) section of the menu, which often includes protein-centered meals without pasta. Go for fish, chicken, or steak with olive oil-dressed vegetables, and skip the bread.

Indian Cuisine:
Tandoori chicken is a standout choice. Add a side of veggies or a small portion of curried chickpeas. Indian dishes often include anti-inflammatory spices, which complement your eating plan.

Pizza Places:
Many spots now offer cauliflower crusts. Load your pizza with vegetables like peppers, onions, and mushrooms. Add olives for a healthy fat boost.

Breakfast Dining:
If your fast is over, stick to eggs, turkey bacon, and a small fruit portion. Veggie-packed omelets are another great pick.

Lifestyle Practices to Support Your Metaboost Diet Habits

Now that you've established the three core habits of the Metaboost Diet, continue to reinforce your progress by focusing on other key lifestyle choices: getting proper sleep, staying active, and practicing mindful self-reflection.

Prioritize Sleep for Long-Term Health

Cutting back on sleep might feel like a productivity hack, but the long-term health costs are steep.

Lack of sleep disrupts your hunger hormones. Ghrelin, which stimulates appetite, increases with insufficient rest—leading to more cravings the next day. At the same time, cortisol rises, which signals your liver to release glucose while lowering insulin response, causing blood sugar spikes and intense cravings—often for refined carbs. Sleep deprivation has also been linked to mood disorders and insulin resistance.

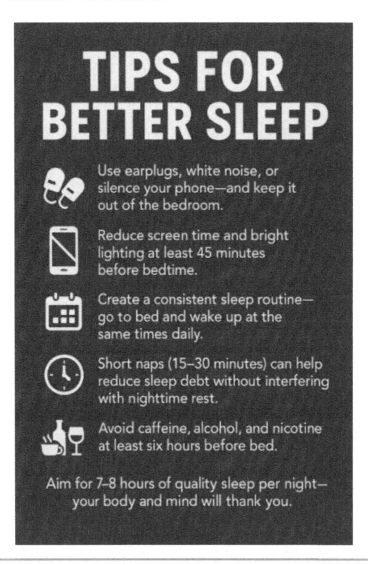

Keep Moving

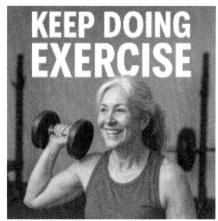

If you began exercising during the Metaboost Diet, now is the time to keep that momentum going. Physical activity supports **weight maintenance** and addresses midlife symptoms in powerful ways.

Exercise reshapes your body composition by increasing **muscle mass** and reducing **fat stores**, helping you maintain a healthy weight. It also improves **bone density**, lowering your risk of osteoporosis—a major concern for women during and after menopause.

Common midlife aches—like joint, back, or hip pain—often respond well to consistent movement. Even areas that feel stiff or sore at first tend to feel better the more you move them.

Exercise also helps redistribute **visceral fat**, which is the dangerous belly fat associated with chronic illness. Combined with anti-inflammatory eating, physical activity protects against conditions like:

- Type 2 diabetes
- High blood pressure
- Heart disease
- Certain cancers
- Fatty liver disease
- Breast cancer

Beyond physical benefits, regular movement elevates your mood, relieves stress, and builds self-confidence. You'll find yourself more energized and productive when you make activity part of your routine.

It's never too late to start. Even if your life is busy or you've been inactive for years, adding just a **20-minute walk**, **yoga class**, or **strength training session** can lead to lasting improvements in health and wellbeing.

Reflect on Your Journey

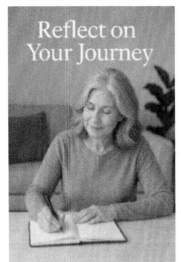

Reflect on Your Journey

Now is a great time to return to the journal you started at the beginning of the Metaboost Diet. Look back on your progress—and look forward to the future. What kind of life do you envision from here?

Ask yourself:

- What does my healthiest, happiest life look like?
- What dreams or goals do I still want to pursue?
- If I couldn't fail, what would I do?

Whether your vision includes stronger relationships, a meaningful career, or simply staying healthy enough to enjoy your grandchildren, allow yourself to dream freely.

This kind of clarity helps anchor your choices and gives you purpose. It reminds you that **something wonderful is always ahead.**

You're entering a new chapter—one filled with confidence, health, and possibility. Embrace it fully.

REFERENCES

Chapter 1

American Heart Association. 2015. "Menopause and Heart Disease." July 31. At www.heart.org.

Chopra, S., et al. 2019. "Weight Management Module for Perimenopausal Women: A Practical Guide for Gynecologists." Journal of Mid-Life Health 10: 165-72.

Dunneram, Y., et al. 2021. "Dietary Patterns and Age at Natural Menopause: Evidence from the UK Women's Cohort Study." Maturitas 143: 165-70.

Malabanan, A. O., and M. F. Holick. 2003. "Vitamin D and Bone Health in Postmenopausal Women." Journal of Women's Health 12: 151-56.

Saccomani, S., et al. 2017. "Does Obesity Increase the Risk of Hot Flashes among Midlife Women?: A Population-Based Study." Menopause 24: 1065-70.

Thurston, R. C., et al. 2008. "Abdominal Adiposity and Hot Flashes among Midlife Women." Menopause 15: 429-34.

Chapter 2

Aune, D., 2017. "Fruit and Vegetable Intake and the Risk of Cardiovascular Disease, Total Cancer and All-Cause Mortality: A Systematic Review and Dose-Response Meta-Analysis of Prospective Studies." International Journal of Epidemiology 46: 1029-56.

Ludwig, D., et al. 2020. "The Carbohydrate-Insulin Model: A Physiological Perspective on the Obesity Pandemic." American Journal of Clinical Nutrition 114: 1873-85.

Misra, S., and D. Mohanty. 2019. "Psychobiotics: A New Approach for Treating Mental Illness?" Critical Reviews in Food Science and Nutrition 59: 1230-36.

Pereira, M., et al. 2005. "Fast-Food Habits, Weight Gain, and Insulin Resistance (the CARDIA Study): 15-Year Prospective Analysis." The Lancet 365: 36-42.

Steptoe, A., et al. 2007. "The Effects of Tea on Psychophysiological Stress Responsivity and Post-Stress Recovery: A Randomised Double-Blind Trial." Psychopharmacology 190: 81-89.

Chapter 3

Egger, G. 1992. "The Case for Using Waist to Hip Ratio Measurements in Routine Medical Checks." Medical Journal of Australia 156: 280-85.

Chapter 4

Alirezaei, M., et al. 2010. "Short-Term Fasting Induces Profound Neuronal Autophagy." Autophagy 6: 702-10.

Baik, S. H., et al. 2020. "Intermittent Fasting Increases Adult Hippocampal Neurogenesis." Brain and Behavior 10: e01444.

Barnosky, A. R., et al. 2014. "Intermittent Fasting vs. Daily Calorie Restriction for Type 2 Diabetes Prevention: A Review of Human Findings." Translational Research 164: 302-11.

Collier, R. 2013. "Intermittent Fasting: The Science of Going Without." Canadian Medical Association Journal 185: e363-64.

de Cabo, R., and Mattson, M. P. 2019. "Effects of Intermittent Fasting on Health, Aging, and Disease." New England Journal of Medicine 381: 2541-51.

Guolin, L., et al. 2017. "Intermittent Fasting Promotes White Adipose Browning and Decreases Obesity by Shaping the Gut Microbiota." Cell Metabolism 26: 672–85.

Hartman, M. L., et al. 1992. "Augmented Growth Hormone (GH) Secretory Burst Frequency and Amplitude Mediate Enhanced GH Secretion during a Two-Day Fast in Normal Men." Journal of Clinical Endocrinology and Metabolism 74: 757–65.

Ho, K. Y., et al. 1988. "Fasting Enhances Growth Hormone Secretion and Amplifies the Complex Rhythms of Growth Hormone Secretion in Man." Journal of Clinical Investigation 81: 968–75.

Horne, B. D., et al. 2022. "Intermittent Fasting and Changes in Galectin-3: A Secondary Analysis of a Randomized Controlled Trial of Disease-Free Subjects." Nutrition, Metabolism, and Cardiovascular Diseases 32: 1538–48.

Jordan, S., et al. 2019. "Dietary Intake Regulates the Circulating Inflammatory Monocyte Pool." Cell 178: 1102–14.e17.

Klempel, M. C., et al. 2012. "Intermittent Fasting Combined with Calorie Restriction Is Effective for Weight Loss and Cardio-Protection in Obese Women." Nutrition Journal 11: 98.

Lean, M. Ej., et al. 2018. "PriMeredithCare-Led Weight Management for Remission of Type 2 Diabetes (DiRECT): An Open-Label, Cluster-Randomised Trial." The Lancet 391: 541–51.

Longo, V. D., et al. 2015. "Interventions to Slow Aging in Humans: Are We Ready?" Aging Cell 14: 497–510.

Longo, V. D., and M. P. Mattson. 2014. "Fasting: Molecular Mechanisms and Clinical Applications." Cell Metabolism 19: 181–92.

Mattson, M., et al. 2014. "Meal Frequency and Timing in Health and Disease." Proceedings of the National Academy of Sciences of the United States of America 111: 16647–53.

Mattson, M. P., et al. 2017. "Impact of Intermittent Fasting on Health and Disease Processes." Ageing Research Reviews 39: 46–58.

Mindikoglu, A. L., et al. 2020. "Intermittent Fasting from Dawn to Sunset for 30 Consecutive Days Is Associated with Anticancer Proteomic Signature and Upregulates Key Regulatory Proteins of Glucose and Lipid Metabolism, Circadian Clock, DNA Repair, Cytoskeleton Remodeling, Immune System and Cognitive Function in Healthy Subjects." Journal of Proteomics 217: 103645.

Nair, P. M., and P. G. Khawale. 2016. "Role of Therapeutic Fasting in Women's Health: An Overview." Journal of Mid-Life Health 7: 61–4.

Natalucci, G., et al. 2005. "Spontaneous 24-h Ghrelin Secretion Pattern in Fasting Subjects: Maintenance of a Meal-Related Pattern." European Journal of Endocrinology 152: 845–50.

Patterson, R. E., et al. 2015. "Intermittent Fasting and Human Metabolic Health." Journal of the Academy of Nutrition and Dietetics 115: 1203–12.

Patterson, R. E., and D. D. Sears. 2017. "Metabolic Effects of Intermittent Fasting." Annual Review of Nutrition 37: 371–93.

Ravussin, E., et al. 2019. "Early Time-Restricted Feeding Reduces Appetite and Increases Fat Oxidation But Does Not Affect Energy Expenditure in Humans." Obesity 27: 1244–54.

Tinsley, G. M., and P. M. La Bounty. 2015. "Effects of Intermittent Fasting on Body Composition and Clinical Health Markers in Humans." Nutrition Reviews 73: 661–74.

Varady, K. A., et al. 2009. "Short-term Modified Alternate-day Fasting: A Novel Dietary Strategy for Weight Loss and Cardioprotection in Obese Adults." American Journal of Clinical Nutrition 90: 1138–43.

Wilkinson, M. J., et al. 2020. "Ten-Hour Time-Restricted Eating Reduces Weight, Blood Pressure, and Atherogenic Lipids in Patients with Metabolic Syndrome." Cell Metabolism 31: 92–104.e5.

Wegman, M. P., et al. 2015. "Practicality of Intermittent Fasting in Humans and Its Effect on Oxidative Stress and Genes Related to Aging and Metabolism." Rejuvenation Research 18: 162-72.

Chapter 5
Au, A., et al. 2016. "Estrogens, Inflammation and Cognition." Frontiers in Neuroendocrinology 40: 87-100.
Bosma-den Boer, M. M., et al. 2012. "Chronic Inflammatory Diseases Are Stimulated by Current Lifestyle: How Diet, Stress Levels and Medication Prevent Our Body from Recovering." Nutrition & Metabolism 9: 32.
Gambardella J., and G. Santulli. 2016. "Integrating Diet and Inflammation to Calculate Cardiovascular Risk." Atherosclerosis 253: 258-61.
Myles, I. A. 2014. "Fast Food Fever: Reviewing the Impacts of the Western Diet on Immunity." Nutrition Journal 13: 61.
Nettleton, J. A., et al. 2006. "Dietary Patterns Are Associated with Biochemical Markers of Inflammation and Endothelial Activation in the Multi-Ethnic Study of Atherosclerosis (MESA)." American Journal of Clinical Nutrition 83: 1369-79.
Rogero, M. M., and P. C. Calder. 2018. "Obesity, Inflammation, Toll-Like Receptor 4 and Fatty Acids." Nutrients 10: 432.
Sears, B., and C. Ricordi. 2011. "Anti-Inflammatory Nutrition as a Pharmacological Approach to Treat Obesity." Journal of Obesity 2011: 431985.
Serafini, M., and I. Peluso. 2016. "Functional Foods for Health: The Interrelated Antioxidant and Anti-Inflammatory Role of Fruits, Vegetables, Herbs, Spices and Cocoa in Humans." Current Pharmaceutical Design 22: 6701-15.
Shieh, A., et al. 2020. "Gut Permeability, Inflammation, and Bone Density Across the Menopause Transition." JCI Insight 5: e134092.
Zhu, F., et al. 2018. "Anti-inflammatory Effects of Phytochemicals from Fruits, Vegetables, and Food Legumes: A Review." Critical Reviews in Food Science and Nutrition 58: 1260-70.

Chapter 6
Arnold, K., et al. 2018. "Improving Diet Quality Is Associated with Decreased Inflammation: Findings from a Pilot Intervention in Postmenopausal Women with Obesity." Journal of the Academy of Nutrition and Dietetics 118: 2135-43.
Lennerz, B., and J. K. Lennerz. 2018. "Food Addiction, High-Glycemic-Index Carbohydrates, and Obesity." Clinical Chemistry 64: 64-71.
Lenoir, M., et al. 2007. "Intense Sweetness Surpasses Cocaine Reward." PLoS ONE 2: e698.
Madsen, H. B., and S. H. Ahmed. 2015. "Drug versus Sweet Reward: Greater Attraction to and Preference for Sweet versus Drug Cues." Addiction Biology 20: 433-44.
Seidelmann, S. B., et al. 2018. "Dietary Carbohydrate Intake and Mortality: A Prospective Cohort Study and Meta-Analysis." Lancet Public Health 3: e419-28.
Tabung, F. K., et al. 2015. "The Association between Dietary Inflammatory Index and Risk of Colorectal Cancer among Postmenopausal Women: Results from the Women's Health Initiative." Cancer Causes Control 26: 399-408.
Wise, P. M., et al. 2016. "Reduced Dietary Intake of Simple Sugars Alters Perceived Sweet Taste Intensity but Not Perceived Pleasantness." American Journal of Clinical Nutrition 103: 50-60.

Chapter 7
Abbasi, B., et al. 2012. "The Effect of Magnesium Supplementation on PriMeredithInsomnia in Elderly: A Double-Blind Placebo-Controlled Clinical Trial." Journal of Research in Medical Sciences 17: 1161-69.

Bacciottini, L., et al. 2007. "Phytoestrogens: Food or Drug?" Clinical Cases in Mineral and Bone Metabolism 4: 123-30.

Barbagallo, M., et al. 2021. "Magnesium in Aging, Health and Diseases." Nutrients 13: 463.

Barnard, N. D., et al. 2021. "The Women's Study for the Alleviation of Vasomotor Symptoms (WAVS): A Randomized, Controlled Trial of a Plant-Based Diet and Whole Soybeans for Postmenopausal Women." Menopause 28: 1150-56.

Cangusso, L. M., et al. 2015. "Effect of Vitamin D Supplementation Alone on Muscle Function in Postmenopausal Women: A Randomized, Double-Blind, Placebo-Controlled Clinical Trial." Osteoporosis International 26: 2413-21.

Chacko, S. A., et al. 2010. "Relations of Dietary Magnesium Intake to Biomarkers of Inflammation and Endothelial Dysfunction in an Ethnically Diverse Cohort of Postmenopausal Women." Diabetes Care 33: 304-10.

Chen, S., et al. 2016. "Dietary Fibre Intake and Risk of Breast Cancer: A Systematic Review and Meta-Analysis of Epidemiological Studies." Oncotarget 7: 80980-89.

Cheng, Y. C., et al. 2020. "The Effect of Vitamin D Supplement on Negative Emotions: A Systematic Review and Meta-Analysis." Depression and Anxiety 37: 549-64.

Durosier-Izart, C., et al. 2017. "Peripheral Skeleton Bone Strength Is Positively Correlated with Total and Dairy Protein Intakes in Healthy Postmenopausal Women." American Journal of Clinical Nutrition 105: 513-25.

Durrant. L. R., et al. 2022. "Vitamins D2 and D3 Have Overlapping But Different Effects on the Human Immune System Revealed Through Analysis of the Blood Transcriptome." Frontiers in Immunology 13: 790444.

Estébanez, N., et al. 2018. "Vitamin D Exposure and Risk of Breast Cancer: A Meta-analysis." Scientific Reports 8: 9039.

Fowke, J. H., et al. 2000. "Brassica Vegetable Consumption Shifts Estrogen Metabolism in Healthy Postmenopausal Women." Cancer Epidemiology, Biomarkers & Prevention 9: 773-79.

Hairston, K. G., et al. 2012. "Lifestyle Factors and 5-Year Abdominal Fat Accumulation in a Minority Cohort: The IRAS Family Study." Obesity 20: 421-27.

Kim, J. M., and Y. J. Park. 2017. "Probiotics in the Prevention and Treatment of Postmenopausal Vaginal Infections: Review Article." Journal of Menopausal Medicine 23: 139-45.

Kroenke, C. H., et al. 2012. "Effects of a Dietary Intervention and Weight Change on Vasomotor Symptoms in the Women's Health Initiative." Menopause 19: 980-88.

Maalmi, H., et al. 2014. "Serum 25-hydroxyvitamin D Levels and Survival in Colorectal and Breast Cancer Patients: Systematic Review and Meta-Analysis of Prospective Cohort Studies." European Journal of Cancer 50: 1510-21.

Masoudi, A. N., et al. 2015. "Fatigue and Vitamin D Status in Iranian Female Nurses." Global Journal of Health Science 8: 196-202.

Mossavar-Rahmani, Y., et al. 2019. "Artificially Sweetened Beverages and Stroke, Coronary Heart Disease, and All-Cause Mortality in the Women's Health Initiative." Stroke 50: 555-62.

Orchard, T. S., et al. 2014. "Magnesium Intake, Bone Mineral Density, and Fractures: Results from the Women's Health Initiative Observational Study." American Journal of Clinical Nutrition 99: 926-33.

Parra, D. et al. 2008. "A Diet Rich in Long Chain Omega-3 Fatty Acids Modulates Satiety in Overweight and Obese Volunteers during Weight Loss." Appetite 51: 676-80.

Parazzini, F. 2015. "Resveratrol, Tryptophanum, Glycine and Vitamin E: A Nutraceutical Approach to Sleep Disturbance and Irritability in Peri- and Post-Menopause." Minerva Ginecologica 67: 1-5.

Piuri, G., et al. 2021. "Magnesium in Obesity, Metabolic Syndrome, and Type 2 Diabetes." Nutrients 13: 320.

Rondanelli, M., et al. 2021. "An Update on Magnesium and Bone Health." Biometals 34: 715-36.

Santoro, N., et al. 2015. "Menopausal Symptoms and Their Management." Endocrinology and Metabolism Clinics of North America 44: 497-515.

Zhang, Y. Y., et al. 2017. "Efficacy of Omega-3 Polyunsaturated Fatty Acids Supplementation in Managing Overweight and Obesity: A Meta-Analysis of Randomized Clinical Trials. Journal of Nutrition, Health, and Aging 21: 187-92.

Chapter 10

Ayas, N. T., et al. 2003. "A Prospective Study of Sleep Duration and Coronary Heart Disease in Women." Archives of Internal Medicine 163: 205-209.

Bayon, V., et al. 2014. "Sleep Debt and Obesity." Annals of Medicine 46: 264-72.

Hanson, J. A., and M. R. Huecker. "Sleep Deprivation." In StatPearls. Treasure Island, FL: StatPearls Publishing, 2022.

Steger, F. L, et al. 2021. "Intermittent and Continuous Energy Restriction Result in Similar Weight Loss, Weight Loss Maintenance, and Body Composition Changes in a 6 Month Randomized Pilot Study." Clinical Obesity 11: e12430.

RESOURCES

The following resources are those I recommend to help your journey on The Metaboost Diet be even more successful.

Books
This Is Your Brain on Food by Dr. Uma Naiboo
The Intermittent Fasting Revolution: The Science of Optimizing Health and Enhancing Performance by Mark P. Mattson
Hooked by Michael Moss
Mini Habits for Weight Loss by Stephen Guise
Untamed by Glennon Doyle
The Obesity Code: Unlocking the Secrets of Weight Loss by Dr. Jason Fung
The Diabetes Code: Prevent and Reverse Type 2 Diabetes Naturally by Dr. Jason Fung
In Defense of Food: An Eater's Manifesto by Michael Pollan
The Longevity Solution: Rediscovering Centuries-Old Secrets to a Healthy, Long Life by Dr. James DiNicolantonio and Dr. Jason Fung
Atomic Habits: An Easy & Proven Way to Build Good Habits & Break Bad Ones by James Clear
Salt Sugar Fat: How the Food Giants Hooked Us by Michael Moss
Metabolical: The Lure and the Lies of Processed Food, Nutrition, and Modern Medicine by Robert Lustig, MD, MSL
Soundtracks: The Surprising Solution to Overthinking by Jon Acuff

Lifespan: Why We Age—and Why We Don't Have To by Dr. David Sinclair and Matthew LaPlante
Podcasts
Weight Loss for Food-Lovers
You Are Not Broken by Kelly Casperson, MD
The Life Coach School
Unlocking Us with Brené Brown
We Can Do Hard Things with Glennon Doyle
The Improvement Project
Tara Brach

Lifespan: Why We Age—and Why We Don't Have To by Dr. David Sinclair and Matthew

ACKNOWLEDGMENTS

I have many people to thank for helping me write this book and, with it, for opening the door to an even wider audience. I am grateful to:

My patients who inspire me every day.

My followers who taught me to be a better advocate and inspired me to fill in the gaps of my training and knowledge.

The early volunteers who tested the program and provided so much feedback.

The early contributors to the program: Cara Coza, Heidi Seigel, Stephanie Vasut, Stephanie Haver, Leah Pastor, and Dr. Alison Warlick.

Those who inspired me: Dr. Kelly Casperson, Dr. Shannon Clark, Dr. David Sinclair and Dr. Tony Youn.

The Metaboost Diet Team: Jen Pearson, Margaret Walsh, Michelle Jones, Ashley Simon, Victoria Thomas, Dawn Drogosch, Jamie Hadley, Sara Joseph, Zach Toth, Ani Hadjinian, Kathy Champagne, Cody Wright, and Judy Corsmeier.

My publishing team: Marnie Cochran, Heather Jackson, and Maggie Greenwood-Robinson

Made in the USA
Columbia, SC
02 July 2025

59900515R00213